Insurance, Regulation, and Hospital Costs

Insurance, Regulation, and Hospital Costs

Frank A. Sloan
Bruce Steinwald
Vanderbilt University

LexingtonBooks
D.C. Heath and Company
Lexington, Massachusetts
Toronto

Library of Congress Cataloging in Publication Data

Sloan, Frank A
  Insurance, regulation, and hospital costs.

  Bibliography: p.
  Includes index.
  1. Hospitals—Economic aspects—United States. 2. Hospitals—Economic aspects—United States—Mathematical models. 3. Hospitals—United States—Cost of operation—Mathematical models. 4. Insurance, Hospitalization—United States—Mathematical models. I. Steinwald, Bruce, joint author. II. Title. [DNLM: 1. Economics, Hospital—United States. 2. Insurance, Hospitalization—United States. 3. Facility regulation and control—United States. WX157 S634i]
  RA981.A2S549   338.4′336211′0973   79-3752

ISBN 0-669-03472-x

Copyright © 1980 by D.C. Heath and Company.

Published simultaneously in Canada.

Printed in the United States of America.

International Standard Book Number: 0-669-03472-x

Library of Congress Catalog Card Number: 79-3752

To our mothers, Edith and Minnie

Contents

Contents

List of Figures
and Tables

Preface

This book is an empirical examination of factors that have influenced hospital costs and employment of inputs during the 1970s. Our research emphasizes the effects of health insurance and regulation, the two most critical—and criticized—influences on the hospital industry during this period. Because analysis of hospital costs alone does not reveal the locus of effects of the many forces that shape hospital behavior, we devote considerable attention to hospital use of labor and nonlabor inputs. It is, after all, hospitals' expenditures on inputs that result in the "bottom line" of costs per admission or patient-day, and a comprehensive examination requires identification of how, not just how much, hospital behavior is influenced by external forces.

This book's empirical approach is matched by its policy orientation—we have striven to design our empirical tests and related discussions to yield information of maximum relevance to current policy deliberations in health care. At the same time, our background discussions attempt to place the research in the context of hospital industry institutions and recent historical developments, theories of hospital behavior, and past research findings. Our effort to touch all the bases has resulted in a rather lengthy book, but we hope that readers of diverse backgrounds and orientations, united by a common interest in the problems and potentials of the hospital industry, can all benefit from the material presented.

Chapter 1 describes the current policy situation vis-à-vis U.S. hospitals and the major issues addressed in ensuing chapters. The first section presents information about the sources and extent of hospital-cost inflation in recent years. The second section provides an overview of issues related to health insurance, regulation, and other factors, including effects of physicians and unions on hospital performance.

Theories of hospital behavior are developed and discussed in chapter 2. We find, as others have found in the past, that formal models provide only a few unambiguous predictions. Nevertheless, working through formal models can be very useful in developing insights about hospital behavior. Chapter 2 contains considerable comparative statics analysis to satisfy more theoretically oriented readers. At the same time, the significance of alternative models and assumptions is discussed in intuitive terms for the less theoretically minded.

Multiple objectives are served in chapter 3. Initially we describe the hospital sample and methods of data-file construction. The bulk of the chapter is devoted to empirical specification, including descriptions of dependent and independent variables. It concludes with sections on econometric properties of the input equations.

Chapters 4 and 5 provide in-depth discussions of third-party reimburse-ment and hospital regulation, respectively. Inclusion of these chapters reflects our view that these two topics are of central importance, from both policy and research perspectives. Chapter 4 presents statistics pertaining to private health insurance, with the household as the unit of observation. While these statistics were generated primarily for development of variables for use in our empirical analyses, we obtained some findings that are of interest in their own right. Chapter 5 presents a detailed overview of current regulatory trends affecting hospitals. Both chapters contain sections on institutions, past research, and issues to be investigated. In conjunction with the specification section of chapter 3, chapters 4 and 5 present our hypotheses regarding effects of the independent variables on hospital costs and input choices.

Chapter 6 is a short chapter containing descriptive evidence. Some statistics on the hospital industry as a whole are included in the text, but the bulk of the chapter is devoted to tables and related discussion pertaining to our 1,228-hospital sample covering the 1970–1975 period.

In chapters 7 and 8, our discussions of empirical findings center on tables 7–1, 8–1, and 8–2, which contain parameter estimates pertaining to the cost and input regressions. Because specifications and hypotheses are presented in prior chapters, these discussions are devoted almost entirely to results, with some reference to past studies for comparative purposes. Chapter 8 is the more complex of the two chapters. It contains additional tables and discussions of indirect effects, interactions, and long-run effects. Both chapters contain summary sections.

Our principal findings are reviewed in chapter 9. In this chapter we focus on the policy relevance of our findings and on remaining questions to be answered by research to assist in formulation of rational public policies toward the hospital industry.

Acknowledgments

We are indebted to a number of individuals who have assisted us in our research and in preparation of the manuscript. Ned Becker, our programmer, has been involved from the earliest stages of creation of raw data files to the final stages of estimation. The manuscript was skillfully typed by Nanette Fancher and Dellinda Henry, who luckily have sharp eyes for split infinitives, inconsistent punctuation, and other assorted linguistic sins. Several research assistants participated in library work, coding, and desk calculations. We thank them collectively because they are too numerous to mention individually.

Part of the material in this book has been published by the University of Chicago Law School in a journal article entitled, "The Effects of Regulation on Hospital Costs and Input Use," *Journal of Law and Economics* (April 1980). Some of the data presented in tables 6-1, 6-3, 6-5, 7-1, 8-1, 8-2, and 8-3 appear in this article. We thank the *Journal of Law and Economics* for granting permission to reprint these findings.

Health insurance data presented in the tables in chapter 4 and appendix H are based on "1970 Survey of Health Services Utilization and Expenditure," by the Center for Health Administration Studies and the National Opinion Research Center of the University of Chicago. We are indebted to Ronald Andersen for releasing these data and related documentation to us.

Our nurse wage variables, which enter into the analysis in chapter 8, are based partly on data from the 1970 U.S. Census. We are grateful to Richard Elnicki of the University of Florida for allowing us to use his computer runs on census data for constructing these variables.

This book represents a major part of the output from "Determinants of Hospital Wage Inflation," Grant 5 R01-HS02590 from the National Center for Health Services Research, Department of Health, Education, and Welfare, to Vanderbilt University. We thank Linda Siegenthaler, our project officer, for her assistance throughout the project.

Insurance, Regulation, and Hospital Costs

1

Setting the Stage

Inflation in the Hospital Industry

In recent years, the U.S. health care system has commanded ever-increasing attention of both policymakers and the public. From the vantage point of government officials at all levels and other persons responsible for health care budgets, such as industry and union officials, rising expenditures on health care services have been a cause for alarm. It is now part of conventional wisdom that, in terms of production costs, health insurance premiums constitute a more important part of a newly produced domestic automobile than steel.

Other health concerns involve access to care and society's seeming inability to realize major improvements in health status in the past twenty-five years or so. Although health status is probably related to the quantity and quality of health services that citizens receive, there is a growing belief that many other factors, including life-style, are perhaps more important. Yet despite a movement in favor of changing priorities toward relatively more emphasis on promoting healthy behavior, at present the concern of policymakers is still focused squarely on improving the ways in which health services are financed and delivered.

The institution most intimately associated with the high rate of increase in the cost of health services is the hospital. In recent years, the cost of a day of hospital care has been increasing at a rate exceeding 15 percent.[1] The rate of growth in the hospital component of the consumer price index (CPI) has led the medical care component of which it is part. Medical care prices, in turn, have risen faster than the overall CPI.[2] Understanding the forces underlying these trends is an important first step in devising appropriate policy remedies.

As it is typically defined, the term *inflation* refers to increases in prices paid by consumers for goods and services. In discussions about the hospitals, inflation takes on other meanings. Some equate it to the growth in aggregate expenditures on hospital services. More often, hospital cost inflation is cast in terms of the growth in expenditure per patient-day or per case (admission or discharge). According to the latter interpretation, inflation results from increases in both costs per unit of input and inputs per unit of output. Patient-days and admissions (discharges) are generally acknowledged as very gross measures of hospital output. Variations in specific procedures per patient-day or case are often referred to as "service intensity." Service intensity is

1

closely related to "input intensity" because more inputs presumably contribute to the production of additional services (for example, X-rays, laboratory tests, physical therapy sessions) per patient-day or case. Probably because of the importance of cost reimbursement insurance, the terms *costs* and *prices* are often used interchangeably in debates over inflation in this sector.

The seeming imprecision of analysts' work on inflation in the hospital sector is at least partially justified in terms of public policy priorities. While price increases per se merit attention in their own right, the dramatic growth in aggregate hospital expenditures is the chief concern of those who pay for hospital service consumption. By 1976, 91 percent of hospital revenues came from third-party sources.[3] Although this figure probably overstates the amount of coverage at the margin, many services are covered in full.[4] Therefore it is not surprising that patients and their physicians have demanded input- (or service-) intensive days and stays.[5] In fact, a recent report published by the U.S. Council on Wage and Price Stability (1977) attributes approximately 75 percent of the rise in daily hospital costs (relative to the inflation rate for the U.S. economy as a whole) to increases in inputs per patient-day and only 25 percent to higher input prices.

Hospitals, of course, have been heavily criticized for their role in expenditure inflation; accusations of both allocative and technical inefficiency in the hospital sector are common. Yet there is some evidence to support industry claims that at least part of the inflationary trend in recent years is due to external influences. Without denying that there has been an increase in hospital inputs, McMahon and Drake (1978), who, as officials of the American Hospital Association (AHA), presumably represent an industry position, concluded that the most recent growth in hospital costs reflects a dramatic rise in the prices of nonlabor inputs used by hospitals. Figure 1–1, taken from McMahon and Drake, suggests that 51.3 percent of the cost increase in 1969 was due to increases in quantities of nonlabor inputs purchased by hospitals. Nonlabor input price increases were relatively unimportant, and wage increases were only moderately important. By contrast, in 1975 the growth in nonlabor input quantities was only a minor contributor to hospital cost inflation; price increases of nonlabor inputs were the major contributor.

Hospitals face a far greater threat of government regulatory intervention if inflation primarily reflects increased input intensity rather than higher input prices, which, to a considerable extent, are beyond the individual hospital's or the hospital industry's control.[6] For this reason, some might question figure 1–1, which relies on AHA data. While we do not endorse the precise numbers, there does appear to have been a shift in importance of the components of inflation during the 1970s in the directions implied by the figure. Yet most hospital regulatory programs that have evolved during this

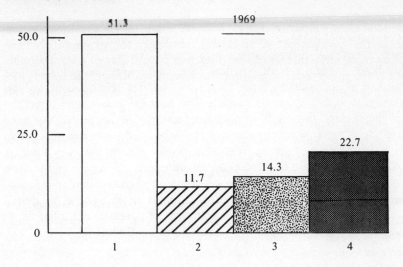

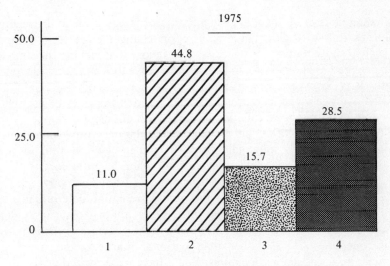

1 = Increases in the quantity of goods and services purchased
2 = Increases in the cost of goods and services purchased
3 = Increases in the quantity of personnel employed
4 = Increases in average wages

Source: J.A. McMahon and D.F. Drake, "The American Hospital Association Perspective," in M. Zubkoff, I.E. Raskin, and R.S. Hanft (eds.), *Hospital Cost Containment* (New York: Prodist, 1978), p. 82; © 1978 by Milbank Memorial Fund.

Figure 1–1. Components of Total Hospital Inflation, 1969 and 1975, by Percentage

period are implicitly based on the presumption that input growth has been an important source of the observed increase in costs and would remain so in an environment without rather stringent regulation.

This book examines both hospital costs and input choices and their determinants. By considering input choices, we cannot help but deal, at least tangentially, with quality issues as well. The hospital is assumed to set the price of its product, but the hospital takes factor prices as given. We have analyzed variations in wages paid to hospital labor and evaluated alternative models of hospital wage setting in another book.[7] We refer to key findings from the other book when they affect the interpretation of our present results. We have separated these works primarily because of the volume of research and descriptive materials involved. This book is more general in that it considers at one time all the major contributors, or potential contributors, to the inflationary trend in hospital costs and input employment.

Research and Policy Issues

In evaluating studies of hospital cost inflation, it is essential to distinguish between descriptive studies that simply report changes in the cost components, such as those reported in figure 1–1, and those that identify the sources of these changes. Descriptions can be useful because they may provide quick clues as to why costs vary. For example, if price increases of nonlabor inputs far exceed average wage increases, it would be inappropriate to ascribe a primary role in hospital cost inflation to the growth of hospital unions. Also, increases in input quantities, either labor or nonlabor, would lead one to question statements by hospital administrators and associations that hospital cost inflation is almost completely beyond individual hospital control.

Yet the number of legitimate inferences possible from descriptive studies is quite limited, primarily because too many potential determinants of hospital behavior change at the same time. One cannot isolate individual influences unless other pertinent factors are held constant. Furthermore, hospitals operate in local rather than national markets, and there are substantial variations among localities. Some have experienced a growth in real per capita income, and others have seen a decline. Both the level and the growth of third-party coverage for hospital services vary geographically and over time. And there is considerable variation in the extent to which states and localities have adopted regulations affecting hospitals. Among regulatory programs of the same type there is substantial diversity in goals, content, and dates adopted. Finally, for purposes of policy making, not only is it important to ascertain that a relationship exists, but also one should know something about the magnitude and timing of hospital responses to exogenous forces. For example, several programs have been developed to control expansion of hospital capital. A thorough evaluation requires knowing not only whether such programs have an effect but also the size of hospital investment response to such programs in equilibrium and how long it takes to get there.

The principal policy instruments that governments possess for affecting hospital behavior encompass third-party reimbursement and regulation. By 1976, 55 percent of hospital revenues came from various levels of government.[8] Governments can vary the specific services covered and, for covered services, the types and levels of expenses allowed. Forms of regulation include tax laws, laws affecting union activity, personnel licensure, hospital licensure and certification, regulation of hospital construction and purchase of equipment, monitoring of financial operations, rate regulation, and utilization-quality controls. Several of these regulatory approaches are intimately related to the government role as a third-party payer. Moreover, large private payers, in particular Blue Cross plans, have implemented various forms of hospital regulation as part of their reimbursement systems.

As already noted, there is a general consensus that the growth in the extent of third-party coverage in the post-World War II period has had a substantial impact on both the size of the hospital sector and the kinds of services provided. The highly sophisticated technological base in even the average hospital of the 1970s probably reflects the extensiveness of third-party coverage. Although we, like others, accept these statements both as working hypotheses and as reasons for emphasizing the role of insurance in research on hospitals, we are also aware that such statements and related conventional wisdom about the effects of third-party coverage on hospital outputs, inputs, and costliness do not rest on a very solid research base. Therefore, our first research priority in this area is to determine to what extent depth of health insurance coverage is responsible for observed levels of hospital inputs and costs associated with the employment of these inputs. In addition to private insurance, our analysis includes the major publicly financed health insurance programs, Medicare and Medicaid.

Our use of the more general term *health insurance* as opposed to *hospital insurance* is by no means accidental. Coverage for physicians' services is also potentially important to hospital behavior for two reasons. First, before being admitted to a hospital, the patient typically sees a physician in a nonhospital setting; therefore, one must be concerned with the patient's incentives to visit a physician in the first place. Second, the patient's expenses incurred for a hospitalization episode consist of separate hospital and physician bills. Although the hospital receives revenue from only the first, decisions about admission, length of stay, and services provided while in the hospital are likely to reflect insurance for both components.

Insurance for hospital services is by no means homogeneous. One important structural characteristic is whether the insurer's reimbursement system is based on hospital charges or costs. The two methods may offer different incentives to the hospital and, depending on associations between reimbursement method and out-of-pocket expenses, to consumers of hospital services as well. Thus, in addition to extent of coverage, this book assesses the relative effects of charge- and cost-based reimbursement on both hospital input demand and average costs.

Many observers of the health care industry see a need for some direct regulatory restraints on hospitals. The hospital is viewed, appropriately in our opinion, as an institution largely isolated from market pressures imposed by price competition. However, evidence pertaining to other regulated industries and our limited experience with contemporary hospital regulatory programs make it clear that controls frequently engender problems. First, they often appear to be ineffective; second, they may produce distortions in the types of outputs produced; third, they sometimes result in inequities in terms of nonneutral treatment of hospitals and consumers; last, controls have frequently worked to the advantage of the regulated group rather than to that of society at large.

Our research adopts the view that regulatory programs are neither good nor bad per se; we seek to determine only their effects on costs and inputs. However, because most current regulatory programs are designed to curtail hospital expansiveness, the absence of negative effects on costs and/or inputs can generally be interpreted as evidence that programs are not fulfilling their intended objectives. We examine governmental and private attempts to implement controls over supply of services, reimbursement, and utilization.

Supply or input controls over hospitals, embodied in state certificate-of-need laws and section 1122 programs under Public Law (P.L.) 92-603, are designed to limit the flow of new capital into the hospital industry as well as the proliferation of sophisticated facilities and services. The rationale for this form of regulation is the view that prevailing hospital reimbursement systems greatly reduce, if not eliminate, the cost to the hospital of new investments. The professional stature of hospital administrators is felt to be related to the size and technical sophistication of the hospital. Moreover, hospitals must compete for medical staff to ensure an adequate supply of patients. In addition to having beds freely available for the admission of patients, physicians often demand to work with the latest equipment. The path of least resistance therefore is purchase and growth of "nothing but the best."

Certificate-of-need and section 1122 programs represent attempts to put a lid on these expansions. In this book we assess the effects of these programs not only on hospital use of capital inputs but also on employment of labor. From the standpoint of public policy, the aim is to restrain not only capital outlays but also hospital expenditures on current accounts. Because capital regulation focuses on one type of hospital input, the potential for bulge effects in other areas cannot be ignored.

Capital regulatory programs have several potential effects on hospital employment of labor. First, some kinds of labor are undoubtedly substitutes for some kinds of capital. For example, some of the hospital's hotel functions can be operated in capital-intensive or labor-intensive modes. There is also evidence that certain architectural designs, which involve additional capital outlays, result in reduced nurse staffing because supervision can be performed more effectively. Second, some forms of labor are complementary with certain forms of capital. These complementary forms often seem to occur in relationship to sophisticated hospital technology. For instance, an open-heart surgery program requires both capital outlays and specific types of skilled labor. In many cases, the incremental cost of staffing a new facility may be higher than the annualized marginal costs associated with the added capital.[9] Third, capital regulation may result in displacements of funds from philanthropic sources, particularly when an investment program is disallowed. In compensation, the hospital might utilize such funds, for example, to upgrade nurse staffing, a type of expenditure that would clearly fall outside the purview of capital expenditure regulation. Restraints on capital inputs could actually stimulate hospital demand for labor for the first and third reasons. Proponents of capital input regulation have emphasized the second reason, the complementarities between labor and capital, rather than the two compensatory responses.

Some Blue Cross plans operate their own capital regulation programs. They disallow operating expenses and depreciation attributable to capital projects that do not meet local planning agency approval. This book also evaluates the effects of these programs on input choices.

In the area of reimbursement controls, several state governments have adopted prospective reimbursement plans. The objective of such plans is to establish reimbursement ceilings that compel hospitals to be cost-conscious without unduly curtailing the quantity or quality of hospital outputs. Existing programs are heterogeneous; about the only feature they have in common is that reimbursement is based on factors other than actual hospital costs or charges. The 1972 amendments to the Social Security Act authorize federal funds for state and regional prospective reimbursement experiments and evaluations of ongoing programs.[10] Although several such evaluative studies have been conducted under Social Security Administration sponsorship, empirical evidence on the multifaceted effects of prospective reimbursement is still inconclusive.[11]

A central issue of this book is whether prospective reimbursement programs, implemented in large part during the late 1960s and early 1970s, have caused a meaningful reduction in the growth of hospital inputs. Because there is substantial variation in these programs, we are also interested in identifying characteristics of the more successful ones. Our research should improve on past evaluations in this area both by incorporating more recent data on a larger and more geographically dispersed sample of hospitals and by holding more factors constant in our empirical analysis of prospective reimbursement.[12]

A form of regulation similar in many ways to prospective reimbursement was the Nixon administration's Economic Stabilization Program (ESP), which was in effect from late 1971 through early 1974. Under ESP, a special set of controls was devised for hospitals. Since the current rate of inflation could, despite contrary statements by government officials, lead to reimposition of controls, an assessment of the recent two-and-a-half-year experience with wage-price controls is timely. In this book, we evaluate the impact of ESP on hospital employment of labor and nonlabor inputs and on hospital costs.[13]

A third form of regulation focuses on utilization and quality of hospital services. In principle, these programs attempt to curtail expenditures on hospital services by reducing "unnecessary" care, without having detrimental effects on the quality of hospital outputs. By and large, these programs are quite new [for example, the nationwide system of Professional Standards Review Organizations (PSROs)], and it is too early to evaluate their effects. Some Blue Cross and Medicaid plans have operated utilization review programs for several years. Our analysis in this area is limited to the latter programs.[14]

Any discussion of utilization of hospital services should properly consider the role of physicians. There is an ongoing debate among economists and others concerning the degree to which physicians can create demand for their own services.[15] Partly because of fears that physicians do have an unusual amount of discretion over the number of types of health care services that patients receive, programs to limit various types of physician workforce are emerging. Probably the best example is the 1976 Health Professions Educational Assistance Act (HPEA), which set limits on the number of residencies in non-primary care specialties and established rigid standards vis-à-vis immigration of foreign medical school graduates.

The debate over physician-created demand has centered on such variables as utilization of physicians' and hospital services per capita population and physicians' fees and earnings. Regardless of their collective ability to generate demand for their services, physicians may have substantial market power in dealing with hospitals. A patient faced with the option of elective surgery may resist what appear to be questionable recommendations for surgery; yet there are certainly good economic and institutional reasons for abiding by the physician's choice of hospital, especially under conditions of nearly complete third-party coverage for hospital services. To our knowledge, no economist would deny that the physician has market power in the choice-of-hospital decision. And to the extent that physicians have an important say in that choice, there is likely to be competition among hospitals in attracting physicians rather than patients.

Unfortunately, empirical research on hospital-physician relationships is

In its infancy. Research by Feldstein (1971a), Salkever (1972), and Pauly (1978) has established links between the mix of physicians in a locality and patient-days demanded per capita population and hospital costs. This book specifically examines the effects of variations in physician availability and specialty mix on hospitals' input choices and costs. To the extent that important links between physician workforce and hospital inputs can be established, there is added rationale for a closer look at both physician education and regulation policies.

Every economic study of an organization's employment of inputs includes measures of input prices, since the underlying theory is quite clear about their role as input determinants. From the vantage point of policy, it is certainly important to know the extent to which a wage subsidy or a change in the minimum wage would have an effect on the demand for labor. On the capital side, policymakers need to have information on the effects of changes in interest rates, allowable depreciation methods, and investment tax credits on investment demand. Policy interest in the effects of changed factor prices on input use is more limited in the health field, but there are exceptions. Such government actions as increases in the federal minimum wage, the 1974 extension of the Taft-Hartley Act to cover nonprofit hospitals, and exemptions of certain classes of hospital employees from wage controls all have potential impacts on wages paid to hospital employees. In this book we assess the impacts of wage changes on demand for labor and nonlabor inputs as well as on hospital costs. Our cost analysis also includes an assessment of the effects of union activity on total and labor costs.

We have attempted to present our theoretical discussion in chapter 2 in such a way that it will be meaningful to readers with different backgrounds and perspectives. We include both intuitive interpretations and equations that constitute our efforts to model hospital response to external forces. Chapters 3 through 5 are composite discussions of data and methodology, health field institutions, past evidence, and current issues. Together these chapters contain our hypotheses and specifications of the models we estimate in the empirical chapters. Chapters 6 through 8 present our empirical findings, beginning with some simple descriptive statistics and ending with more complex findings related to model dynamics. The concluding chapter synthesizes our findings and discusses implications of the research.

Notes

1. U.S. Council on Wage and Price Stability (1977).
2. U.S. Bureau of the Census (1977).
3. Gibson and Mueller (1977).
4. Approximately three-quarters of these third-party payments are made

under "service benefit" plans, both private and public, which essentially eliminate any cost sharing by consumers for covered services at the margin (see chapter 4). The remaining one-quarter of the payments involve some cost sharing, but many of these plans offer considerable reimbursement at the margin (for example, major medical plans).

5. Several writings attribute a major role to the physician. See, for example, Fuchs (1974) and Redisch (1978).

6. There would be no disagreement with this statement with regard to most nonlabor inputs. On the labor side, however, some would argue that hospitals possess monopsony power in markets for the more hospital-specific occupations (Altman 1970; Yett 1970). Moreover, there is the "philanthropic wage hypothesis" advanced by Martin Feldstein. For a detailed discussion of the structure of hospital labor markets, see Sloan and Steinwald (1980).

7. Sloan and Steinwald (1980).

8. Gibson and Mueller (1977). The proportion is even higher if one counts the tax benefits associated with the purchase of private health insurance.

9. In a study of Boston hospitals, Cromwell, Ginsburg, and Hamilton (1975) found that labor costs were three times as large as equipment depreciation and maintenance costs.

10. The 1972 Social Security Act amendments also gave the Department of Health, Education, and Welfare (HEW) authority to limit cost reimbursement under Medicare and Medicaid. This program became effective in 1976, too late to be included in our analysis.

11. These studies are reviewed at length in chapter 5.

12. This is important because omitted explanatory variables can cause substantial bias in estimated parameters, in this case pertaining to the effects of prospective reimbursement on hospital costs. See Theil (1971).

13. Sloan and Steinwald (1980) present evidence on the effect of ESP on hospital wages.

14. We have excluded from consideration in our analysis the older forms of quality-oriented regulation, such as hospital licensure and certification by the Joint Commission on Accreditation of Hospitals. Such programs may be important, but they have been universally in existence for so long that the chances of detecting effects with current data are slight.

15. See Sloan and Feldman (1978), Reinhardt (1978), and Yett (1978).

2 Theory

Factors that have placed hospitals at the forefront of many policy debates in recent years have also elicited a spate of articles by economists attempting to model the U.S. hospital. Several of these studies are purely conceptual; and because the hospital industry is dominated by nonprofit organizations, there has been considerable controversy over the relative merits of alternative objective functions that formally describe what hospitals attempt to accomplish. Typically, economists pay much more attention to a decision-maker's constraints than to his objectives—assumptions about an organization's objectives are merely a means toward the end of generating empirically verifiable hypotheses. But, in regard to hospitals, constraints are often given short shrift. One of us was made aware of this during a recent conference of health economists when several participants expressed doubts that hospitals face any budget constraints!

This book's emphasis is on empirical evidence; yet without reference to an underlying theory, presentations of empirical results readily become disorganized and difficult to interpret. Ideally, one would start with a hospital preference function and a set of constraints and then deduce a series of unambiguous predictions about the effects of changes in selected exogenous variables on specific hospital decision variables (for example, prices, outputs, amenities, inputs, and costs). This would leave the dual tasks of formally testing these qualitative predictions and obtaining estimates of the underlying parameters to the empirical stage.

Often, as is illustrated later, theory does not yield unambiguous predictions of hospital responses to external influences because of offsetting effects. Indeed, as a casual perusal of any advanced microeconomics text would show, this limitation is not confined to analysis of hospitals. But, among other things, theory can be used to organize the exogenous variables and to show the general form of behavioral relationships to be estimated. Moreover, theory has a useful negative role of showing what cannot be deduced. This is especially relevant to illustrating the dangers of attempting to deduce consequences of alternative public policies based on commonsense reasoning. Thus, theory has its uses; yet because of its limitations a sense of modesty in theorizing about hospital behavior is appropriate.

Our discussion of theory continues in the first section with an examination of conceptual contributions to understanding hospital behavior by sociologists and experts in hospital administration. It would be excessively

11

chauvinistic to ignore such contributions, and they provide a useful contrast to economic theory in this area, the topic of the second section. Unlike hospital-oriented studies by noneconomists, most economic theories of hospitals are based on the assumption of a single hospital preference function. Although there is reason to doubt that hospitals, in fact, operate as single-mindedly as the models reviewed in this section imply, the models have the advantage of generating some testable hypotheses about hospital behavior in response to external forces. This and the third section, which deals with output measurement in the hospital context, lead us to the economic model of the unregulated hospital in the fourth section. Theoretical effects of various forms of hospital regulation on hospital behavior are considered in the fifth section, and effects of cost-based reimbursement are treated in the sixth section. The final section summarizes the chapter and discusses implications for empirical analysis.

Hospital Organization and Objectives: Perspectives from the Organizational Literature

The question, Who makes what decisions affecting hospital inputs and outputs? interests policymakers and scholars alike. A related but more policy-oriented question was recently raised by Zubkoff (1978, p. 246): "Are tools to contain costs actually within the grasp of an individual hospital administrator?" If the locus of decision making is elsewhere, perhaps in the hands of medical staff, or if certain "decisions," such as factor prices, are exogenous to the individual hospital or to the hospital industry as a whole, then cost containment policies that depend on hospital administrator responses may seriously miss the mark.

Among sociologists and specialists in organizations, issues related to decision making within hospitals have scholarly interest. By contrast, with a few exceptions, economists have little interest in complex organizations in general or in hospitals as a special case.[1] In fact, they are typically quick to assume that organizations possess an objective function with a very limited number of arguments to make the theory that follows, once constraints are added, as simple as possible. Reasons for economists' proclivities include a penchant for formal modeling, a general lack of interest in conflict within decision-making units,[2] and disinterest in how preferences are formed.

A large number of noneconomic studies assess relative power of three groups within the hospital: the physicians, the trustees, and the administration.[3] These studies agree that although administrators may influence the development of guidelines and procedures regarding patient utilization of hospital resources, physicians have almost exclusive jurisdiction over strictly medical matters (see, for example, Kovner 1972). A number of studies imply that physician control over utilization, including the ordering of laboratory tests and X-rays and length of stay, is greater on average than is their control over hospital efficiency per se.

A well-known sociological study by Perrow (1961) developed a multi-stage theory of hospital power. Traditionally, when voluntary general hospitals depended on community funds for an important part of their capital and operating budgets, trustees dominated hospital decision making. Trustee domination was allegedly most common during the late 1800s and early 1900s.[4] The increasing technical sophistication of medicine, knowledge which the trustees did not possess, led to domination by medical staff. More recently, according to Perrow, the power of hospital administrators has grown and in some cases now dominates the trustee and physician groups. Sources of administrative power are hospital needs for (1) coordinating increasingly complicated, nonroutinized functions; (2) managing large numbers of nonphysician personnel, sometimes shielding nonphysicians from unreasonable demands of medical staff; and (3) relating to outside groups, including third-party payers and community agencies.

Sometimes none of the three power groups dominates—this is the multiple-leadership case. When the goals of the three parties diverge, not an infrequent occurrence, a considerable amount of time is devoted to decision making in multiple-leadership hospitals. Although the Perrow study lacks a substantial empirical base, it does suggest that physician dominance is by no means universal in hospital settings. Strong trustees and administrators, in some cases, have a leading role in hospital decision making.

More recently, Roemer and Friedman (1971) devoted an entire book to doctor-hospital relations and internal hospital organization. To illustrate the range of possible relationships, they developed the concept of medical staff organization (MSO), which depends on such dimensions as composition of medical staff (including credentials required for medical staff membership), appointment procedures (including requirements to attend meetings and participate in intramural programs), commitments (including contractual arrangements and policies on practice in other hospitals), departmentalization (authority and reporting systems), and so on. The authors illustrated and elaborated on the MSO concept with a series of case studies describing the MSO in nine hospitals. There was notable variation among the nine. Which types of MSOs are most prevalent and specifically how the MSO relates to hospitals' input choices were not addressed by Roemer and Friedman. Further consideration of MSOs could be very worthwhile, but data limitations preclude such analysis in this book.[5]

Two policy-oriented articles have questioned whether hospital managers have the power to constrain costs. Allison (1976) and Zubkoff (1978) voiced a concern, one widely shared by many experts in the health field, that many attempts to contain the growth of hospital costs may be ineffective because they do not affect physician behavior.

Allison surveyed hospital administrators in Michigan. The administrators were asked to assess the cost-saving potential of several variables relating to hospital behavior and performance. For example, if savings could be realized through improvements in hospital productivity or efficiency, how much of an impact would this have on increases in hospital costs? As seen in table 2–1, administrators saw reduction in length of stay and admissions as having the greatest potential for cost savings. They were also asked to gauge the power of administrators and physicians in affecting levels of the cost-influencing variables. Not too surprisingly, the administrators felt they have power over variables that mattered the least. Physicians allegedly have correspondingly more power in areas that mattered the most.

The rankings presented in table 2–1 emphasize the limitations of administrator authority and, by inference, of cost control programs that exclude the physician. However, some of the variable categories are quite general. Whether or not efficiency gains have the potential of reducing hospital expenditures depends on the specific type of efficiency gain under consideration. Whether or not the administrator has control over input prices depends

Table 2–1
Cost-Influencing Variables

Variable	Cost-Saving Potential[a]	Administrator's Power	Physician's Power
Length of stay	1	5	5
Admissions	2	6	2
Quality[b]	3	7	6
Intensity[c]	4	9	4
Teaching[d]	5	4	7
Efficiency	6	3	8
Scope of services	7.5	8	3
Input prices	7.5	2	9
Case mix	9	10	1
Investments[e]	10	1	10

Source: R.F. Allison, "Administrative Responses to Prospective Reimbursement," *Topics in Health Care Financing*, vol. 3, no. 2 (Winter 1976): 103. © 1976 by Aspen Systems Corporation, reprinted with permission.
[a]All three columns show rank orders based on responses of hospital administrators.
[b]*Quality* was defined by respondents themselves. Most saw quality as a combination of scope of services and efficiency.
[c]*Intensity* refers to the kinds of diagnostic and therapeutic procedures performed on patients.
[d]Defined by the authors to include both in-service and occupational educational programs.
[e]Includes investments in labor and capital and policies regarding plant maintenance, in-service and professional education, and so on.

on the competitiveness of the input market. One of the most surprising features in the table is the low ranking in importance for cost savings given to investments. Perhaps this reflects a reaction toward the considerable amount of regulatory activity in hospital investment control during the period of study.

Zubkoff (1978), using his own experience in hospital administration as a guide, asked whether hospital administrators have control over the several alternative tools of cost containment. He claimed that hospital administrators have "no control" over wage rates or prices of supplies. These presumably are exogenous to the hospital. They have "partial control" over the selection of supplies through an active therapeutics committee supported by an effective hospital formulary program, and they have "minimal control" over utilities and equipment purchases. In Zubkoff's (1978, p. 247) view, staffing is the one area among those listed over which the administration has control. Savings in staffing may be accomplished "through good personnel selection procedures, proper motivation of employees, and effective utilization of all manpower resources."

Based on review of the hospitals-as-organizations literature and our own observations, we offer the following generalizations. Some of these will be reflected in empirical specifications and in later discussions.

First, the relative power of administrators, trustees, and medical staff varies over time and at any given moment. Certainly the locus of decision making varies according to hospital ownership. Government bodies, for example, are effectively the trustees of government hospitals.

Second, irrespective of what one believes about the physician's power over patient demand, hospitals per se have no ability to generate demand except by varying the technological sophistication or quality (however defined) of their outputs. It is difficult to determine empirically to what extent physicians are attracted by a hospital's technology base and to what extent hospital selection is made by patients or by physicians acting in their patients' interests. In any case, such determinations are not essential for conceptual work on hospitals.[6]

Third, except in those situations where utilization review is effective, administrators and trustees have at best a minimal *direct* influence on admissions, length of stay, services utilized, and case mix. This is probably the most important deficiency of the model developed later in this chapter to gauge hospital responses to selected exogenous stimuli; the alternatives, however, have other weaknesses.

Fourth, the issue of locus of control over hospital investment in plant and equipment is rather confused in much of the literature. In the sense that there frequently is nonprice competition among hospitals for staff physicians and their patients, hospitals are motivated to provide technically sophisticated equipment and readily available beds. Yet it is hard to believe that such decisions, at the margin, have a dramatic effect on a hospital's viability. Individual hospitals probably have *some* monopoly power that allows administrators latitude in varying equipment and capacity, thereby influencing utilization of services.[7]

Fifth, one may safely assume that hospitals are price takers in factor markets. Where the literature suggests that administrators control wages, there appears to be confusion about the meaning of the term *control*. Moreover, the literature suggesting that hospitals possess monopsony power in markets for highly skilled personnel, such as professional nurses, has failed to present very convincing empirical evidence.[8]

Economic Models of Hospital Behavior

A comprehensive review of economic theories of hospital behavior by Davis (1972) provides a description of hypothesized hospital objective functions used by economists in early (pre-1970) research on hospitals, particularly nonprofit hospitals. The objectives include (1) recovery of costs, according to which the hospital's main concern is to set prices to cover average costs (Ingbar and Taylor 1968); (2) output maximization subject to a deficit constraint (Long 1964; Klarman 1965; and Reder 1965); (3) quality and quantity maximization subject to a break-even constraint, where quality is defined in terms of the quantities of inputs used in producing any given level of output (Newhouse 1970; Feldstein 1971b); (4) utility maximization, in which measures of case complexity or inputs (for example, hospital capital, size of medical staff) comprise the arguments (Reder 1965); and (5) cash flow or profit maximization, where cash flow excludes the economic return on equity capital (Davis 1969).

Davis (1972) evaluated the above alternative objective functions using several tables containing descriptive information on hospital revenue, expenses, net income, plant assets, labor and capital inputs per patient-day, and specialized facilities and services. Although these data did not permit definitive conclusions, a few noteworthy findings were suggested. Most important, Davis found that nonprofit hospitals make sizable profits, implying that models specifying an objective subject to a break-even constraint are inconsistent with available evidence, at least in the short run. From examination of aggregate financial data pertaining to hospitals over the 1960s, Davis reported that profits actually increased throughout the decade. Of course, this may have been a disequilibrium phenomenon arising from outward shifts in hospital demand curves during the period. Nevertheless, Davis' conclusion that positive net income is sought by nonprofit hospitals is well taken.

Some of the more recent conceptualizations of hospital behavior merit a closer look. Newhouse (1970), Feldstein (1971b), and Ginsburg (1976) developed models of the nonprofit hospital in which a coalition of the hospital's trustees, the administrator, and the medical staff possesses a common preference function with quantity and quality of hospital care as arguments. A break-even constraint allowing the hospital to run a deficit on current operations (if compensated with funds from noncurrent operating sources) was specified. Quality was defined in terms of input intensity rather than treatment effectiveness.

Newhouse and Feldstein presented their models graphically. With quantity held constant, an implication of both studies is that quality, inputs, and costs rise with increased insurance. More generally, these variables increase as a result of any outward shift in the patient's demand curve. If output quantity is allowed to vary, predictions about the effect of demand-curve shifts require specification of the properties of the hospital preference function.

Ginsburg, and Evans (1970) before him, introduced the notion of "organizational slack" as an argument in utility functions of nonprofit hospitals. Such hospitals have no shareholders, so no one has property rights to the dollars saved by controlling costs. Extensive third-party financing further dilutes incentives for hospitals to be technically efficient. Being cost-conscious is burdensome to managers, and the returns to them (in salary and promotions) may be very low.[9]

In Ginsburg's extension of the Newhouse-Feldstein type of model, it is assumed that (1) hospitals are product price takers, which includes regulated price situations, and (2) price does not enter the demand function, which is valid if insurance covers all expenditures on hospital services. Ginsburg found that an increase in the exogenous price raises quality and quantity (which is obtained once quality is known), but the impact on slack is ambiguous because of offsetting income and substitution effects. Intuitively, as the controlled price rises, the opportunity cost of slack rises, causing hospitals to want to reduce it; on the other hand, if one assumes (as is plausible) that slack is a normal good, the added revenue from the price rise motivates hospitals to "purchase" additional amounts of slack.

An alternative model of hospital behavior has been developed by Pauly and Redisch (1973). According to their model, a physicians' cooperative sets levels of nonphysician labor, nonlabor inputs, and the number of medical staff consistent with maximization of the physicians' collective money income. The hospital itself is assumed to break even, with residual income (the difference between total expenditures for physician and hospital services and the hospital bill) going to the doctors.[10]

The first-order conditions for nonphysician labor and nonlabor inputs from Pauly and Redisch's model imply simply that the marginal revenue (or value) products of the inputs equal their respective marginal supply prices.

The condition on medical staff states that the marginal revenue product of staff physicians equals their net (of the hospital price) average revenue product.

As long as doctors in Pauly and Redisch's cooperative act collectively (explicitly or implicitly), there is no room in their model for organizational slack. After all, residual money income is maximized by minimizing unnecessary hospital costs. However, as they noted, policing individual physician behavior may be costly; therefore, it may pay the individual doctor to cheat the system. That is, he may attempt to secure the use of hospital inputs that serve his individual practice but not the hospital's medical staff as a whole. As all physicians in the cooperative begin to engage in such activities, the sum of their individual incomes falls below the level obtainable by setting inputs in a manner consistent with joint income maximization. Pauly and Redisch conjectured that imperfect cooperation becomes more likely as concentration of hospital output among medical staff members decreases.[11] Although this seems plausible, it also is plausible that physicians in hospitals where output is indeed diffuse would decide to develop appropriate policing mechanisms. Evidence presented by Roemer and Friedman (1971) supports this view.

Pauly and Redisch's model is an interesting attempt to capture some of the institutional features of the hospital sector. As specified, it characterizes some types of hospitals very well, but is probably inappropriate for others, such as large government, teaching, and chain proprietary hospitals. Models of the Newhouse-Feldstein-Ginsburg variety are far more general.

According to a model developed by Harris (1977), the hospital is organized as two separate firms: medical staff (the demand division) and the administration (the supply division). Allocations within the hospital take place through a complicated set of nonprice rationing rules [for example, procedures for sharing operating-room time, waiting lists, "shouting and screaming" (p. 478)]. Although cast in economic jargon, this model is actually more in the tradition of the noneconomic models reviewed above, and because of its complexity it practically defies formalization. As stressed later, more investigation of behavioral relationships among various parties within the hospital would be worthwhile. An important barrier to us and to previous authors has been adequate data on internal hospital functions.

Output Measurement in the Hospital Sector

In chapter 1 we noted that the terminology used by analysts of the hospital industry is subject to ambiguities—the term *inflation*, as applied in this sector, is a good example. In this chapter we have already used several terms related to hospital output without defining them, and we must say more before turning to our own conceptual modeling in the next section. In particular, we consider the concepts of quantity, quality, and amenities.

Hospitals are complex organizations rendering a variety of services: hotel, including food and laundry; ambulatory care, both by clinic departments which produce an overlapping set of services for inpatients and outpatients and by emergency rooms; diagnostic and therapeutic, including laboratory and radiology; outreach, including social services; research; and training. Although inpatient services generally are emphasized in discussions of hospitals, outpatient visits have been growing at a much more rapid pace than admissions.[12] To exclude everything but inpatient care is to greatly understate hospital output. Most recent analyses use alternative quantity measures based on patient-days or admissions[13] and outpatient visits. Our empirical work on hospital costs also adopts this approach, but we recognize that not all important sources of variation in hospital services are captured.

While there are certainly problems involved in measuring quantity of hospital services, quality is a more difficult concept to deal with both theoretically and empirically. The most common treatment of quality in hospital research is to equate it to *service intensity*, the amount of services provided per unit of output. Thus defined, quality is characterized in terms of the process of care rather than in terms of outcome. Current methods of evaluating patient outcomes are not sufficiently well developed to be used as the basis of measuring hospital quality, at least for empirical research. In spite of the lack of conclusive empirical evidence regarding the relationship between process measures and patient outcomes, experts in the field are more confident in using process criteria.

For analytic purposes, parsimony in the choice of variables is crucial. Thus, rather than define separate variables for quantity and quality as others have done, for some analytic purposes it is useful to define a single composite measure of patient care services X. In this way, one avoids the amorphous term *quality*.[14] But this approach has deficiencies. The importance of specific services within X may not be invariant with respect to key exogenous variables. For example, as patient income and third-party reimbursement increase, demand for certain ancillary services may rise in relative importance. And use of clinic services may decline in absolute terms as the patient's ability to pay improves. Changes in output composition should, in turn, affect hospital demand for specific labor and nonlabor inputs. Quality is assumed to be especially responsive to growth in such variables as patient income and insurance coverage in models having a distinct term representing quality.

Policy discussions have often emphasized that hospitals may offer particular services as a competitive response.[15] We concur. Physicians generally want to associate with hospitals offering a full range of services as well as various perquisites. Such factors tend to increase practice incomes without increasing costs to the physician. Moreover, with complete or nearly complete hospital insurance coverage, physicians seldom face complaints about costs from patients who are placed in "Cadillac" hospitals. For various reasons, including travel time, physicians find it optimal to practice in only a few hospitals,[16] and hospitals may engage in competition for medical staff in innumerable ways.

Hospitals have increasingly moved away from the use of an all-inclusive daily rate. Nevertheless, many items of potential value to patients and their physicians are not billed separately, but rather are reflected in the daily room-and-board charge and other billable expenses. A partial list includes attractive rooms and good meals; fast nurse response time when the nurse is called by inpatients; excess bed capacity, which shortens the expected wait for admission; good parking facilities for medical staff; few physician committee assignments or rotation responsibilities; coverage of the attending physician's inpatients at night and on weekends by residents; and physician offices near the hospital at low or no cost. Amenities such as these tend to make the hospital relatively attractive to patients *and* physicians. It is worth emphasizing that even a profit-maximizing hospital would offer some of these amenities. The extent to which such amenities are (optimally, from the hospital's standpoint) provided depends on relative magnitudes of the marginal costs of providing them versus associated marginal revenues.

As noted above, the notion of organizational slack has been applied to the hospital industry. It implies that there are wasted resources in equilibrium because there is a positive cost to eliminating slack. Ginsburg (1976) extended the concept to encompass perquisites offered to attending physicians. It is doubtful that many of these would be eliminated, even if enforcement of efficiency standards were costless. However, a regulatory agency, by prohibiting hospitals from offering some types of perquisites and amenities, could rule out certain forms of nonprice competition altogether.

In the theoretical work presented in the following sections, amenities (including perquisites to physicians) are represented by the variable Y. Our empirical work does not investigate relationships between pertinent exogenous variables and amenities; rather these relationships are reflected in variations in hospital inputs and costs. An in-depth investigation of hospitals' amenity offerings would certainly be a worthwhile undertaking.

A Model of the Unregulated Hospital

This section presents a simple model of hospital behavior in the absence of regulation. Its purpose is (1) to show how exogenous product demand, factor price, and other exogenous variables shifting the hospital's cost function affect key hospital decision variables and, when possible, (2) to identify directions of influence. Tables summarize the comparative statics results.

Our model of hospital behavior starts with the assumption that the hospital possesses a single preference function U with a service composite X, amenities Y, and profits π as arguments. This model follows the tradition of previous theoretical research on hospitals by Feldstein (1971b), Newhouse (1970), and Ginsburg (1976), with the exception that π appears as an argument in the preference function rather than as a constraint.[17] As discussed above, the service composite X incorporates both quantity and quality dimensions of output.

As specified, the objective function is quite general. Hospitals in different ownership categories may place different weights on the three objectives. For-profit hospitals may place exclusive emphasis on π; public hospitals stress X rather than π. Private nonprofit hospitals may offer higher levels of Y than profit maximizers or government hospitals would.

$$U = U(X, Y, \pi) \qquad (2.1)$$

All three arguments are "goods" (that is, $U_X, U_Y, U_\pi > 0$), but subject to diminishing marginal utility (that is, $U_{XX}, U_{YY}, U_{\pi\pi} < 0$). Further, X, Y, and π are substitutes (that is, $U_{X\pi}, U_{XY}, U_{Y\pi} > 0$).

The hospital faces a downward-sloping demand curve in the market for its product which contains Y as well as X as arguments:

$$P = P(X, Y; M) \qquad (2.2)$$

where $P =$ hospital's price[18] and $M =$ any exogenous demand determinant. Very general (and commonplace) restrictions on the demand function are $P_X < 0$, $P_Y > 0$, and $P_M \gtrless 0$.

The hospital's cost function is

$$C = C(X, Y; N) \qquad (2.3)$$

where $N =$ any exogenous determinant of costs, *including* factor prices.

Let $\pi = P(\cdot)X - C$. Then, π may be expressed in terms of X and Y. The first-order conditions are

$$U_X = U_X + U_\pi \pi_X = 0 \qquad (2.4)$$

and

$$U_Y = U_Y + U_\pi \pi_Y = 0 \qquad (2.5)$$

According to equations 2.4 and 2.5, the hospital sets levels of output and amenities so that the marginal utilities of output and amenities equal the marginal disutility of profit losses resulting from extending output and amenities beyond their profit-maximizing levels. Given positive U_X, U_Y, and U_π, then π_X and π_Y must be negative if the first-order conditions are to be satisfied. Under simple maximization of profits, $\pi_X = 0$ and $\pi_Y = 0$. But assuming the hospital values X and Y for their own sake, as opposed to what the market is willing to pay them, it will give up some net revenue, setting X and Y at levels where the marginal net revenues π_X and π_Y are negative. Figure 2–1 illustrates the profit-maximizing point A and the utility-maximizing point B, which is at the tangency of a curve indicating alternative profits for various levels of X and the hospital's indifference curve between X and π, with Y held constant. A similar diagram can be constructed for Y and π, with X held constant. In effect, the hospital purchases additional units of X and Y with π.

The second-order conditions require that U_{XX} and U_{YY} be negative and that the determinant H, given by equation 2.6, be positive:

$$H = \begin{vmatrix} U_{XX} & U_{XY} \\ U_{YX} & U_{YY} \end{vmatrix} \qquad (2.6)$$

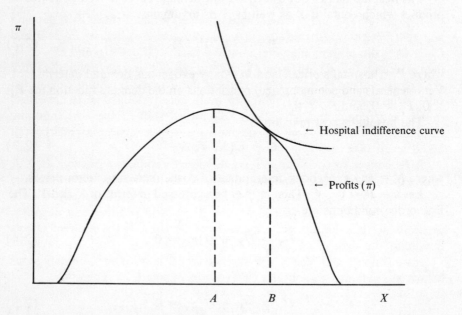

A = profit-maximizing level of output
B = utility-maximizing level of output

Figure 2–1. Profit- versus Utility-Maximizing Levels of Output X, with Amenities Y Held Constant

We follow standard convention and assume that the necessary and sufficient conditions for a maximum are satisfied.[19] Then one can evaluate the effects of changes in exogenous demand and cost determinants on X and Y and, by substitution, on P, C, and π.

$$\frac{dX}{dM} = -\frac{U_{XM}U_{YY} - U_{XY}U_{YM}}{H} \tag{2.7}$$

$$\frac{dY}{dM} = -\frac{U_{XX}U_{YM} - U_{XM}U_{YX}}{H} \tag{2.8}$$

$$\frac{dX}{dN} = -\frac{U_{XN}U_{YY} - U_{XY}U_{YN}}{H} \tag{2.9}$$

$$\frac{dY}{dN} = -\frac{U_{XX}U_{YN} - U_{XN}U_{YX}}{H} \tag{2.10}$$

Variable H is defined by equation 2.6.

If we assume M and N represent exogenous variables shifting the demand and cost functions outward and upward, respectively (that is, $P_M > 0$ and $C_N > 0$),[20] diminishing marginal utility of profits ($U_{\pi\pi} < 0$), and $U_{XY} \geq 0$, then it follows that dX/dM and dY/dM are positive and dX/dN and dY/dN are negative. That is, an outward shift in the demand function, caused by, say, an increase in patient income or more generous third-party coverage, raises both output and amenities. An upward shift of the cost function, resulting, for example, from a wage increase, which raises marginal cost at initial levels of X and Y, has the opposite effect.

A tenuous assumption underlying the above results is a positive U_{XY}. A strong income effect (the marginal utility of profits is strongly diminishing) would contribute to a negative U_{XY}. If U_{XY} is negative, the direct effects on X and Y of the above changes in M and N are still positive and negative, respectively, but the indirect effects are offsetting.[21] If the indirect effects dominate, the signs of dX/dM through dY/dN reverse.

If we simplify and specify a preference function in X and π, unambiguous results are obtained without the necessity of signing U_{XY}. Then

$$U = U(X, \pi) \tag{2.1'}$$

$$P = P(X; M) \tag{2.2'}$$

$$C = C(X; N) \tag{2.3'}$$

The first-order condition then is

$$U_X = U_X + U_\pi \pi_X = 0 \tag{2.11}$$

which has the same interpretation as equations 2.4 and 2.5. Since the hospital values X for its own sake, it will purchase additional units of X with profits. Now the effects of M and N on X are given by

$$\frac{dX}{dM} = -\frac{U_{XM}}{U_{XX}} \tag{2.12}$$

and
$$\frac{dX}{dN} = -\frac{U_{XN}}{U_{XX}} \tag{2.13} [22]$$

For the kinds of shifts in M and N considered above, dX/dM and dX/dN are unambiguously positive and negative, respectively. An outward shift in demand for the hospital's product expands output; an upward shift in its cost function lowers it. Since

$$\frac{dC}{dM} = \frac{\partial C}{\partial X}\frac{dX}{dM} \quad \text{and} \quad \frac{\partial C}{\partial N} = \frac{\partial C}{\partial X}\frac{dX}{dN} + \frac{\partial C}{\partial N},$$

outward shifts in demand unambiguously raise hospital costs, if a positive marginal cost $\partial C/\partial X$ is assumed. The effect of an upward shift in the hospital cost function has an ambiguous impact on total costs. The term $\partial C/\partial N$ is positive; but if services fall ($dX/dN < 0$) and the marginal-cost curve has a positive slope, there is an offsetting negative effect.

Up to now, our theoretical analysis has subsumed the hospital production function in a cost function. Since much of our empirical research involves analysis of hospital use of specific labor and nonlabor inputs, it is useful to examine the effects of selected exogenous variables on demand for specific inputs conceptually. We retain the preference and demand functions, equations 2.1' and 2.2', and add a production function and a cost identity:

$$X = f(K, L) \tag{2.14}$$

where $K =$ nonlabor inputs and $L =$ labor inputs. And

$$C = rK + wL \tag{2.15}$$

where $r =$ price of nonlabor inputs and $w =$ wage rate. Since there are only two inputs, they must be substitutes (that is, $f_{KL} > 0$). In empirical work with more inputs, some inputs may be complements. Substituting equations 2.14, 2.15, and 2.2' into equation 2.1' and differentiating, one obtains the first-order conditions (with R, hospital revenue)

$$U_K = U_f f_K + U_\pi R_f f_K - U_\pi r = 0 \qquad (2.16)$$

and $$\qquad U_L = U_f f_L + U_\pi R_f f_L - U_\pi w = 0 \qquad (2.17)$$

From equations 2.16 and 2.17, one can readily devise familiar textbook conditions for optimal input ratios, which are unaffected by our specification of a preference function with X and π as arguments:

$$\frac{r}{w} = \frac{f_K}{f_L} \qquad (2.18)$$

According to equation 2.18, capital and labor are employed in amounts at which the ratio of the two marginal products equals the ratio of the two factor prices.

Again, using comparative statics analysis, one can assess the effects of an outward shift in the hospital's demand curve and increases in factor prices on hospital input use.

Changes in labor and nonlabor inputs in response to changes in w and M are, respectively,[23]

$$\frac{dL}{dw} = -\frac{\bar{U}_{KK}\bar{U}_{Lw} - U_{KL}\bar{U}_{Kw}}{H} \qquad (2.19)$$

$$\frac{dK}{dw} = -\frac{\bar{U}_{Kw}\bar{U}_{LL} - \bar{U}_{Lw}\bar{U}_{LK}}{H} \qquad (2.20)$$

$$\frac{dL}{dM} = -\frac{\bar{U}_{KK}\overset{+}{U}_{LM} - U_{KL}\overset{+}{U}_{KM}}{H} \qquad (2.21)$$

We have placed pluses or minuses over terms that are readily signed.[24] The problem in signing equations 2.19 and 2.20 lies in the ambiguous sign of U_{KL}. If U_{KL} is positive, both dL/dw and dK/dw are unambiguously negative, but a negative U_{KL} produces ambiguous predictions. A negative U_{KL} may reflect strongly diminishing marginal utilities of X and π and/or strongly diminishing marginal revenue. Even in the standard profit-maximizing case in which the firm sets the product price, the sign of dK/dw is indeterminate. However, the law of demand, $dL/dw < 0$, applies under conditions of monopoly as it does under competition when marginal revenue is constant.[25]

The sign of dL/dM (and likewise of dK/dM) is unambiguously positive if U_{KL} is positive; if the sign of U_{KL} is negative, dL/dM is indeterminate. As with dL/dw (and by analogy dK/dr and dL/dr), the theory based on a two-argument preference function does not yield refutable hypotheses; either sign is consistent with the underlying theory.

Table 2–2 summarizes predicted effects of changes in selected exogenous variables on hospital output, amenities, costs, and employment of labor and nonlabor inputs. The first column lists the exogenous change. We then list assumptions about hospital objectives and the structure of the hospital's product market. Finally, we show the predictions. As seen in the table, there are many A's for ambiguous predictions. However, there are also some arrows, which serve as a guide for the empirical research presented in later chapters. Predictions on L and K are based on a two-input model. In the empirical work, several labor and nonlabor inputs are specified. Hence the predictions on K and L in table 2–2 are, if anything, overly strong. All effects in table 2–2 are symmetric. Decreases in product demand, for example, would reverse the arrows; ambiguous predictions would still apply.

Hospital Responses to Regulation

This section examines potential effects of three types of regulation of hospitals: rate regulation, revenue regulation, and input regulation. As in the previous section, comparative statics analysis is our evaluative tool.

Table 2–2
Predicted Effects of Changes in Exogenous Variables: Unregulated Hospital

	Assumptions about		Predicted Effect on				
Exogenous Change	Hospital Objective(s)	Product Market	X	Y	C	L	K
Outward shift in demand	$U(X, Y, \pi)$	Monopolistic	A	A	A	n.a.	n.a.
Upward shift in cost curve	$U(X, Y, \pi)$	Monopolistic	A	A	A	n.a.	n.a.
Outward shift in demand	$U(X, \pi)$	Monopolistic	↑	n.a.	↑	n.a.	n.a.
Upward shift in cost curve	$U(X, \pi)$	Monopolistic	↓	n.a.	A	n.a.	n.a.
Increase in wage	$U(X, \pi)$	Monopolistic	A	n.a.	A	A	A
Increase in wage	π	Monopolistic	A	n.a.	A	↓	A
Increase in wage	π	Competitive	↓	n.a.	↓	↓	↓
Outward shift in demand[a]	$U(X, \pi)$	Monopolistic	A	n.a.	A	A	A
Outward shift in demand[a]	π	Monopolistic	A	n.a.	A	A	A
Outward shift in demand[a]	π	Competitive	↑	n.a.	↑	↑	↑

A = ambiguous effect; n.a. = not applicable to specific model evaluated.
[a]Model contains a production function with K and L as inputs (as opposed to cost function above).

All our analysis is static, although in reality there may be important dynamic effects. If, for example, the revenue limit in year $t + 1$ depends on revenues and expenditures in year t or $t - 1$, a hospital may be willing to run a deficit in the short run to boost subsequent ceilings.[26] Likewise, with input regulation, hospitals may accumulate inputs in anticipation of controls.[27] For now, the static effects seem sufficiently complex without explicit consideration of the dynamics in our formal work.[28] In later chapters we assess dynamic effects of regulation empirically.

Rate Regulation

Under rate regulation, government fixes the price of X at P^*. Assume for now that every patient has complete insurance. Then the demand curve becomes $X = X(Y; M)$. In effect, the only way the hospital can secure additional patients is by raising Y:

$$U = U(X(Y; M), Y, P^*X(Y; M) - C(X(Y; M), Y; N)) \quad (2.22)$$

The first-order condition is

$$U_Y = U_X X_Y + U_Y + U_\pi(P^*X_Y - C_X X_Y - C_Y) = 0 \quad (2.23)$$

According to equation 2.23, the hospital equates the marginal utilities of extra X and Y with the marginal disutility of the loss of profits associated with producing above the profit-maximizing levels of X and Y.

The effect of changes in the regulated price on Y is given by

$$\frac{dY}{dP^*} = -\frac{U_{YP^*}}{U_{YY}} > 0 \quad (2.24)$$

since U_{YP^*} is positive under plausible assumptions.[29] Therefore, as the reimbursement rate per unit of output rises, say for a patient-day, the amounts of both output and amenities rise (since $X_Y > 0$) as do outlays for hospital care C. State rate-review programs that effectively constrain P should lower X, Y, and C. Further,

$$\frac{dY}{dN} = -\frac{U_{YN}}{U_{YY}} < 0 \quad (2.25)[30]$$

Thus, as the hospital's cost function shifts upward, amenities fall, as does output. If factor as well as product prices are regulated, as under the Nixon administration's Economic Stabilization Program, there are offsetting effects of regulation on Y and X.[31] The effects of changes in M on Y (and hence also on X) are ambiguous and are not pursued here. Since we assume complete health insurance coverage, exogenous demand-curve shifts, by and large, reflect nonpolicy developments (say, growth in patient income).

An alternative formulation assumes incomplete third-party coverage; then the demand function becomes $X = X(Y; P^*, M)$. Although the impact of a cost-function shift on Y and X can still be evaluated, with the more general formulation, it is impossible to sign dY/dP^*. To state that a higher regulated price would increase X, Y, and C requires an assumption of complete coverage.

Total Revenue Regulation

Under revenue regulation, total hospital revenue from patients R^* is set by an outside agency.[32] Again, assuming a downward-sloping demand curve in X, we have

$$R^* = P(X, Y; M)X \qquad (2.26)$$

The hospital maximizes

$$U = U(X, Y, P(X, Y; M)X - C(X, Y; N)) + \lambda[P(X, Y; M)X - R^*] \qquad (2.27)$$

Moving directly to the total effects of changes in the revenue ceiling, we can easily show that

$$\frac{dY}{dR^*} = - \frac{-U_{YX}^{?}[P_X X \overset{+}{+} P(\cdot)] + U_{XX}^{-}(P_Y^{+} X)}{H} \qquad (2.28)$$

and
$$\frac{dX}{dR^*} = - \frac{-U_{XY}^{?}(P_{YY}^{+} X) + U_{YY}^{-}[P_X X \overset{+}{+} P(\cdot)]}{H} \qquad (2.29)$$

The signs of dY/dR^* and dX/dR^* are positive if U_{XY} is positive; that is, output, amenities, and costs rise in response to an increase in the revenue limitation. But two underlying forces potentially contribute to a negative U_{XY}: diminishing marginal utility of profits and/or negative π_{XY}, the impact of changes in Y on the marginal profitability of X.[33] Under a standard profit-maximizing assumption, one may argue convincingly that π_{XY} is positive,[34] but if one assumes non-profit-maximizing behavior, one cannot be so sure this is so.

Input Regulation

Forms of input regulation, especially certificate of need, attempt to restrain the growth of the hospital sector by controlling expansion of capital. Assume the hospital maximizes

$$U = U(f(K^*, L), P(f(K^*, L; M))f - wL - rK^*) \quad (2.30)$$

With K fixed at K^*, the hospital's sole decision variable involves labor:[35]

$$U_L = U_f f_L + U_\pi[P_f f_L f + P(\cdot)f_L - w] = 0 \quad (2.31)$$

According to equation 2.31, the hospital employs more labor than it would if output were not an argument in the utility function.

It is of interest to know how the amount of L purchased varies with the amount of capital allowed:

$$\frac{dL}{dK^*} = -\frac{U_{LK^*}}{U_{LL}} \quad (2.32)$$

$$U_{LK^*} = U_{ff}f_{K^*}f_L + U_f f_L f_{K^*} + U_{f\pi}[P_f f_L f + P(\cdot)f_L - w] + U_f f_L f_{LK^*}$$

$$+ U_{\pi\pi}[P_f f_L f + P(\cdot)f_L - w] [P_f f_{K^*} f + P(\cdot)f_{K^*}]$$

$$+ U_\pi[\underbrace{f_{LK^*}(P_f f + P(\cdot))}_{\substack{\text{marginal} \\ \text{revenue}}} + \underbrace{f_L f_{K^*}(P_{ff}f + 2P_f)}_{\substack{\text{derivative of} \\ \text{marginal revenue}}}) \quad (2.33)$$

Equation 2.33 contains the usual offsetting effects that are due in part to diminishing marginal utilities in output and profits. To sign equation 2.33, it would be necessary to assume both profit maximization and a perfectly competitive product market. Then U_{LK^*} would be positive, and decreasing a hospital's allowable capital would decrease both labor and output. With the objective function given by equation 2.30, a decrease in K^* could raise L. This would occur if the marginal utility of output and/or marginal net revenue rose so rapidly with decreases in output that the hospital wanted to boost it back up, and the only way it can do this under a regulatory capital constraint is to raise L. The effects of varying the capital constraint on employment of labor inputs must be ascertained empirically.

Table 2–3 summarizes results from the comparative statics analysis of the regulated hospital. As in table 2–2, there are several ambiguous pre-

Table 2–3
Predicted Effects of Changes in Exogenous Variables: Regulated Hospital

Exogenous Change	Assumptions about		Predicted Effect on				
	Hospital Objective(s)	Product Market	X	Y	C	L	K
Rate regulation							
Increase in regulated price P^*	$U(X, Y, \pi)$	Binding price constraint[a]	↑	↑	↑	n.a.	n.a.
Upward shift in cost curve	$U(X, Y, \pi)$	Binding price constraint	↓	↑	A	n.a.	n.a.
Total revenue regulation							
Raise revenue constraint R^*	$U(X, Y, \pi)$	Monopolistic	A	A	A	n.a.	n.a.
Raise revenue constraint R^*	π	Monopolistic	↑	↑	↑	n.a.	n.a.
Input regulation (constrain K)							
Raise capital constraint	$U(X, \pi)$	Monopolistic	A	n.a.	A	A	↑[b]
Raise capital constraint	π	Monopolistic	n.a.	n.a.	A	A	↑[b]
Raise capital constraint	π	Competitive	↑	n.a.	↑	↑	↑[b]

A = ambiguous effect; n.a. = not applicable to specific model evaluated.
[a]Assumes all patients have complete insurance; otherwise, results are ambiguous.
[b]By assumption.

dictions; yet we are able to establish signs on a number of influences exogenous to the hospital.

Hospital Responses to Different Reimbursement Methods

Alternative reimbursement methods may produce incentives for hospitals to perform in different ways. In this section, we assess possible effects of cost-based reimbursement on hospital decision making. It is the first time we explicitly consider methods of third-party payment. A more comprehensive review of pertinent literature is presented in chapter 4.

In a departure from previous sections, we assume that hospitals maximize profits π. Although it is not a realistic assumption for the nonprofit hospital, a more realistic specification would greatly complicate this discussion, given the complexities of reimbursement, and would lead to even weaker predictions than those presented here.

Assume that the hospital has two types of patients. One type has no insurance, and the other has complete service benefit, cost-based reimbursement insurance. Let $P = P(\tilde{X}, Y)$ and $X(Y; M)$ be the demand curves facing the hospital for its uninsured and insured patients, respectively. Variables $\tilde{X}$ and X are output delivered to the two types of patients, respectively. According to the first demand curve, patients are willing to pay more if they are offered extra amenities. Presumably, various exogenous factors also affect demand, but we have suppressed the demand shift term to simplify the analysis. Since the second group has complete coverage, price does not enter $X(\cdot)$. To attract such patients, hospitals must engage in nonprice competition.

The hospital maximizes

$$\pi = P(\tilde{X}, Y)\tilde{X} + \gamma X(Y; M)AC(\tilde{X} + X, Y; N)$$
$$- AC(\tilde{X} + X, Y; N)(\tilde{X} + X(Y; M)) \qquad (2.34)$$

where $AC(\cdot) = $ hospital's average cost function and $\gamma = 1 + $ a plus factor (a fraction) offered by the insurer on top of allowable average costs. Several features about equation 2.34 are noteworthy. First, for patients covered by cost-based reimbursement insurance, costs generate revenues. In fact, if $\tilde{X}$, the number of uninsured patients, were zero, π would be $(\gamma - 1)X(\cdot)AC(\cdot)$. The hospital would earn a profit of $\gamma - 1$ per dollar of expense, an amount equal to the plus factor. But, as Davis (1973) has noted, with uninsured patients having a downward-sloping demand curve, a high price may drive away such patients. For this reason, ever higher prices may not be consistent with profit maximization.

The first-order conditions are

$$\pi_{\tilde{X}} = P_{\tilde{X}}\tilde{X} + P + \gamma XAC_{\tilde{X}} - AC - (\tilde{X} + X)AC_{\tilde{X}} = 0 \quad (2.35)$$

and

$$\pi_Y = P_Y\tilde{X} + \gamma X_Y AC + \gamma X(AC_X X_Y + AC_Y)$$
$$- X_Y AC - (AC_X X_Y + AC_Y)(\tilde{X} + X) = 0 \qquad (2.36)$$

According to equations 2.35 and 2.36, $\tilde{X}$ and Y are set where marginal revenue (for $\tilde{X}$ and Y) equals marginal cost (for $\tilde{X}$ and Y). If $\tilde{X} = 0$ (that is, there are no uninsured patients), equation 2.35 does not apply, and equation 2.36 becomes

$$\pi_Y = (\gamma - 1)(X_Y AC + XX_Y AC_X + XAC_Y) \qquad (2.36)'$$

Since the terms AC, AC_X, AC_Y, and X are positive,[36] equation 2.36' implies that the hospital will increase Y until X_Y becomes negative. Of course, as Y becomes large, so does AC. And costs tend toward infinity! The restraining force in this model is the presence of uninsured patients.

Returning to the specification implied by equations 2.35 and 2.36 and assuming that the second-order conditions for a maximum are satisfied, one can evaluate the effects of changes in γ, M, and N on $\tilde{X}$ and Y and, by substitution, on X, P, and AC. Only changes in γ and M are discussed here.

As above, an important cross partial is $\pi_{\tilde{X}Y}$, the effect of changes in Y on marginal profits from $\tilde{X}$. To obtain some conclusive results, $\pi_{\tilde{X}Y}$ must be positive. Increases in Y must increase $MR_{\tilde{X}}$ more than it does $MC_{\tilde{X}}$, a condition that may not hold.[37]

Impacts of changes in the plus factor are evaluated from

$$\frac{d\tilde{X}}{d\gamma} = -\frac{\overset{+}{\pi_{\tilde{X}\gamma}}\overset{-}{\pi_{YY}} - \overset{?}{\pi_{\tilde{X}Y}}\overset{+}{\pi_{Y\gamma}}}{H} \tag{2.37}$$

$$\frac{dY}{d\gamma} = -\frac{\overset{+}{\pi_{\tilde{X}\tilde{X}}}\overset{+}{\pi_{Y\gamma}} - \overset{+}{\pi_{\tilde{X}\gamma}}\overset{?}{\pi_{YX}}}{H} \tag{2.38}[38]$$

If $\pi_{\tilde{X}Y}$ is positive, both $d\tilde{X}/d\gamma$ and $dY/d\gamma$ are positive. An increase in the plus factor raises output to *both* insured and uninsured patients. Average costs rise because of increases in output and amenities. If $\pi_{\tilde{X}Y}$ is negative, direct effects are still positive, but there are offsetting indirect effects. If the number of uninsured patients is small relative to the number with cost-based insurance, a positive $\pi_{\tilde{X}Y}$ is more likely, but this is not a sufficient condition for a positive $\pi_{\tilde{X}Y}$. We cannot say for sure that an increase in this plus factor will necessarily boost AC.

Now consider the effects of a growth in the number of persons in the hospital's market area with cost-based insurance:[39]

$$\frac{d\tilde{X}}{dM} = -\frac{\pi_{\tilde{X}M}\overset{-}{\pi_{YY}} - \pi_{YM}\pi_{\tilde{X}Y}}{H} \tag{2.39}[40]$$

$$\frac{dY}{dM} = -\frac{\pi_{\tilde{X}\tilde{X}}\overset{-}{\pi_{YM}} - \pi_{\tilde{X}M}\pi_{Y\tilde{X}}}{H} \tag{2.40}[41]$$

For positive $\pi_{\tilde{X}Y}$ and an $\tilde{X}/X$ ratio less than or equal to $\gamma - 1$, $\pi_{\tilde{X}M}$ and π_{YM} are negative and positive, respectively. Then the growth in cost-based enrollments lowers output to uninsured patients and raises amenities and output to insured patients. If aggregate output also rises, average cost should rise as well. These predictions hold only for low $\tilde{X}/X$, that is, a low ratio of uninsured patients to patients with cost-based insurance. The signs of equations 2.39 and 2.40, at markedly higher values of $\tilde{X}/X$, could reverse.

Thus, it is not necessarily true that an influx of patients with cost-based coverage would necessarily raise output to insured patients X and hospital amenities. Also the effect on average cost AC is uncertain. The ratio $\tilde{X}/X$ is a key element.

Two themes emerge from this discussion. First, the exercise shows conditions under which cost-based insurance leads to hospital cost inflation. The relationships are not as simple as most policy discussions would lead one to believe. Second, the existence of patients without cost-based insurance serves as a restraint. Under complete coverage, there should be an explosive rise in costs. Why not raise wages, for example, if for each $1.00 increase the insurer pays $1.05?

Third-party payers would be quick to add that they do not consider every conceivable cost reimbursable. "Unreasonable" costs are disallowed. To the extent that this is so (and the extent currently is unknown), one should specify a term $\gamma X(\cdot) AC_A(AC(\cdot))$ to replace $\gamma X(\cdot) AC(\cdot)$, where AC_A refers to allowable average costs. If $\partial AC_A/\partial AC$ is far less than 1, hospitals should become more cost-conscious since they may have to pay some of the costs attributable to cost-based patients from other sources.[42]

Up to now, we have distinguished between persons without insurance and those with full-coverage, cost-based reimbursement. More realistically, most persons without cost-based reimbursement have some other form of insurance for hospital care. We consider this matter again in chapter 4, so our discussion of alternative types of insurance here is very brief.

A form of insurance, originally offered by commercial insurers and more recently by Blue Cross-Blue Shield, is major medical insurance. It pays a high proportion of "reasonable" charges (typically 75 to 80 percent). Large expenses may be covered in full. As the percentage of paid major medical approaches 100, this insurance, too, has an explosive effect on provider costs. And so does full-service, charge-based insurance if everyone has it. The underlying analyses, with a profit maximization assumption, have been worked out by Frech and Ginsburg (1975) and Sloan and Steinwald (1975). Qualitatively speaking, past results are similar to those of this section. The culprit seems to be full coverage rather than cost-based reimbursement per se. Emphasis on the inflationary effect of a particular type of coverage has probably been misplaced. We evaluate the effects of cost-based insurance in our empirical work for the sake of completeness (albeit reluctantly).

Summary, Conclusions, and Implications

Conceptual research on hospitals by now has spanned more than a decade. There have been various attempts to analyze hospital behavior by using traditional economic approaches. Accordingly, various types of hospital

preference functions and constraints have been proposed, and some implications about hospital responses to selected exogenous factors have been
derived. In many instances, these studies have not derived their results
formally. Unfortunately, this has led to a false sense of security. When
formalized, these models offer few implications about hospital behavior, far
fewer than figures and charts, based on less formal reasoning processes, have
suggested. For example, Dowling (1974) presented a table showing an array
of expected responses to alternative forms of prospective payment to
hospitals. Unlike table 2–3, the Dowling table shows no ambiguous predictions. Yet without a model of hospital behavior and a method for deducing
implications from the model, many of the predictions are misleading at best.

The principal uses of theory are that (1) it forces one to be explicit about
underlying assumptions, (2) it allows one to deduce some likely responses to
exogenous stimuli, (3) it serves as a means for classifying variables, both
endogenous and exogenous, (4) it identifies offsetting effects underlying
ambiguous predictions, and (5) it compels researchers and policymakers
alike to be more cautious about deductions based on common sense. Only
empirical research has the potential of settling many of the issues this chapter
has addressed in addition to other issues, such as dynamic responses, which
this chapter has neglected.

Since the central results of the comparative statics analysis have been
summarized in tables 2–2 and 2–3, there is no need to repeat these
theoretical findings here. The principal result of the theoretical analysis of
cost-based reimbursement is to question the notion that this reimbursement
approach is innately inflationary.

Although the comparative statics of this chapter are complex enough,
they do not capture several important dynamic effects that should be
considered in any assessment of regulation. For example, "grandfather"
clauses contained in certificate-of-need laws may greatly affect the timing of
hospitals' capital expenditure decisions, and capital hoarding may dominate
observed hospital responses for a number of years. Under prospective
reimbursement, hospitals may increase future rate bases by exceeding
reimbursement limitations in the short run. Hospitals may react differently if
they believe a given regulation will be temporary. During the years of the
Nixon administration's Economic Stabilization Program, hospitals may have
been willing to forgo profits; however, over a longer period, they might have
made more pronounced adjustments in input and output levels.

Substantial measurement problems pose serious obstacles to theoretical
as well as empirical work. There is a virtual tautology between quality,
defined in terms of input intensity, and input use. Organizational slack, which
in some models yields utility to management but not to consumers, is difficult
to distinguish from various amenities, which determine the position of the
hospital demand curve. The Pauly-Redisch model is distinguished from its

predecessors in that it predicts no organizational slack under conditions of perfect physician cooperation. But, to the extent that organizational slack remains an amorphous concept, this prediction cannot be refuted empirically.

Experts in organizational behavior, rather than specifying an overall preference function for the hospital, have emphasized conflict among hospital decision makers—administrators, trustees, and doctors. Although the ideas of organizational theorists coincide with the reality many of us have observed, at the same time they greatly complicate any attempt to develop explicit models of hospital behavior. For this reason, with some reservations, we have devoted most of this chapter to the traditional economic approach. The notion that parties within the hospital may not agree lends further support to the view that hospitals' responses should be evaluated empirically. Combined with a thorough examination of important institutions within the health field, empirical analysis can advance understanding of hospital behavior far beyond the boundaries of available theoretical deductions. Following chapter 3, which considers our data base and methodology, the remainder of this book is devoted to institutions and empirical evidence.

Notes

1. An important exception is a recent article on hospitals by Harris (1977) discussed later in this chapter.

2. There are some notable exceptions.

3. Our general comments are based on a reading of Guest (1972), Kovner (1972), Bates and White (1961), Coser (1958), Goss (1961), Perrow (1961), Pfeffer (1972), Roos, Schermerhorn, and Roos (1974), and Shortell and Brown (1976).

4. The use of philanthropic funds for hospital operations currently is negligible. The proportion of funds for hospital construction from philanthropic sources has been declining over time. By 1976, only 7.5 percent of funds for hospital construction came from this source. See Lightle (1978).

5. We shall examine physician-hospital relationships more closely in future research, using data from the American Hospital Association.

6. On the "agency" relationship in which the doctor acts *for* the patient, see Feldstein (1974).

7. For a more detailed discussion of competition among hospitals, see Salkever (1978a).

8. See Sloan and Steinwald (1980).

9. This concept has been developed at length by Leibenstein (1966, 1976), Williamson (1967, 1975), and others.

10. Detailed comparative static results from the cooperative model (as applied to Soviet agriculture) are reported in Domar (1966).

11. In a later article, Pauly (1978) quantified this relationship.

12. Between 1970 and 1975, admissions and outpatient visits in hospital settings grew 14 and 41 percent, respectively, according to data provided in American Hospital Association (1977). The growing importance of ambulatory care in hospitals is also apparent from surveys of patients. See Sloan and Bentkover (1979).

13. For a useful discussion of the advantages and disadvantages of admissions as opposed to patient-days as hospital output measures, see Feldstein (1967).

14. Suppose that one had a single, but vaguely defined measure of quality. Then one can presume that there are several alternative quality measures which are monotonic transformations of the first. But beyond determining the sign of the first partials between the former and the latter measures (that is, stating that the latter are monotonic transformations of the first), nothing is known; the second partials are left unspecified. With a number of such possible transformations, the analytics becomes a mess and/or the necessary assumptions become quite numerous. Without finding a measure of quality that is generally accepted, one is wide open to the charge that "plausible" signs on specific second-degree terms cannot be determined. A comprehensive review of studies on this topic is found in Berki (1972).

15. For a more extensive discussion of competition in the hospital sector, see Salkever (1978a).

16. Salkever (1978a).

17. The fact that private nonprofit hospitals persistently earn profits on current operations seems inconsistent with the types of budget constraints specified in past research; these allowed the hospital to run deficits that are made up with revenue from nonpatient sources. There are numerous accounts of the importance of profits to nonprofit hospitals in addition to the sources cited above (such as American Hospital Association 1976).

18. Economists have typically assumed that hospitals are price setters in their product markets. See Salkever (1978a).

19. Variables U_{XX} and U_{YY} are negative, given the assumptions in the text:

$$U_{XY} = \overset{+}{U}_{XY} + \overset{+}{U}_{X\pi}\overset{-}{\pi}_{Y} + \overset{-}{U}_{\pi\pi}\overset{-}{\pi}_{X}\overset{-}{\pi}_{Y} + \overset{+}{U}_{\pi Y}\overset{-}{\pi}_{X} + \overset{+}{U}_{\pi}\overset{?}{\pi}_{XY}$$

Expected signs are shown above each term. A positive π_{XY} implies that further additions of quality raise marginal revenue $R_X (= P_X X + P)$ more than marginal cost C_X. Sloan and Feldman (1978) have argued that π_{XY} is likely to be positive over a considerable range of X and Y, but a negative π_{XY} cannot be ruled out.

20. If $P_M < 0$ and $C_N < 0$, the signs of equations 2.7 through 2.10 are reversed.

21. See note 19.

22. Note:

$$U_{XM} = U^+_{X\pi}\overset{+}{\pi}_M + U^-_{\pi\pi}\overset{+}{\pi}_M\overset{-}{\pi}_X + U^+_{\pi}\overset{+}{\pi}_{XM} > 0$$

$$U_{XN} = U^+_{X\pi}\overset{-}{\pi}_N + U^-_{\pi\pi}\overset{-}{\pi}_N\overset{-}{\pi}_X + U^+_{\pi}\overset{-}{\pi}_{XN} < 0$$

23. There is no need to write out the expression for dK/dM since dL/dM tells the whole story.

24. Negative U_{KK} and U_{LL} and a positive H are required for the existence of a maximum. Also, $U_{Lw} = -U_\pi - U_{\pi\pi}L\,(\,R_f f_L - w\,) - U_{f\pi}f_L L$ and $U_{Kw} = U_{\pi\pi}L\,(\,r - R_f f_K\,) - U_{f\pi}f_K L$. Under the plausible assumption of diminishing marginal utility of profits, U_{Lw} is negative since $R_f f_L - w$ is negative from the first-order condition and, with two arguments, $U_{f\pi}$ must be positive. For an analogous reason, U_{Kw} is negative as well. Now, $U_{KL} = U_{LK} = U_{f\pi}(R_f f_L - w)f_K + f_{LK}(U_f + U_\pi R_f) + U_{\pi\pi}(R_f f_k - r)\cdot (R_f f_L - w) + U_\pi(R_{ff}f_K f_L + R_f f_{LK})$. Under plausible assumptions, the first, third, and fourth products of U_{LK} are negative and the second product is positive.

25.
$$\frac{dL}{dw} = -\frac{\begin{vmatrix} \pi_{KK} & 0 \\ \pi_{LK} & -1 \end{vmatrix}}{H}$$

One does not have to sign π_{LK} because it is multiplied by zero. Under utility maximization, U_{Kw} is nonzero.

$$\frac{dK}{dw} = -\frac{\begin{vmatrix} 0 & \pi_{KL} \\ -1 & \pi_{LL} \end{vmatrix}}{H}$$

To sign dk/dw, one must sign π_{KL}. Under perfect competition, $\pi_{KL} > 0$ and $dK/dw > 0$. These results are found in standard microeconomics texts. See, for example, Hadar (1971).

26. See, for example, Worthington (1976).

27. Blumstein and Sloan (1978) and Lewin and Associates (1975a, 1975b).

28. Dynamic responses to prospective reimbursement are amenable to analysis by using techniques from optimal control theory.

29. Note:

$$U_{YP*} = X^+_Y[\overline{U^+_{X\pi}X_Y} + U^+_{Y\pi} + U^-_{\pi\pi}(\overline{P^*X_Y - C_X X_Y - C_Y}) + U^+_\pi]$$

30. Note:

$$U_{YN} = U_{\pi}^{+}(\overbrace{-C_{XN}\overset{-}{X_Y} - C_{YN}}) + U_{\pi\pi}^{-}(\overbrace{P^*X_Y - C_X X_Y - C_Y}) \cdot$$

$$(\overbrace{-C_{XN}\overset{-}{X_Y} - C_{YN}}) - C_N^{+}(\overbrace{U_{X\pi}X_Y + U_{Y\pi}}^{+})$$

31. We have also assessed the effects of wage control on the use of nonlabor inputs. To do this, one must assume that the individual hospital faces an upward-sloping labor supply curve rather than the horizontal supply curve assumed elsewhere in this chapter. This modification per se is not particularly troublesome since the regulated industry facing a competitive labor market would probably be able to retain some labor for a while, especially if important competing sectors are also regulated. Of course, some workers would simply decide to work less. To obtain unambiguous predictions about the effects of a change in the regulated wage W^* on K and Y, again one needs to make an assumption about the strength of the income effect as reflected in $U_{\pi\pi}$. The derivation is available from the authors on request.

32. Our models permit using accumulated profits from previous periods to finance losses on current operations; but if we assume diminishing marginal utility of profits, there is a penalty to increasing the deficit (or, for that matter, moving away from profit-maximizing levels in Y and X).

33. Note:

$$U_{XY} = U_{YX} = U_{XY}^{+} + U_{\pi\pi}^{-}(\overbrace{P_X X + P - C_X}^{-}) \, (\overbrace{P_{YX} - C_Y}^{-})$$

$$+ \overset{\pi_{XY}?}{\underset{+}{U_{\pi}(\overbrace{P_{XY}X + P_Y - C_{XY}})}} + \lambda X(\overbrace{P_{XY}X + P_Y}^{+})$$

The expressions $P_X X + P - C_X$ and $P_{YX} - C_Y$ are negative from the first-order conditions (not shown).

34. See Sloan and Feldman (1978).

35. One could allow the capital constraint to be nonbinding, but for purposes of this discussion a binding constraint is sufficiently realistic.

36. For large X, AC_X is likely to be positive. Throughout this section, we assume that $AC_X = AC_{\tilde{X}} > 0$ and $AC_{XX} = AC_{\tilde{X}\tilde{X}} > 0$.

37. Note:

$$\pi_{\tilde{X}Y} = \overset{MR_{\tilde{X}Y}}{\overbrace{P_{\tilde{X}Y}\tilde{X} + P_Y + \gamma(X_Y AC_{\tilde{X}} + X AC_{\tilde{X}Y} + AC_{\tilde{X}\tilde{X}}X_Y)}}$$

$$\underset{MC_{\tilde{X}Y}}{\underbrace{- AC_Y - (\tilde{X} + X)AC_{\tilde{X}\tilde{X}}X_Y - X_Y AC_{\tilde{X}} - (\tilde{X} + X)AC_{\tilde{X}Y}}}$$

38. Now, $\pi_{\tilde{X}\gamma} = XAC_{\tilde{X}} > 0$ and $\pi_{Y_\gamma} = X_Y AC + X(AC_X X_Y + AC_Y) > 0$. Both expressions are positive for $AC_{\tilde{X}} = AC_X > 0$.

$$\pi_{\tilde{X}Y} = P_{\tilde{X}Y}^+ \tilde{X} + \overbrace{(P_Y - AC_Y)}^{?} + X_Y^+ [\overbrace{AC_{\tilde{X}}(\gamma - 1) - AC_X}^{-}]$$

$$- AC_{XY}\overbrace{[X(\gamma - 1) - \tilde{X}]}^{?}$$

The sign of $\pi_{\tilde{X}Y}$ depends on P_Y versus AC_Y, $\gamma - 1$ versus $\tilde{X}/X$, and more.

39. We assume no shifts in $P(\cdot)$. If $P(\cdot)$ shifted inward, the qualitative results would be the same.

40. Since $\pi_{\tilde{X}M} = (\gamma - 2)X_M AC_{\tilde{X}} + (\gamma - 1)XAC_{\tilde{X}X}X_M - \tilde{X}AC_{\tilde{X}X}X_M \lesseqgtr 0$, a sufficient condition for a negative $\pi_{\tilde{X}M}$ is $(\gamma - 1) < \tilde{X}/X$. Within the range of plausible values of γ (approximately $1 < \gamma < 1.08$), $\gamma - 1$ can never be much larger than $\tilde{X}/X$. And $\pi_{\tilde{X}M}$ is probably negative. If we had specified a simultaneous inward shift in P, a negative $\pi_{\tilde{X}M}$ would have been even more likely.

41. Since $\pi_{YM} = (\gamma - 1)Z_1 + [(\gamma - 1)X - \tilde{X}]Z_2$, where $Z_1 = X_{YM}AC + X_Y AC_X X_M + X_M(AC_X X_Y + AC_Y)$ and $Z_2 = AC_{XX}X_M X_Y + AC_{YX}X_M$, a sufficient condition for a positive π_{YM} is $(\gamma - 1) > \tilde{X}/X$. For values of $\tilde{X}/X$ less than but in the neighborhood of $\gamma - 1$, π_{YM} is positive. For values far below this, π_{XM} could be negative.

42. This point is developed by Evans (1970).

3

Data and an Empirical Approach

As seen in the previous chapter, theory alone does not take one very far toward understanding forces underlying variations in hospital costs and input use. Although theory per se might prove to be the basis for a few leads about the nature of hospital responses, ultimate judgments must be based on the empirical evidence. This chapter provides a large part of the groundwork necessary for understanding our empirical approach and results.

The following sections cover sample selection procedures and data file construction, empirical specifications, functional forms (including methods for obtaining reduced forms from structural parameter estimates), details concerning the dynamic properties of our input model, and the method used to estimate parameters of our dynamic model. These discussions provide pertinent background information about the specification of average cost and input equations. Because both types of equations share a common data base as well as most explanatory variables, they are considered together. The input equations involve several additional complexities. For this reason, after the empirical specification section, remaining discussions deal exclusively with the input equations.

Data

The Sample

The observational unit for our empirical analyses is the individual hospital. The following selection criteria were applied to public-use data supplied by the American Hospital Association (AHA):

1. Only nonfederal, short-term general hospitals were selected.[1]
2. Hospitals were confined to those located within primary sampling unit (PSU) areas developed by the National Opinion Research Center (NORC) of the University of Chicago.
3. Hospitals meeting the above criteria were discarded from the sample if they did not exist in *each* of the seven years from, 1969 to 1975 *or* if they existed but did not respond to AHA survey questionnaires in any one of the seven years.

This selection process yielded a sample of 1,228 hospitals, which represents 21.3 percent of all nonfederal, short-term general hospitals and

41

Table 3–1
Selected Characteristics of Sample Hospitals and of All Nonfederal, Short-Term General Hospitals, 1975

Characteristic	Sample Hospitals		All Nonfederal, Short-Term General Hospitals	
	Mean	Standard Deviation	Mean	Standard Deviation
Proportion controlled by state or local government	0.146	—	0.307	—
Proportion for profit	0.136	—	0.132	—
Proportion with medical school affiliation	0.250	—	0.102	—
Proportion with nursing school affiliation	0.156	—	0.077	—
Total beds	268	213	163	173
Full-time-equivalent employees per bed	2.51	0.71	2.17	0.67
Total expenses per bed	$43,707	15,147	$32,400	14,735
Total admissions per bed	35.7	8.43	35.5	10.1
Outpatient visits per bed	239	176	199	167
Occupancy rate (percent)	75.3	12.0	70.5	13.3
Average length of stay (days)	7.93	2.29	7.53	2.97

17.0 percent of all U.S. hospitals as of 1975. Omission of federal, long-term, and specialty hospitals from the sample is common practice and has the advantage of homogenizing the hospital "product" under study. Although there is still considerable variation among sample hospitals in the nature and mix of services provided, the selection process reduces this variation to a manageable level. Moreover, most policy interest is focused on this type of hospital where the mainstream of hospital services in the United States is provided.

Use of the PSU framework for sample selection results in a cluster sample. This is a sensible approach for our purposes because of the necessity of merging large quantities of data pertaining to the geographic locations—counties and standard metropolitan statistical areas (SMSAs)—of our sample hospitals. Random selection of U.S. hospitals would have increased the time and computer costs of merging area data to prohibitive levels without adding much to our empirical analysis.[2] The PSU framework is based on 1970 census data and was designed for sampling households.

The sample includes hospitals from thirty-four states (including the District of Columbia) and 250 countries throughout the United States.[3] Table 3–1 compares selected characteristics of sample hospitals and the universe from which they were drawn. Compared to the sampling universe, sample hospitals are larger on average, more likely to have medical and nursing school affiliations, and less likely to be controlled by state or local government. Sample hospitals have more full-time-equivalent employees, expenses, and outpatient visits per bed, higher occupancy rates, and longer average lengths of stay. Most of, if not all, these differences reflect the fact that sample hospitals tend to be located in more highly urbanized areas than universe hospitals. In essence, our sampling methodology assigns weights to hospitals based on the populations using them, making it more likely for hospitals in heavily populated areas to be selected. Therefore, our sample is representative of the patient populations served by hospitals rather than of hospitals themselves. From the standpoint of statistical inferences to be drawn from our empirical estimates, we regard this as appropriate, and given that these differences have been made explicit, we do not view sample and universe differences as consequential.[4]

The Pooled File

Our primary data source is the AHA annual survey of U.S. hospitals for 1969 to 1975 inclusive. These surveys have been conducted by the AHA since the 1940s. A wide range of information is collected, including hospital facilities and services mix, utilization, staffing, expenses, assets, and revenues. Survey tapes made available by the AHA do not contain revenue data because this information is regarded as too sensitive for distribution, even for purposes of scholarly research. In addition to the annual general survey, the AHA conducts periodic surveys on topics of special interest. For our purposes special surveys pertaining to the years 1973 and 1975 were utilized to construct variables pertaining to hospital unionization.[5]

American Hospital Association data pertaining to the 1,228 sample hospitals were supplemented with community data from a variety of sources, identified in Appendix A. Area data pertaining to counties, SMSAs, or (in some cases) states were merged with AHA data via locational identifiers contained on the AHA files. All hospitals and years were then pooled into a time series of cross sections, yielding a single file with 7,368 observations. The pooled file was used for all the empirical work in this book (with the exception of chapter 4).

The empirical methodology requires that all dependent variables have merged lagged values; that is, dependent variable values for 1974 had to be merged with the 1975 portion of the file, values for 1973 merged with the 1974 portion of the file, and so on. Data for 1969 were used only for lagged values. Because there are ten dependent variables, there are ten lagged value variables.

Remaining file construction tasks are described in the appendixes. Our attention now turns to examining the variables constructed for purposes of our empirical research.

Empirical Specification

Overview

The empirical specification follows the general form of the theoretical analysis in chapter 2. Average costs and input levels depend on exogenous variables reflecting hospital product demand, factor supply input prices, hospital characteristics, regulation and reimbursement programs, and response lags. Although there are some differences in specifications between average cost and input regressions that we mention later, the similarities outweigh the differences. For this reason, both types of equations are described within a single section.

Our specification follows the lead of most recent research in this area, which views cost and input use as behavioral responses to a number of exogenous forces. In contrast to a few studies [for example, Baron (1974) and Pauly (1978)] which study hospital cost variations subject to exogenously determined levels of output and factor prices, we retain the assumption of exogenous factor prices but allow output to be endogenous. With output endogenous, costs and input use depend on a number of forces, such as hospital product demand variables, which are excluded in specifications with exogenous output.

Dependent Variables—Average Costs

Estimation of hospital cost functions has a long tradition in economics.[6] Emphasis on this topic reflects the facts that production theory is a reasonably well-developed part of economics and that hospital cost data have been readily available to researchers. Initially, economists focused on determining whether there are economies of scale in the production of hospital services. Beyond this, early economic research on hospital costs contributed little to the public-policy debate. More recently, studies have recognized that hospital costs reflect a number of behavioral responses. But, to our knowledge, no large-scale studies of hospital costs have attempted to measure the impact of regulatory programs and reimbursement methods to the extent of this book.

Four dependent variables relating to hospital costs have been defined: total expenses per adjusted patient-day (EXPAPD) and per admission (EXPADM) and labor expenses per adjusted patient-day (LPBAPD) and per admission (LABADM). The AHA provides data on "adjusted" as well as raw patient days. The adjustment, albeit crude, converts outpatient visits into patient-day equivalents, on the basis of relative costs, and adds the converted outpatient series to the raw patient-day series. Particularly because the number of outpatient visits has been rising dramatically in recent years, some adjustment for the outpatient component of hospital product is desirable.

We used alternative output denominators with the expectation that comparisons might yield some insights that a single measure would not permit. Adjusted patient-days and admissions measure somewhat different phenomena, and there is no agreement among economists on which of the two is the better output measure. Moreover, in some cases, one might hypothesize different effects of independent variables on costs depending on which output measure is used.[7] For example, as discussed in chapter 5, existing formula prospective reimbursement programs tend to produce an incentive for hospitals to increase length of stay, which might result in different cost consequences when patient-days and admissions are used as alternative output measures.

Given this book's emphasis on the hospital labor force, we estimate separate regressions for the labor cost component. Aside from being able to focus directly on factors affecting hospital labor costs, we are also able to compare parameter estimates from our labor cost regressions to corresponding estimates pertaining to labor input regressions. From such comparisons inferences may be drawn about the degree to which determinants of labor input intensity are also factors underlying labor costliness.[8] The cost variables reflect input prices as well as input quantities, and the cost regressions are in several respects more easily interpreted than the input regressions. However, the latter are useful in determining the manner in which exogenous forces affect hospital behavior and in distinguishing between input quantity and input price contributions to cost changes.

Dependent Variables—Labor Inputs

Our labor-input dependent variables are full-time-equivalent (FTE) registered nurses (RNs) per bed (RNBED), licensed practical nurses (LPNs) per bed (LPNBED), and "other" employees per bed (OTHBED).[9] To obtain structural estimates, we have used beds as the denominator in all our input regressions. These estimates can readily be combined with estimates from a regression with beds as the dependent variable to yield reduced-form estimates with input levels (rather than ratios) as dependent variables.[10] Specification of the input dependent variables in terms of ratios rather than levels greatly reduces multicollinearity resulting from the inclusion of several explanatory variables related to hospital size.

Our specification of labor-input variables reflects staffing data availability from the AHA. Data are given on full- and part-time RNs, LPNs, interns and residents, employed physicians, and total employees, from which FTEs have been calculated. The "other" employee category is total FTE employees minus the sum of the specified employee types. Interns and residents and employed MDs are not included in the analysis because they cannot be regarded simply as inputs in the production of hospital services. Employment of interns and residents and often salaried MDs involves production of educational services. Moreover, the methods of compensating many hospital-based physicians, particularly those in radiology and pathology, are the result of bilateral negotiations between physicians and hospitals rather than input choice decisions on the part of hospitals above. Thus, analysis of physician employment is best left to studies specifically tailored to account for these factors.[11]

As specified, our labor-input regressions will enable us to draw inferences regarding labor substitution possibilities and "normalcy" or "inferiority" of specific labor inputs. Given that the hospital production function incorporates quality, the notion of input inferiority in hospital service production, particularly with regard to less skilled labor categories, becomes a real possibility.[12] Negative signs on such variables as per capita income in LPN staffing regressions reported by Levine and Phillip (1975) suggest that hospital quality is relatively income-elastic, and comparatively fewer LPNs are required in the production of high quality. The possibility of input inferiority is a major source of ambiguity in comparative statics analysis of hospital behavior.

Dependent Variables—Nonlabor Inputs

Three nonlabor-input variables have been defined: estimated value of net plant assets per bed (ASSETB), nonlabor expenses per bed (NLEXP), and the hospital's bed supply (BDTOT).

Estimation of ASSETB is described in full in Appendix C. Predicted rather than actual values of net plant assets were employed primarily because variations in hospital asset vintage and depreciation methods would impart a serious errors-in-variables bias if hospital-reported dollar assets were used.[13] For example, two identical facilities, one built in 1970 and the other in 1975, could report vastly different asset values to the AHA because plant valuation is typically in terms of original costs and inflation in construction costs has been rapid in recent years.

The asset index was obtained by regressing 1975 net plant assets per bed, deflated by an area price index, on a comprehensive list of binary variables representing hospital facilities and services (for example, cobalt therapy program, premature nursery, family planning service, home care department) and a few other standardizing variables which, with one or two small exceptions,[14] remain constant from year to year (say, region, city size). The estimated parameters from this asset regression indicate the amount of fixed capital associated with specific facilities and services. Since facilities and services vary over time and, of course, among hospitals, so does the index. When used as an explanatory variable in our average-cost regressions, predicted assets per bed (ASSETB) represents the sophistication of the asset base, case mix, and, in total expense regressions, associated interest costs.[15] As a dependent variable, ASSETB is intended as a measure of fixed capital input that is purified of the effects of asset vintage and depreciation accounting variations.

Our current nonlabor variable, NLEXP, measures yearly hospital expenditures per bed on noncapitalized items such as supplies, food, energy, minor equipment, and contract purchases.[16] This variable excludes depreciation and interest expenses. Like ASSETB, NLEXP is measured in real monetary terms,[17] for there is no good way to measure current nonlabor inputs in physical units.

Hospitals face multiple opportunities for trade-offs between current labor and nonlabor expenses, particularly with regard to choices of whether to provide laundry, housekeeping, dietary, and other labor-intensive services internally or to purchase such services externally on a contract basis or via sharing arrangements with other hospitals. Virtually no research has been done to determine whether exogenous forces influence such trade-off decisions. If they do, the influences should be discernible by comparing parameter estimates from the NLEXP regression with other input regressions. Aside from potential trade-offs, general discussions of hospital behavior (rather than formal theory) lead us to expect NLEXP to respond positively to demand pressure on the hospital to upgrade the "quality" of the hospital product or, alternatively, to increase the amount of "slack" in hospital operations.[18]

Our final input is hospital beds. Typically, one thinks of changes in bed supply in terms of long-run additions to hospital plant or, less frequently, retirement of existing capacity. However, hospitals also have the option of some short-run change in bed supply by decreasing the number of "setup and staffed" beds or by adding beds to fill existing underutilized space. Because of high fixed costs and the inflexibility of space, such options tend to be limited. Nevertheless, we observe some changes in bed complements of individual hospitals; major changes tend to represent the fruits of building programs or, in isolated instances, retirement of large sections of the hospital plant. Thus, we expect both short- and long-run bed supply responses to changes in demand for hospital services and other exogenous factors.

Product Demand Variables

The first category of explanatory variables pertains to exogenous factors that influence demand for the hospital's product, thereby affecting its production-input choices. Our demand variables are measures of community characteristics (PERCAP, DENS), county physician and hospital bed supply characteristics (POPMD, GPPROP, POPBD), and third-party reimbursement (MCARE, MCAID, INS).

Per capita income (PERCAP) has been shown to have a positive impact on hospital patient-days.[19] Past empirical research on hospital costs, however, has not consistently demonstrated a substantial effect of income (Salkever 1972), and its impact on input use has varied by input. For example, positive effects have been reported on employment of RNs and negative effects on employment of LPNs (Levine and Phillip 1975; Sloan and Elnicki 1978).

The expected effect of population density DENS on hospital demand is uncertain. Because traveling for medical care is likely to be more substantial in low-density areas, hospitalization may be a more attractive alternative to ambulatory care, for both physicians and patients, in cases where inpatient and outpatient care are plausible alternatives (in a medical sense). However, as Feldstein (1971b) noted, there may be a tendency for a higher proportion of serious illnesses to be admitted in high-density areas; he found that density had a negative impact on admissions but a positive impact on mean stay. This suggests that hospital care received in high-density areas may be more input-intensive than care received in low-density areas. Both the number and the difficulty of cases should be reflected in hospital costs and input use. Salkever (1972) found that density had a weak negative impact on costs in his study of hospitals in New York State.

The availability of physicians in the hospital's market may affect the demand for hospital services in several ways. Increased availability of physicians may cause a shift from hospital care toward ambulatory care, thus reducing the demand for the former. Although inpatient and ambulatory care are substitutes in this sense, hospitalization may also be seen as complementary to physician's services in that patients are admitted to a hospital only on a physician's recommendation. Thus, where physicians are relatively numerous, there may be a greater propensity to recommend treatment, including hospitalization. Evidence from previous studies of the effect of physician availability on hospital use is mixed. Both positive and negative signs have been reported in hospital demand studies (Davis and Reynolds 1976; Feldstein 1971b; and Newhouse and Phelps 1976).[20]

Population per office-based, patient-care MD in the hospital's county (POPMD) represents the overall influence of physician supply. Because of offsetting effects discussed in chapter 2, the expected sign of this variable on product demand, let alone on costs and inputs, is ambiguous. However, rigorous theorizing aside, we expect the variable representing the proportion of these physicians who are general practitioners (GPPROP) to exert a negative impact on costs and the use of "sophisticated" inputs. General practitioners are much less likely to rely on the hospital for complementary inputs than specialists. Furthermore, a patient requiring specialized treatment is probably more likely to cross county boundaries for medical services, including hospitalization, than a patient with a relatively uncomplicated illness. Not only could this lead to a large quantity of hospital services demanded in countries with high specialist ratios, but also the mean case complexity is likely to be greater in such areas as well.

As the number of beds in other hospitals in the county increases relative to population (POPBD falls), the demand schedule facing our sample hospital should shift inward. Under the standard set of assumptions economists typically propose for firms, this increase should reduce output, and if we assume positively sloped cost curves, average costs and inputs should fall. But the standard theory of the firm does not suffice. First, the underlying model must take account of idiosyncratic characteristics of this industry and hence loses predictive power. Second, much of the competition in the hospital sector is nonprice, and thus costs and input intensity may be *higher* when a hospital faces competitors in its market area. For this reason, effects of POPBD in our regressions may well be negative.

Our three insurance variables are MCARE, the proportion of county population age sixty-five and over; MCAID, the proportion of under-sixty-five state population eligible for Medicaid benefits; and INS, an estimate of depth of coverage under private health insurance measured for counties. Construction of these variables is described fully in chapter 4 and Appendix H. Past research and policy discussions lead one to expect increased insurance coverage to raise product demand. However, variations in institutional features of different insurance programs provide the basis for tempering this prediction somewhat. These institutional variations, and related hypotheses, are described in chapters 4 and 5.

Factor Supply Variables

Factor price variables consist of measures of area unit prices of labor and nonlabor inputs (RNWG, LPNWG, OTHWG, CAP, CPI) and relative price variables constructed from these variables. Variable construction is explained in detail in Appendixes A through F. These variables are used primarily in the input regressions, although OTHWG is used as a single labor price variable in the cost regressions. Hourly wages for RNs and LPNs (RNWG, LPNWG) were derived from Bureau of Labor Statistics (BLS) and census data pertaining to SMSAs and census "county groups." The estimate of average hourly wage for "other" hospital employees (OTHWG) is based on payroll data provided in the AHA surveys. To purge the other employee wage of measurement errors, an instrumental-variables approach has been utilized. Because the instruments used to estimate OTHWG are area variables, OTHWG, like the other factor prices with the exception of CAP, measures area wage effects on our dependent variables.

Our cost-of-capital variable (CAP), the input price of our fixed capital measure (ASSETB), is based on construction cost and interest rate data provided in *Statistical Abstracts of the U.S.* Unlike the other input price measures, which are area-specific, we assume that the market for capital is nationwide. While construction costs vary geographically, costs of special hospital equipment do not. Thus, there is a case for either an area-specific or a national measure, and we have opted for the latter. Finally, the consumer price index (CPI) variable, the price of current nonlabor inputs, is based on cost-of-living data provided by the BLS.[21]

In the traditional theory of the firm, all input prices exert a negative impact on employment of their associated inputs. With the types of models explored in chapter 2, one can devise circumstances under which even this inference is violated. Neither textbook nor chapter 2 theory allows the signs of cross-input-price variables to be deduced a priori. As explained later, cross input prices enter the input equations as ratios of cross prices to "own" prices.

The cost regressions contain three binary measures of unionization activity. Hospital-specific wage and other effects of collective bargaining (for example, on turnover, staffing, job satisfaction, and productivity) are captured by these variables. Variable COLREQ identifies hospitals that have had a formal request from a union for recognition as a collective-bargaining agent within the twelve months preceding the survey date. This variable is a measure of the threat effect of unionization. That is, do hospitals alter their behavior in measurable ways to forestall or respond to union recruitment of hospital employees? Variable UNION identifies hospitals with signed collective-bargaining agreements with at least one union; STRIKE identifies hospitals that have had a strike or other work stoppage during the twelve-month period preceding the survey date. These variables are gross measures because they do not indicate the degree of union activity in hospitals, only its presence.[22] Nevertheless, past research on hospital costs has not attempted to measure union influences, and our specification represents an initial attempt to investigate the cost consequences of unionization. Moreover, because of the changes in the Taft-Hartley Act enacted in 1974, which require hospitals to recognize collective-bargaining units chosen by hospital employees, these consequences are likely to grow in importance as increasing proportions of hospital employees become the subject of union attention.

Hospital Characteristics Variables

Certain characteristics of hospitals may reflect preferences for the production of different types of outputs or may be related to the efficiency of production. Variables falling into this category are ASSETB, GOVT, PROP,

MEDSCH, NURSCH, SIZE1, and SIZE2, and SIZE3. The latter three variables, which are measures of hospital bed size, are included in the cost regressions only.

The variable ASSETB was described above as a nonlabor input. It is also included as an independent variable in the cost, labor input, and current nonlabor expense regressions to account for variations in case and service mix among hospitals. As noted above, ASSETB has been estimated from variables reflecting primarily the hospital's facilities and services mix.[23] Relatively high values of ASSETB thus reflect a high degree of service intensity, that is, more services available per bed than in hospitals with relatively low values of ASSETB. Lave and Lave (1978), in their study of hospital costs per admission and per patient-day in a random sample of U.S. hospitals in the late 1960s and early 1970s, found that the number of facilities and services exerted a substantial impact on costs.[24] We expect a positive impact of ASSETB in both input and cost regressions.[25]

In view of our inclusion of ASSETB as a dependent variable, one can very reasonably argue that ASSETB is endogenous when it appears as an explanatory variable. Even so, given our negative past experience and that of others with the use of simultaneous-equation techniques on cross-sectional data, we decided to eschew these methods in favor of single-equation estimation. We consider this simultaneity issue again in evaluating our empirical results.

Binary variables GOVT and PROP identify government (nonfederal) and proprietary (for-profit) hospitals, respectively. These variables adjust for probable differences in hospital objectives. If arguments regarding "cream skimming" are correct, proprietary hospitals tend to seek simple cases and employ fewer inputs, holding other factors constant, for reasons unaccounted for by the product demand variables.[26] Government hospitals, like other government institutions, are thought by many to be inefficient. If this is so, we would expect such hospitals to employ more inputs and have higher unit costs, *ceteris paribus*, than other hospitals.

Binary variables MEDSCH and NURSCH identify hospitals with medical school affiliations and with professional schools of nursing, respectively. Hospitals with such training programs use low-paid (interns and residents) and unpaid (nursing students) inputs in the production of hospital services. Also, medical school-affiliated hospitals derive benefits from treating patients with complex illnesses because of their value in the training process. Hospitals with nursing schools are likely to incur lower search and recruitment costs for staff nurses. On the whole, these factors do not suggest unambiguous hypotheses regarding the impact of these variables on hospital costs and input employment. However, we may expect the presence of medical or nursing school affiliations to be reflected in unit cost measures. This is especially true of physician training, particularly if educational requirements result in a more complex case mix.

Three binary variables indicating hospital bed-size class have been defined: SIZE1 for hospitals of less than 100 beds, SIZE2 for hospitals of 100 beds or more but less than 250 beds, and SIZE 3, for hospitals with 250 beds or more but less than 400 beds. The largest size class—hospitals with 400 beds or more—represents the excluded category in the cost regressions. In the past researchers have attempted to detect economies of scale in the production of hospital services. This has been a difficult task because of the association between bed size and the complexity of hospital services. If complexity is not accounted for sufficiently well, empirical results may spuriously indicate diseconomies of scale. However, even in studies where complexity measures have been entered into the empirical specifications, evidence in favor of economies of scale has been fairly weak (Lave and Lave 1970; Evans and Walker 1972; and Salkever 1972).

Regulation and Reimbursement Method Variables

Because we devote separate chapters to insurance and regulation (chapters 4 and 5, supplemented by Appendixes I and J), the present discussion is brief. We have constructed five variables pertaining to certificate of need (CON) alone (CCON1, CCON2, NCON1, NCON2, and PRECON). In the past several years, CON legislation has proliferated at the state level with obvious federal approval and legislative support. Our empirical estimates will attempt to discern effects of CON on hospital performance and dimensions of timing of CON programs vis-à-vis hospital anticipatory, compensatory, and lagged responses. We also distinguish between programs that focus primarily on bed growth and more comprehensive programs that scrutinize service and facility expansion in addition to bed growth.

Our reimbursement variables set (S1122, BCPAA, COSTB, FPR, BPR, UR, ESP) also contains measures of programs designed to curb hospital capital expansion. Even though these variables pertain to programs with differing objectives, their common denominator is that they all relate to third-party reimbursement. They measure programs that use reimbursement restrictions and incentives as a regulatory device. The exception, COSTB, measures fundamental differences in reimbursement method without necessarily relating to regulatory initiatives.

Static Properties of the Input Model

Functional Form

Ideally, input equations would be derived directly from hypothesized hospital preference and production functions. Unfortunately, even with comparatively straightforward assumptions (say, a multiplicative utility function with output and profits as arguments, a downward-sloping demand function for the hospital's product, exogenous input prices, and a Cobb-Douglas production function with two inputs), the resulting input equations contain important nonlinearities. Our experience with nonlinear regression techniques, coupled with dynamic estimation complexities and the large number of explanatory variables and observations, led us to the conclusion at an early stage in our research that nonlinear regression would not be worth the cost. Rather, if input demand equations are based on assumptions of profit maximization, price taking in factor markets, and price setting in product markets, then the resulting input employment equations are easy to estimate. These simplifying assumptions do not seriously impede our analysis; they result in a form of behavioral model which, as discussed above, has an established tradition in economic research.

If the demand curve for the hospital's product is

$$P = BX^\theta \tag{3.1}$$

where P = price, X = service composite, and B and θ are constants, and the production function is

$$X = AL^\alpha K^\beta \tag{3.2}$$

The profit function to be maximized is

$$\pi = BA^{(1 + \theta)}L^{\alpha(1 + \theta)}K^{\beta(1 + \theta)} - wL - rK \tag{3.3}$$

After some manipulation, the derived demand-for-labor equation is

$$\ln L = \frac{\beta(1 + \theta)[\ln w - \ln r] - \ln w - C}{[\alpha(1 + \theta) - 1][\beta(1 + \theta) - 1] - \beta\alpha(1 + \theta)^2} \tag{3.4}$$

where C is a constant containing, *inter alia*, exogenous variables and associated parameters reflecting shifts in the product demand function, equation 3.1. The corresponding equation for capital is similar, with reversals in the positions of the w and r terms (that is, r appears where w appears in equation 3.4, and vice-versa).

According to equation 3.4, the own factor price enters by itself (in absolute terms—represented by $\ln w$ in equation 3.4) and as the numerator of ratios which are divided by other factor prices (represented in general form in equation 3.4 by $\ln w - \ln r$). The denominator of equation 3.4 is positive, if we assume $-1 < \theta < 0$ or, equivalently, the product price elasticity $(1/\theta)$ is less than -1 (that is, the demand curve has a greater than unitary elasticity for all levels of X). For all positive output elasticities β within the unit interval, the own-wage elasticity is negative. Under these conditions the cross-price elasticity is also negative for product price elasticities within the admissible unit interval range. Under product price setting, derived demand equations are not homogeneous of degree zero with respect to prices as under competitive product market conditions. As already noted, exogenous demand shift variables are included in the general term C in equation 3.4.

Equation 3.4 is generalizable to several inputs. The own price of each input enters as w in equation 3.4, and there are terms for each pair of input prices, like $\ln w - \ln r$. The Cobb-Douglas production function rules out inferior inputs. As long as inputs are defined as broad categories, this restriction is plausible.

The use of the profit function in equation 3.3 means that we omit explicit consideration of variations in quality, amenities, and styles of care in obtaining equation 3.4. Because of this compromise and the ambiguities noted in chapter 2's theoretical discussion, we use two-tailed tests of significance to evaluate our empirical results.

Method for Obtaining Reduced-Form Estimates

The six input equations are interrelated in static and dynamic senses. In this section, we consider static relationships. All labor input equations and one nonlabor input equation (for current nonlabor expense) contain the fixed-asset measure as an independent variables. Furthermore, beds enter these four equations and the fixed-asset equation because the dependent variables include beds in the denominator. For some purposes, it is useful to gauge the indirect effect of an exogenous variable on input employment operating through effects on assets and beds, as well as the direct effect.

Suppose, for example, that the coefficient of PERCAP in the equation for RNs per bed is 0.2. Then 0.2 is the direct effect. Further, assume that PERCAP has coefficients of 0.3 and 0.05 in the ASSETB and beds equations, respectively, and ASSETB has a coefficient of 0.1 in the equation for RNs per bed. Then the total effect of PERCAP on input employment of RNs, if we neglect dynamic effects, is calculated as follows:

$$\ln\left(\frac{RNs}{beds}\right) = 0.1 \ln(ASSETB) + 0.2 \ln(PERCAP) + \text{other variables}$$

$$(3.5)$$

$$\ln\left(\frac{assets}{beds}\right) = 0.3 \ln(PERCAP) + \text{other variables} \qquad (3.6)$$

$$\ln(beds) = 0.05 \ln(PERCAP) + \text{other variables} \qquad (3.7)$$

Then, substituting equation 3.7 into 3.5 and neglecting other variables which do not enter this calculation, one obtains

$$\ln(RNs) = 0.1 \ln(ASSETB) + 0.25 \ln(PERCAP) + \ldots$$

$$(3.8)$$

Substituting equation 3.7 into 3.6 and the result into equation 3.8 yields

$$\ln(RNs) = 0.285 \ln(PERCAP) + \ldots \qquad (3.9)$$

The 0.285 elasticity represents the total effect of PERCAP on RN employment; the elasticity is composed of a 0.2 direct effect (from equation 3.5) and a 0.085 indirect effect. These hypothetical parameter estimates imply that per capita income affects RN employment both directly and indirectly via its positive effects on fixed asset and bed use.

Dynamic Properties of the Input Model

Rationale

Static variants of the input model, which use ordinary least squares, are estimated in this book. We also devote considerable attention to dynamic relationships among inputs. Possible interrelationships among various factors of production have been stressed by Nadiri and Rosen (1973) and provide a convincing rationale for our empirical approach. As Nadiri and Rosen (1973, p. 38) noted,

> A priori, logic suggests that the lags in production worker employment should be substantially shorter than for capital, since adjustment costs to the firm are probably smaller. Thus, the long lags estimated for [both] capital and employment have been something of an empirical puzzle. However, if one accepts the basis of the current [Nadiri-Rosen] model, the puzzle disappears.... [Accordingly,] anything producing long lags in the system as a whole tends to produce a long lag for each and every input. Thus, the adjustment process for employment and hours might display long lags, simply because the adjustment for capital—probably the ultimate source of lags—displays long lags. *If the firm is not in long-run equilibrium with respect to capital stock for very long periods, a complementary disequilibrium must appear elsewhere in the system*, if factor demand functions are time-interrelated and firms operate near their production possibility frontiers.

Another way to look at possible interrelationships among inputs is seen in figure 3–1, which depicts two inputs, labor and capital. The firm (it could be a

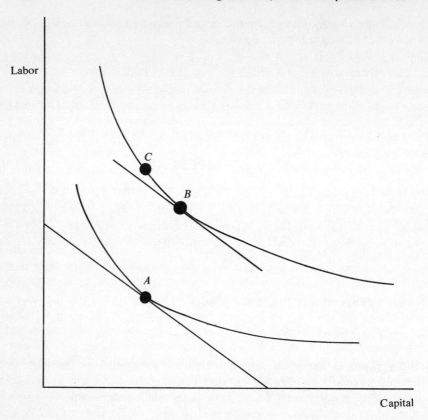

Figure 3–1. Expansion of Labor and Capital in the Short and Long Run

hospital) experiences a growth in demand for its product and therefore desires to increase its output. Referring to figure 3–1, we see that in the long run the firm would like to move from *A* to *B*, where, given factor prices for labor and capital, it can produce the new output at minimum cost. However, given the relative fixity of capital in the short run, it may be advisable to first move from *A* to *C*, which involves a substantial increase in labor and hardly any increase in capital. Although *C* does not correspond to an efficient labor-capital ratio in the long run, it may be appropriate in the short run if one considers the relative transactions costs involved in rapid expansion of capital versus labor inputs. This type of time path can be approximated in input equations for labor *and* capital in period *t* if *both* contain variables for labor and capital in period $t - 1$ as explanatory variables.

  More formally, consider two inputs, capital and labor. (The underlying principles are easily extended to a greater number of inputs.) Let

$$K_t - K_{t-1} = \beta_{11}(K_t^* - K_{t-1}) + \beta_{12}(L_t^* - L_{t-1}) \quad (3.10)$$

and $\quad L_t - L_{t-1} = \beta_{21}(K_t^* - K_{t-1}) + \beta_{22}(L_t^* - L_{t-1}) \qquad (3.11)$

where β_{ij} are fractions relating the change in capital and labor between $t-1$ and t to the difference between desired levels of capital and labor (K_t^* and L_t^*) at time t and actual levels at time $t-1$. The differences $K_t^* - K_{t-1}$ and $L_t^* - L_{t-1}$ may be positive or negative. If, for example, $L_t^* - L_{t-1}$ is positive, then there is a short-run labor "shortage." Conversely, a negative $L_t^* - L_{t-1}$ reflects a short-run labor "surplus." If one assumes the equation system is stable, imbalances between actual and desired stocks are eliminated in the long run. The "own" adjustment coefficients β_{11} and β_{22} lie between 0 and 1. The "cross" adjustment coefficients may be positive or negative. A negative sign implies that excess demand for the "other" factor has a negative impact on the change in the input in question between $t-1$ and t. Suppose, to cite a nonhospital example, an automobile factory is unable to secure tires in the short run; then it may decide to lay off some of its workers. To see the effect of a positive β_{ij}, for $i \neq j$, consider the following example from the hospital industry. Hospitals frequently report they are experiencing an RN "shortage," and as a result, they take certain actions (for example, close down beds, assign non-RNs to tasks traditionally performed by RNs, and so on).[27] Explicit considerations of interrelationships among inputs allows one to give statements such as these a formal meaning.

To continue the model, let

$$K_t^* = aM_t \qquad (3.12)$$

and $$L_t^* = bM_t \qquad (3.13)$$

where M_t represents exogenous (in this case, demand) variables, even though determinants of K_t^* and L_t^* could include other factors as well. Then

$$K_t = \beta_{11}aM_t + (1 - \beta_{11})K_{t-1} + \beta_{12}bM_t - \beta_{12}L_{t-1} \quad (3.14)$$

and $\quad L_t = \beta_{21}aM_t - \beta_{21}K_{t-1} + \beta_{22}bM_t + (1 - \beta_{22})L_{t-1} \quad (3.15)$

In matrix form,

$$\begin{bmatrix} K_t \\ L_t \end{bmatrix} = \begin{bmatrix} \beta_{11} & \beta_{12} \\ \beta_{21} & \beta_{22} \end{bmatrix} \begin{bmatrix} aM_t \\ bM_t \end{bmatrix} + \begin{bmatrix} 1 - \beta_{11} & -\beta_{12} \\ -\beta_{21} & 1 - \beta_{22} \end{bmatrix} \begin{bmatrix} K_{t-1} \\ L_{t-1} \end{bmatrix}$$

$$(3.16)$$

Estimated coefficients show $1 - \beta_{11}$, $1 - \beta_{22}$, $-\beta_{12}$, and $-\beta_{21}$, from which the underlying adjustment parameters can be obtained.

If we let the input vectors in equation 3.15 be Q_t, Q_t^*, and Q_{t-1}, equation 3.15 may be rewritten in matrix notation as

$$Q_t = \beta Q^* + (I - \beta)Q_{t-1} \qquad (3.17)$$

where I is an identity matrix. In equilibrium, inputs converge to a level $\bar{Q}$ so that

$$\bar{Q} = \beta Q^* + (I - \beta)\bar{Q} \qquad (3.18)$$

which establishes equality between desired and actual (equilibrium) levels of the inputs.

One might question whether a stable equilibrium exists. Necessary and sufficient conditions for a stable equilibrium are that all characteristic roots of β lie within the unit circle. If some roots lie slightly outside the range, Nadiri and Rosen (1973) show that the system will not demonstrate explosive oscillations immediately. But larger roots (in absolute value) do indicate that the system, once disturbed by an exogenous force, will not converge to a new equilibrium.

Estimation of Dynamic Models

With a dynamic specification, it is mandatory to use a method of time-series cross-sectional pooling. Otherwise, one could be certain that the estimated parameters on our lagged dependent variables would incorporate unspecified "state" effects (in this application, hospital effects). Moreover, if the state effects are not purged, readers would have reasonable grounds for doubting our conclusions about the effects of specific forms of regulation on input choice. After all, areas containing hospitals that are profligate users of inputs may be the first to implement various forms of regulation.

Alternative econometric methods could be used, but according to Nerlove (1971), the method described here showed least bias, lowest mean-square error, and greatest overall robustness against specification error. The procedure involves two rounds. In the first, an estimate of ρ, a parameter reflecting the importance of time-invariant effects, is derived. Let y_i. be the mean value of the dependent variable for the ith hospital over all T years and $x_i.(k)$ be the corresponding mean for the kth explanatory variable. A regression is run on the deviations between actual annual values and the means for the observations over all years. The regression is of the following form:

$$y_{it} - y_{i\cdot} = b_1(x_{1t} - x_{1\cdot}) + b_2(x_{2t} - x_{2\cdot}) + b_3(x_{3t} - x_{3\cdot}) + \cdots$$
$$+ b_k(x_{kt} - x_{k\cdot}) \tag{3.19}$$

Let $\hat{b}_1$ through $\hat{b}_k$ be the estimated parameters from equation 3.19 and s^2 be the sum of squared residuals from this regression. The estimated ρ will reflect the importance of the state effect in the equation's error team. In analysis of variance, ρ is often called the *intraclass correlation coefficient* ($\rho = \sigma_\mu^2/\sigma^2$).
To obtain $\hat{\rho}$, form

$$\hat{\sigma}_\mu^2 = \frac{1}{N} \sum_{i=1}^{N} \{y_{i\cdot} - y_{\cdot\cdot} - \sum_k \hat{b}_k[x_{i\cdot}(k) - x_{\cdot\cdot}(k)]\}^2 \tag{3.20}$$

where N stands for the number of observations in any year (in our case, either communities or hospitals), $y_{\cdot\cdot}$ and $x_{\cdot\cdot}(k)$ are grand means [means over all communities (hospitals) and years], and $\hat{b}_k$ are estimated parameters from the first-stage regression, equation 3.19. If there are no state effects, $y_{i\cdot}$ will tend to $y_{\cdot\cdot}$ and the same is true for $x_{i\cdot}(k)$ and $x_{\cdot\cdot}(k)$; $\hat{\sigma}_\mu^2$, which is based on squared deviations, will be small.
An estimate of ρ is then

$$\hat{\rho} = \frac{\hat{\sigma}_\mu^2}{\hat{\sigma}_\mu^2 + s^2/(NT)} \tag{3.21}$$

In the absence of state effects, $\hat{\rho} = 0$. Conversely, if state effects dominate, $\hat{\rho}$ approaches 1.
Using $\hat{\rho}$, one calculates estimates of $\hat{\varepsilon}$ and $\hat{\eta}$, which are characteristic roots of the variance-covariance matrix of the disturbance terms:

$$\hat{\varepsilon} = 1 - \hat{\rho} + T\hat{\rho} \qquad \hat{\eta} = 1 - \hat{\rho} \tag{3.22}$$

where T is the number of periods (years) in the time series.
As $\hat{\rho}$ approaches 0, both $\hat{\varepsilon}$ and $\hat{\eta}$ are 1. Conversely, as $\hat{\rho}$ becomes nearly 1, $\hat{\varepsilon}$ approaches T and $\hat{\eta}$ approaches 0.
Given $\hat{\varepsilon}$ and $\hat{\eta}$, one estimates a second regression:

$$\frac{y_{it} - y_{i\cdot}}{\sqrt{\hat{\eta}}} + \frac{y_{i\cdot}}{\sqrt{\hat{\varepsilon}}} = \alpha \left[\frac{y_{it-1} - y_{i\cdot}(-1)}{\sqrt{\hat{\eta}}} + \frac{y_{i\cdot}(-1)}{\sqrt{\hat{\varepsilon}}} \right]$$
$$+ \beta \left(\frac{x_{it} - x_{1\cdot}}{\sqrt{\hat{\eta}}} + \frac{x_{i\cdot}}{\sqrt{\hat{\varepsilon}}} \right) + \frac{\gamma}{\sqrt{\hat{\varepsilon}}} + \frac{u_{it} - u_{i\cdot}}{\sqrt{\hat{\eta}}} + \frac{u_{i\cdot}}{\sqrt{\hat{\varepsilon}}} \tag{3.23}$$

where, assuming a Koyck distributed lag, $y_i.$ (-1) is the mean of the lagged dependent variable for observational unit (hospital) i.

If $\hat{\rho}$ is nearly zero (the case of essentially no state effects), $\sqrt{\hat{\eta}}$ and $\sqrt{\hat{\varepsilon}}$ are nearly 1. Then the terms representing observational means nearly disappear, and one is left with an ordinary least squares regression. If $\hat{\rho}$ is nearly 1, the items containing $\sqrt{\hat{\eta}}$ in the denominators become very large, resulting essentially in a regression with all variables expressed as differences between actual and mean values (over all years) for the observational unit. In this case the persistent state effects are eliminated by subtraction.

To illustrate, assume $\hat{\rho} = 0.95$ and $T = 8$. Then $\sqrt{\hat{\eta}} = 0.22$ and $\sqrt{\hat{\varepsilon}} = 2.77$. The terms containing $\sqrt{\hat{\eta}}$ receive about ten times as much weight. Say $\hat{\rho} = 0.5$ and $T = 8$. Then $\sqrt{\hat{\eta}} = 0.71$ and $\sqrt{\hat{\varepsilon}} = 2.12$, and the terms containing $\sqrt{\hat{\varepsilon}}$ gain in importance. Finally, say $\hat{\rho} = 0.05$ and $T = 8$. Then $\sqrt{\hat{\eta}} = 0.97$ and $\sqrt{\hat{\varepsilon}} = 1.16$, and the means of the variables nearly cancel.

Although the time-series cross-sectional estimates are preferable, we also estimate static input regressions using ordinary least squares (OLS). The pooling method is especially hard on the few variables which by necessity had to be constructed in part by linear interpolation. The OLS estimates are particularly useful in such cases.

Notes

1. Short-term hospitals are defined by the AHA as those where over 50 percent of all patients admitted stay less than thirty days. General hospitals provide general medical and surgical care as opposed to specialty (for example, orthopedic, geriatric) services only.

2. Data-merging tasks were substantial, even with a cluster sample.

3. See Appendix F.

4. In any case, only under specific, infrequent circumstances will alternative sample selection and weighting schemes affect the estimated parameters. See Porter (1973). By contrast, estimates of variable means and standard deviations are highly dependent on sample selection and weighting.

5. In earlier years, the AHA asked information on special topics as part of its annual survey. We also use hospital-specific data on unionization available from the 1970 AHA survey.

6. See, for example, Feldstein (1967), Berry (1967), Lave and Lave (1970), Evans (1971), Evans and Walker (1972), and Salkever (1972). See Berki (1972) for a review of the earliest studies.

7. On this point, see Lave and Lave (1970).

8. As a hypothetical example, suppose that we find that a specific explanatory variable exerts a statistically and economically (that is, relatively high-elasticity) significant impact on RNs per bed, but not on labor

cost per admission or per patient-day. One plausible interpretation of this result would be that the impact of the variable on nursing intensity is compensated by reduced intensity in another labor input. Because our data do not permit examination of a wide range of specific labor inputs, we are unable to identify such substitutions through input analysis alone.

9. We assume, as does the AHA, that all part-time employees are equivalent to half a full-time equivalent.

10. See the discussion later in this chapter and in chapter 8 for additional detail.

11. In preliminary analysis, a variable representing interns and residents per bed was defined for only hospitals which had at least five FTE interns and residents in 1970. This reduced our sample for analysis of this type of input from 1,228 to 444. Hospital demand for interns and residents is an exceedingly complex issue because, unlike other labor inputs, these employees both contribute to the production of hospital services and are the recipients of medical education which, in turn, involves a commitment of other hospital resources. This goes far beyond the typical on-the-job training received by most types of employees—interns and residents are in training for their entire tenure of employment. Our preliminary research yielded very few conclusive results, and we thought it best to defer further inquiry for future research.

12. See Hadar (1971) for a discussion of input inferiority.

13. It is often noted in the hospital literature that variations in methods of evaluating assets and depreciation are substantial among hospitals. See, for example, Cleverley (1978).

14. For example, beds and beds squared in the asset regressions. The area price index is described in Appendix B.

15. We recognize that facilities and services variables have not been validated as case-mix variables. Further, binary variables do not account for variations in facility or service scale. Berry (1970) used these variables in a manner similar to ours. Also see Lave and Lave (1978).

16. An anomaly of the AHA data is that fringe benefits are recorded as a nonlabor expense. We have therefore deducted fringes from our nonlabor-expense variables.

17. As indicated in Appendix B, our area price deflator relies extensively on the consumer price index. We selected this deflator on the basis of a statement in U.S. Council on Wage and Price Stability (1977) that the CPI is almost perfectly correlated ($r = 0.98$) with a hospital price index developed in Feldstein (1974). After we completed the bulk of our empirical research, comparisons of an AHA input price index and the CPI came to our attention (McMahon and Drake 1978). This source indicates that while the CPI followed the AHA index fairly closely over 1970–1973, by 1975 the AHA index was clearly higher, principally because of rises in prices of such

items as malpractice insurance. To account for this and other time-related anomalies, we have included a trend variable (TIME) in the input regressions.

18. As stated in chapter 2, some economists have specified hospital objective functions with organizational slack as an argument, following recent industrial organization literature on non-profit-maximizing behavior of firms. Empirically, it is very difficult to distinguish between quality enhancement and reduced efficiency. Additions to quality may be reflected in improvements in patient chances of recovery or reduction in patient disutility associated with being hospitalized. Because these factors cannot be measured accurately at the micro level, we are forced to accept the ambiguity of a measured increase in expense per bed.

19. See Davis and Reynolds (1976), Feldstein (1971b), and Newhouse and Phelps (1976). Patient-days are the product of the number of admissions and the length of stay per admission. Income elasticities associated with admissions are always lower than those for length of stay. In fact, in two studies—Davis and Russell (1972) and Rosenthal (1964)—income has a negative impact on admissions. However, as Davis and Russell note, the negative sign on income may reflect the absence of adequate health-status measures in these studies.

20. Issues concerning the relationship between physician availability and performance in health-related markets are discussed at length in Sloan and Feldman (1978). Also, see Reinhardt (1978).

21. The CPI is the same as COL72, our variable used to deflate all monetary dependent and independent variables. See Appendix B.

22. See Sloan and Steinwald (1980) for data on union effects on wages paid to specific classes of hospital employees.

23. Construction of ASSETB is described in Appendix C.

24. The Lave and Lave (1978) measure was simply the sum of facilities and services provided. This has the disadvantage that all facilities and services are given equal weight, whereas our method attempts to estimate the contribution of each facility and service to the hospital's asset base.

25. Service intensity is clearly related to hospital case mix, which is a likely determinant of costs per unit of output. Some past studies of hospital costs have used direct measures of case mix (say, distribution of patients by type of diagnosis) and generally have found such measures to be important in explaining hospital cost variations. See, for example, Evans (1971), Evans and Walker (1972), Lave, Lave, and Silverman (1972), and Lee and Wallace (1973). Lipscomb, Raskin, and Eichenholz (1978) provide a general discussion of issues associated with accounting for case-mix variations in hospital cost studies.

26. See Steinwald and Neuhauser (1970), Rafferty and Schweitzer (1974), and Bays (1977) for discussions of the cream-skimming issue. The latter two sources provide evidence of systematic differences in case mix between for-profit and nonprofit hospitals.

27. We discuss this point in greater detail in chapter 8.

4

Third-Party Reimbursement for Hospital Services

This chapter has a dual purpose. First, it describes in detail the procedures employed to construct third-party reimbursement variables to be used in the empirical analyses of hospital costs and inputs. These variables gauge the extent of coverage under the major publicly financed reimbursement programs, Medicare and Medicaid, and the extent of coverage under private health insurance. Past treatments of private health insurance in empirical work on hospital behavior often relied on state aggregate data on proportions of populations insured. This approach, while understandable in light of limitations on data availability, disregards substantial variation among states and among insurance programs. Because of the importance of health insurance to the hospital industry, we made a concerted effort to develop a variable that more accurately reflects depth of coverage and is measured at aggregation levels more closely approximating hospital market areas.

The second purpose is more general. Despite the fact that the vast majority of people in the United States are insured for hospital services, some hospitalized patients incur relatively large out-of-pocket expenses arising from coverage limitations of their insurance policies. In this chapter we describe important characteristics of health insurance policies and identify sources of variation in depth of coverage.

Next we discuss health insurance institutions and provide illustrative statistics. Then details of the construction of our private health insurance variable are presented. The chapter concludes with a brief section on hypothesized effects of insurance variables on hospital costs and input choices and a summary of our findings pertaining to the demand for private health insurance.

Insurance for Hospital Services: Institutions and Evidence

Overview

By the end of 1975, roughly 81.3 percent of the U.S. civilian population under age sixty-five had private health insurance coverage for hospital care.[1] About 98 percent of the over-sixty-five population were covered by the Medicare program, and roughly 63 percent of the aged had private health insurance, usually to supplement Medicare benefits. Of the estimated 35 million persons under age sixty-five without private health insurance for hospital care, most had coverage under a variety of publicly financed programs, chiefly Medicaid. Approximately 19 million persons were eligible for hospitalization benefits under the Medicaid program in 1975 (National Center for Social Statistics 1976). Additional coverage was provided to the nonelderly by Medicare, the Maternal and Child Health program, and other federal, state, and local programs. It is difficult to determine the precise number of persons without any public or private health insurance coverage. According to the 1976 household interview survey conducted by the National Center for Health Statistics, 22.8 million persons under age sixty-five were without any coverage (Carroll and Arnett 1979), somewhat higher than conventional wisdom would suggest.

The distribution of persons enrolled in private hospitalization insurance programs among different types of insurers was as follows in 1975: approximately 40.2 percent of enrollees were covered by Blue Cross-Blue Shield, 55.3 percent were covered by commercial insurance companies, and 4.3 percent were covered by "independent plans."[2] The last category consists of health maintenance organizations (HMOs) and other plans that combine insurance with the provision of hospital and other services. Although important from a public-policy standpoint, these plans represent a relatively small share of the hospital insurance market and are conveniently ignored in the present context. Thus, our discussion of private hospitalization insurance is confined to Blue Cross and commercial insurance companies.

Similarly, our discussion of public programs is confined to Medicare and Medicaid. For Medicare, we simply took population age distribution data by county to construct a variable representing the proportion of population over age sixty-five, MCARE. This introduces a very slight error by ignoring under sixty-five Medicare beneficiaries and the very few elderly not eligible for Medicare. However, because Medicare is a uniform program nationwide in structural terms, its impact on hospital performance is well represented by MCARE.[3] Relative to private hospital insurance, Medicare is a comprehensive program in that a wide range of hospital services are covered. But there are significant limitations in coverage, including deductibles, coinsurance, and service maximums. This is why many elderly choose to supplement their coverage with private health insurance.

With regard to hospital services, Medicaid is also a reasonably uniform program.[4] Medicaid is generous in that services are provided to eligible persons with little or no out-of-pocket cost. From the hospital standpoint, however, the generosity of Medicaid is not so clear-cut. Complaints regarding amounts and timeliness of payments to hospitals tend to be more frequent with Medicaid than with other types of insurers.[5] Most of the variations in Medicaid importance to hospitals derives from state variations

In eligibility requirements vis-à-vis family or individual income levels. Some states have relatively liberal requirements; others are more stringent. In the former, Medicaid is likely to be a relatively more important force in hospital behavior.

We were forced to use state data to estimate population proportions eligible for Medicaid because smaller-area data are unavailable. In addition, Medicare coverage takes precedence over Medicaid. In the case of persons eligible for both programs, Medicare pays hospital expenses, but Medicaid often covers some expenses not reimbursed by Medicare. To avoid double counting, our Medicaid variable (MCAID) subtracts the county proportion of persons sixty-five and over from the state proportion of population eligible for Medicaid.[6] Because different population bases are used, this introduces some tolerable error into our Medicaid variable series.

Depth of Coverage under Private Health Insurance

Depth of coverage refers to the purchasing power of a given health insurance policy for hospital and other health services. There are three primary components of depth of coverage: which benefits are covered, how generous the benefits are, and how much patient copayment is required.

Most health insurance policies specify the benefits to which the insured is entitled. Virtually all policies include inpatient hospitalization benefits. However, variations in depth of coverage can be partially attributed to the extent to which other services are covered, such as X-rays and laboratory tests, outpatient ambulatory care, and so on.

In terms of generosity of benefits, most policies specify limitations on reimbursement for covered services. Such limitations may be monetary (say, daily hospital room-and-board dollar limits) or related to the extent of use (for example, a maximum number of days of hospitalization coverage per year). In addition, stipulations frequently limit the applicability of benefits (for example, exclusion of coverage for services obtained for treatment of "preexisting conditions").

Patient copayments consist primarily of deductibles, amounts paid for services prior to the insurance becoming effective, and coinsurance, a specified percentage of charges paid by the insured.[7] There is relatively little variation in copayment amounts. Deductibles tend to be on the order of $100 in most private insurance programs, and the coinsurance rate is typically 20 percent. However, there is considerable variation among insurance programs as to when copayment provisions are applied, if at all.

Several specific characteristics of health insurance policies are related to depth of coverage. First is the type of insurance—basic benefit, major medical, or combined. Basic insurance features "first dollar" coverage.

There tends to be relatively little patient out-of-pocket payment *unless* benefit limitations are exceeded, which is not uncommon. In contrast, major medical insurance tends to have deductibles that must be paid by patients until covered expenses exceed the specified amount, and coinsurance is typically associated with this form of insurance. Major medical insurance is designed to protect against relatively large health service expenditures, and then benefits usually are associated with periods of time rather than specific episodes of care.

A priori it is impossible to determine whether basic or major medical insurance provides greater depth of coverage. The tendency for basic-insurance subscribers to exceed benefit limitations offsets the built-in copayment provisions of major medical insurance. Many insured persons have combined basic and major medical coverage, in which major medical benefits are effective for services not covered by basic benefits or when basic benefits for covered services are exhausted. In recent years, major medical has been the fastest growing type of health insurance. By the end of 1976, nearly 100 percent of commercial health insurance subscribers with hospitalization coverage had major medical (Health Insurance Institute 1978).[8] Blue Cross writes less, but also a growing amount, of this type of insurance.

A second feature of health insurance policies related to depth of coverage is whether benefits are the indemnity or service variety. This is particularly relevant to coverage for inpatient hospitalization. Because there is some confusion in the literature regarding definitions of these concepts, we provide our own definition that dichotomizes all benefits as either service or indemnity. Under *service* benefits, the subscriber is insured for the service rather than for expenditures. This means that regardless of the provider's charge for the service, the individual is fully covered. There may be some limitations (for example, a Blue Cross subscriber may have to obtain services at a Blue Cross-participating hospital to be ensured full coverage), but generally the insured is entitled to receive the covered service at no out-of-pocket cost. Any disputes over the amount of the charge (or cost) are a matter for negotiation between the insurer and the provider. Service benefits is a concept employed principally by Blue Cross and Blue Shield plans (collectively referred to below as "the Blues").

Under *indemnity* benefits, the insured is indemnified against covered expenses, but the extent of indemnification is limited. In its simplest form, an indemnity policy will pay a specified amount (say, $50 per day hospitalized), regardless of expenses actually incurred. Other forms of indemnity coverage are linked to the hospital's charge or cost structure, for example, daily reimbursement for costs not to exceed 90 percent of the hospital's most common semiprivate room rate. Under this type of arrangement, the insured will typically incur some out-of-pocket expense. Indemnity plans, particularly the first variety, are much more common among commercial insurance programs than the Blue Cross. Moreover, this concept is most relevant to basic insurance for hospitalization episodes.[9]

Another factor is the loading charge of the health insurance policy. The *loading* is the difference between the premium and the expectation of benefits payments. All policies have some loading to cover insurance program administrative and claims review costs and company profits in the case of profit-seeking commercial firms. If the premium is held constant as loading increases, depth of coverage should decrease because there is less residual premium available to cover health service expenditures.

The amount of loading on health insurance policies is extremely variable and strongly related to several insurance policy characteristics. The most important is whether the policy is group or individual. Group policies are written for groups or enrollees, usually associated with a single employer; individual policies are written separately for single individuals or families. During the 1968–1970 period, commercial insurers collected roughly 19 percent more in group policy premiums than was paid out in health insurance benefits, while the excess of premiums over benefits paid for individual policies was about 47 percent (Blair and Vogel 1975). This discrepancy is mainly due to the fact that group policies are far less costly to market and administer than individual policies. The vast majority of health insurance policies are group policies.

Another factor related to loading is the type of insurer—commercial or Blue. In 1974, commercial insurance companies collected about $18.5 billion in health insurance premiums and paid out about 74 percent in benefits while Blue Cross, Blue Shield, and other hospital and medical plans collected about $14.5 billion in premiums and paid out about 94 percent.[10] One explanation for the difference in benefits-to-premiums ratios is that the commercial companies sell a higher proportion of individual health insurance policies. Other potentially important factors include the following: (1) The Blues tend to be taxed at lower rates than the commercial companies. (2) Commercial firms retain a higher proportion of earnings for distribution as profits or to finance future growth. (3) Commercial firms are subject to more cost-increasing regulatory attention than the Blues.

The extent of importance of these factors is uncertain. Frech and Ginsburg(1978) asserted that the tax and regulatory advantages of the Blues are of sufficient magnitude to question why the commercial firms are able to compete and retain their market shares. Their explanation was that the Blues use their competitive advantage to "purchase" the ability to provide more complete health insurance than is warranted by market demand and to have substantial managerial slack in plan administration.[11] Blair and Vogel's (1975) empirical evidence gives support to the view that there is a managerial slack in Blue Cross-Blue Shield operations. They observed that there is evidence of significant economies of scale in the provision of commercial insurance but no evidence of such economies in Blue plan operations. Their explanation was that the Blues tend to be less inclined to minimize costs as plan size grows. Blair and Vogel also observed that Blue Cross and Blue Shield plans are reluctant to merge even though there is evidence that such mergers tend to reduce unit costs in sale and administration of health insurance policies.

A final topic related to depth of coverage pertains to regulation of health insurance and reimbursement. Health insurance regulation traditionally has been conducted at the state level and has been oriented toward consumer protection.[12] Such regulations have been concerned primarily with protection against fiscal insolvency of insurers with resultant loss of coverage for the insured; review of complaints regarding settlement of claims and other transactions between insurers and the insured; and protection against fraud and insufficient value in insurance purchases, particularly in the case of insurance policies sold to individuals.

Until recently, regulations falling under these three categories accounted for the bulk of activities of state health insurance regulatory agencies. Within the past several years, the focus of health insurance regulation has changed somewhat, owing to the combined effect of increased government health insurance purchases and inflation in hospital and other health service expenditures. Insurers have been criticized for not monitoring more closely their reimbursements to hospitals for claims incurred by policyholders. Indeed, because insurer-instituted controls over hospital expenditures would appear to be in the economic interests of insurers (for example, effective monitoring could theoretically allow reduced prèmiums and increased sales), inflation in hospital expenditures has led to allegations of collusion between insurers and hospitals. This is especially true of Blue Cross which, because of its nonprofit status and presumed public-service orientation, has been open to considerable reproach for contributing to the inflationary trend in hospital costs.[13] Consequently, several recent regulations have been promulgated which intervene in transactions between insurers and providers by limiting methods and amounts of hospital reimbursement.

Descriptive Evidence

Industry and government sources do not provide much detail on characteristics of health insurance policies. A household survey conducted by the Center for Health Administration Studies (CHAS) and the National Opinion Research Center (NORC) in 1971 provides comprehensive data on characteristics of health insurance policies. This survey collected detailed data on health insurance premiums, benefits, and payments *and* verified and expanded the data base by surveying respondents' insurance organizations on specific features of policies held by respondents. All the remaining empirical evidence in this chapter is based on the CHAS-NORC survey.[14]

Tables 4–1 and 4–2 present data on private health insurance policies illustrating some of the dimensions of depth of coverage. Table 4–1 shows coverage distributions for several insurance benefits by type of insurer and type of insurance. Nearly all insured persons were covered for inpatient hospital benefits in 1970, and proportions having coverage for surgery and other hospital services were not much lower. Comparison of commercial and Blue coverage proportions reveals a slight tendency for the Blues to emphasize coverage of services performed in the hospital, while the commercial companies tended to have a greater proportion of subscribers eligible for noninstitutional benefits. However, one could not conclude from Table 4–1 that either type of insurer tends to provide more thorough benefits. Although not exhaustive, this list represents the vast majority of health insurance benefits payments.

The second part of table 4–1 gives the coverage type distribution for each covered benefit. (The four row percentages in the second part add to 100 for each benefit.) These data show that roughly two-fifths of benefits pertaining to services performed in the hospital tend to be covered under basic-only plans, and a slightly higher proportion are covered under combined basic and major medical. However, the coverage proportions for major medical plans increase substantially for services performed outside the hospital, and the coverage proportions for basic-only and combined plans tend to be correspondingly less.

The significance of these data relates to their implications for coverage of the marginal dollar of health service expenditure. Basic plans provide thorough coverage (that is, little or no patient out-of-pocket expense) up to the point where coverage limits are exceeded. If such limits are exceeded, the marginal rate of patient payment may be 100 percent. This seldom happens with major medical coverage (major medical policies tend to have limits that are exceeded only in cases of catastropic illness), but patient payment rates are 100 percent prior to satisfaction of the deductible and seldom fall below 20 percent after that. Even combined basic–major medical policies, which are the most thorough type, tend to have "corridor" deductibles that require patient out-of-pocket payment when basic benefits are exhausted before major medical coverage becomes effective. Thus, type of health insurance influences both average and marginal out-of-pocket payments by insured consumers, and the relationship between average and marginal payments varies with insurance type.

Table 4-1
Benefits Available to Under-sixty-five Insured Household Heads in 1970, by Type of Insurer and Type of Coverage

Benefit	Percentage of Insured Persons with Benefit Covered by Type of Insurer			Percentage Distribution of Coverage Type for Those with Benefit Covered			
	Commercial	Blue Cross-Blue Shield	Total[a]	Basic Only	Major Medical	Combined	Other
Inpatient hospital care	99.2	99.7	99.4	42.3	7.5	47.0	3.1
Treatment in outpatient department or emergency room of hospital	91.2	99.5	95.7	40.4	7.9	49.4	2.3
In-hospital surgery	98.9	93.6	96.0	40.2	7.3	49.2	3.3
Surgery in a doctor's office	98.7	91.1	95.2	39.7	9.4	47.6	3.3
Doctor visits in a hospital	85.9	89.8	88.5	35.2	14.4	46.9	3.6
Doctor visits in a private office, clinic, or patient's home	71.2	56.5	65.2	11.6	61.4	21.1	5.9
X-ray and laboratory tests	86.7	84.0	86.3	40.0	18.5	38.1	3.4
Nursing home care	22.6	27.0	24.6	24.6	54.5	17.6	3.2
Out-of-hospital prescribed drugs	68.4	47.8	57.6	2.2	87.1	6.1	4.5
Dental care outside a hospital	10.8	7.1	9.8	6.6	50.7	22.1	20.6
(n)	(624)	(650)	(1,388)				

Source: CHAS-NORC Household Survey, 1971.
[a]Includes 114 persons covered by other (noncommercial, non-Blue Cross-Blue Shield) private insurance plans.

Table 4–2
Selected Characteristics of Blue Cross-Blue Shield and Commercial Health Insurance Policies of Under-sixty-five Insured Household Heads, 1970

Characteristic	Commercial		Blue Cross-Blue Shield		All[a]		
	Family	Nonfamily	Family	Nonfamily	Family	Nonfamily	Total
Mean total premium	$295	$106	$355	$148	$326	$135	$277
Percentage group	82.6	44.4	86.0	78.5	85.0	63.2	79.7
Percentage with major medical covering hospitalization	72.7	50.4	46.1	38.6	58.2	42.5	54.6
Percentage with major medical covering surgery	72.1	52.6	50.1	41.8	59.9	45.0	56.5
Percentage with service benefit for hospital room and board	30.7	12.8	80.9	71.2	58.0	46.2	55.3
Percentage with service benefit for appendectomy	28.8	25.9	47.2	34.3	38.1	32.3	36.8

Source: CHAS-NORC Household Survey, 1971
[a]Includes approximately 8 percent persons covered by other (noncommercial, non-Blue Cross-Blue Shield) insurance plans.

The low proportions of benefits covered by other insurance reflect the relatively low market penetration of HMOs and other "independent" health insurance plans in 1970. A notable feature of these data is the relatively high proportion of dental benefits covered by this type of plan. In general, the independent plans tend to be more comprehensive than those of the Blues or commercial firms, and out-of-pocket payment for health services consumed tends to be low under independent plans.

Table 4–2 reveals major differences between family and nonfamily health insurance and between commercial and Blue policies. As one would expect, family policy premiums are much higher than those of individual policies. In this sample, they differ by a factor of about 2.4[15] In addition, a higher proportion of family policies are group policies, and a higher proportion of family subscribers have major medical coverage and are eligible for service benefits. These factors suggest that family policies tend to provide more comprehensive coverage as well as covering more persons than individual policies.

There are significant differences between commercial and Blue policies pertaining to nearly all characteristics reported in table 4–2. The Blue plans return a higher proportion of premium income to subscribers in the form of benefit payments, but their premiums tend to be higher than those of commercial firms. Blue and commercial plans tend to market roughly equal proportions of group family coverage, but those of the Blues have a much higher proportion of nonfamily policies sold on a group basis. Commercial insurers sell a greater proportion of major medical insurance than the Blues, but there is relatively little difference between the two in major medical coverage for hospitalization and surgical benefits.

The most striking difference between commercial firms and Blue plans pertains to the incidence of service benefits, which can be viewed as a measure of generosity or thoroughness of covered benefits. The Blues provide far greater service benefits than do commercial companies, especially in the case of inpatient hospital care. Because the insurer pays a higher proportion of health care expenses incurred under service benefit programs, this is likely to account for a large part of the difference in premiums between Blue and commercial plans.

To this point, our treatment of depth of coverage under health insurance has been entirely descriptive. Our view is that an understanding of health insurance institutions is essential to an examination of health insurance effects on provider and consumer behavior. The next section presents an empirical investigation of determinants of variations in depth of coverage among population groups. This investigation is a part of the process of constructing a private health insurance variable to be used in our analysis of hospital costs and inputs.

Development of a Measure of Depth of Private Health Insurance Coverage

Overview

A private health insurance variable (INS) has been derived from a three-stage process, by using verified health insurance premium data from the CHAS-NORC survey. First, we regressed health insurance premiums, measured for family household heads, on twenty-four binary variables describing the insurance policy's benefit structure and other variables associated with interplan and interarea differences in loading. The resulting parameter estimates on the insurance policy variables represent the value that the (marginal) consumer places on each insurance benefit characteristic. We summed the variables and their respective coefficients to form a depth-of-coverage index for each insured household head in the sample. Second, we regressed the predicted index on variables hypothesized to affect the demand for insurance (including age, income, and family size), again with the family head as the observational unit. Finally, estimated parameters from this regression were used in combination with county estimates of the insurance demand variables to predict depth of coverage for counties for 1970 to 1975. Comparisons between the growth in our predicted series and the actual growth in real premiums showed that our series understated the growth, probably reflecting unspecified year effects (which clearly cannot be captured by a single cross section). We therefore scaled the predicted values to make the growth in our series equal the aggregate U.S. growth in real (deflated by the CPI) premiums. These stages are descibed in greater detail.

Stage One: Determinants of Variations in Premiums

An adequate description of our specification of the first-stage regression would necessarily require a substantial amount of space. Because this estimation process is a means toward an end (that is, construction of INS), details of the first stage have been placed in Appendix H. However, some important features of model specification and statistical results merit consideration here.

In the first stage, the family's health insurance premium is the dependent variable. For any given premium, the following identity holds:

$$\text{Premium} \equiv \text{expected benefit} + \text{loading} \qquad (4.1)$$

The insurer's expected benefit, or payout, reflects the policy's benefit structure as well as the health status of the insured. In the health insurance field, risk discrimination on the basis of the individual's or family's health status, or related factors, is quite rare. This factor can be neglected in an equation explaining variations in premiums. Loading includes administrative costs and profits of the insurers. As stated earlier, it is likely to depend on such variables as the type of insurer, individual versus group policies, group size (for group policies), and various forms of insurance regulation.

The regressions presented in Appendix H explain about 40 percent of the variation in family health insurance premiums and about 28 percent of the variation in individual premiums. Most of the parameter estimates had the expected signs, but there were a few anomalous results. The benefits variables were the most consistent determinants of premium variations, but variables related to loading tended to be inconsistent with regard to sign and magnitude and were most often statistically insignificant.

Among the benefits variables, those pertaining to inpatient hospitalization had the strongest effect on premiums. The findings indicated a substantial impact of generosity of inpatient benefits (daily room-and-board dollar maximum and maximum days of care per year) on premiums. To illustrate, those with family coverage under a basic-only plan with generous daily room-and-board benefits (more than $55 per day or reimbursement at the most common semiprivate room rate or higher) paid about $145 more in premiums, *ceteris paribus*, than those with similar coverage with low-level benefits ($25 per day or less). As noted in Appendix H, because of collinearity among the benefits variables, these results should not be accepted uncritically.

Several dummy variables were included in the regressions to represent combinations of commercial or Blue coverage, group or individual insurance purchases, and states with or without authority to regulate health insurance premiums. These factors were combined in this way because the regulatory authority tends to vary among states according to type of insurer and type of insurance purchase. Based on past research [for example, Phelps (1973) and Frech and Ginsburg (1978)], we expected the Blues' premiums to be lower than those of commercial firms, group premiums to be lower than individual premiums, and regulated premiums to be lower than nonregulated premiums. However, parameter estimates on these variables did not support our expectations—once benefit structure is accounted for, no consistent pattern was discernible. This result is particularly surprising with regard to the lack of difference between Blue and commercial insurance, in light of the fact that the Blues tend to return a higher proportion of premium income in benefit payments than the commercial companies. It may be true, however, that this factor is offset by a tendency for the Blues to enroll populations with a higher incidence of illness than the commercial firms do.[16] Alternatively, it may be true that our list of benefits variables, despite its comprehensiveness, does not fully capture depth-of-coverage differences between the Blues and commercial companies.

State health insurance regulation variables were constructed from information presented in Lewin and Associates (1975a).[17] Results pertaining to these variables are generally unfavorable to our hypotheses. For example, while there is some evidence that state authority to regulate health insurance premiums and consumer health insurance education programs exert a depressing effect on premiums, the positive sign of the utilization review variable and the negative sign on the premium tax variable are implausible.[18] On the whole, these parameter estimates do not convey much useful information about the effect of state health insurance regulatory programs on premiums,[19] and at the same time they emphasize the danger of policy statements without research.

Stage Two: Demand for Health Insurance Coverage

In the second stage, we estimated determinants of the demand for private health insurance coverage. Two dimensions of demand were examined: the demand for *any* insurance (that is, the presence or absence of private coverage), represented by a binary dependent variable, and the health insurance premium, given that coverage is obtained. The latter measure was expressed in three different ways: (1) as the total actual health insurance premium; (2) as the predicted total premium obtained from parameter estimates of regressions presented in Appendix H; and (3) as the predicted hospital component of the total premium, also obtained from regressions presented in Appendix H. The predicted hospital premium uses the same parameter estimates as the predicted total premium, *excluding* those pertaining to benefits for services outside the hospital, plus a proportion of the constant term corresponding to the national proportion of private health insurance benefits payments paid for hospital care.[20]

Our interest centers on the predicted premium series; regressions with actual premium data have been estimated for comparative purposes. The predicted series are superior to the actual in the present context for two reasons. First and foremost, predicted premiums approximate depth of coverage more closely. For purposes of prediction, the nonbenefit variables were set equal to the sample means and multiplied by their respective parameter estimates. The products were summed and added to the constant term. This effectively purifies the predicted premium series of the influences of loading and regulation and at the same time preserves variation that is due to insurance benefits and reimbursement characteristics. Second, predicted premiums eliminate much of the "noise" present in actual premium data (present although the insurance data come from insurers rather than households).

As with the first-stage regressions, data were obtained from the 1971 CHAS-NORC survey. The sample includes household heads with and without private health insurance in 1970.[21] Independent variables representing determinants of demand for insurance, as discussed below, reflect a mixture of individual characteristics, locational attributes, and characteristics of local health services markets.

The hypothesized effects of age on health insurance purchases reflect a combination of factors. Because illness risks increase with age, the probability of being insured and benefits demanded (conditional on the insurance purchase) are expected to increase with age. Potentially offsetting the risk effect are cases where insurance premiums increase with age (primarily individual insurance) and the fact that group-insurance enrollees typically do not have many options to vary the amount of insurance purchased. In addition, the availability of Medicare coverage to persons over 65 reduces the expected probability of having private coverage and the expected amount of private coverage once insured. Three variables representing age classes of household heads are included in the regressions: Age 1 represents persons under twenty-five years of age; AGE3, persons forty-five to sixty-four; and AGE4, persons sixty-five and older. The omitted category corresponds to persons twenty-five to forty-four.[22]

The expected effect of the variable FEMALE, which takes the value 1 if the household head is a woman, is negative in both the insured/uninsured and amount-of-coverage (premium) regressions. First, women are less likely to be employed, and once employed, they are less likely to be in employment positions where health insurance benefits are subsidized. Second, they are more likely to have health insurance benefits available to them from other sources (say, separated husbands and programs designed for widows).

The variable WHITE equals 1 if the household head's race is white. In part, this variable acts as a proxy for demographic characteristics not fully captured by remaining variables in the equation. These characteristics tend to be related with lower consumption patterns for goods and services in general. Race also signifies differences in health service utilization patterns which have persisted over time. In general, nonwhites have utilized fewer private physicians and less nonurgent medical care and have relied more heavily on clinics and emergency rooms, with other factors held roughly constant. For these reasons, the predicted effect of WHITE in all regressions is positive.

In general, education produces more informed consumers—those who are able to satisfy their wants most efficiently in the marketplace. Grossman (1972) and Michael (1972), among others, have asserted that educated persons are more efficient "producers" of health than the uneducated; that is, *ceteris paribus*, they are able to achieve a higher level of health status with a given commitment of household resources to health services. The effect of greater efficiency in household production on the demand for health services is indeterminant a priori, as is the propensity to purchase health insurance. But more educated persons are more likely to be employed in occupations where health insurance purchases are subsidized by employers.[23] One potential offsetting effect is that if educated persons are better able to obtain insurance purchases at the lowest price, this may exert a negative impact on premiums. Therefore, the expected effects on the variable EDUC, the number of school years completed, cannot be determined in advance.

The impact of income on health insurance purchases has been shown to be positive in past research.[24] The variable FAMINC measures family income of the household head in thousands of dollars. Its expected effect is positive in all regressions. The variable measuring family size (FAMSIZE) is also expected to have an unambiguously positive effect on the insurance demand, because of both the higher risk of illness in the family as family size grows and the absence of discrimination in (benefit structure-adjusted) premium determination on the basis of family size (other than in individual versus family policies).

Remaining variables in the regressions represent characteristics of areas of residence of the family heads. The variable METRO equals 1 if the respondent lives in a metropolitan area. In such areas, household heads are more likely to have employment in which insurance purchases are subsidized, and health insurance markets may be more efficient (in matching prospective health insurance purchasers with sellers). The expected effect is therefore positive in all regressions. The variable FARM equals 1 if the household head is in a farming-related occupation. Because such occupations are less likely to have subsidized insurance and some respondents are likely to be located in less efficient rural market areas, the expected sign in all regressions is negative.

The next three dummy variables, NEAST, MWEST, and SOUTH, represent respondents located in Northeast, North Central, and Southern United States, respectively, with the omitted category being the Western census area. From other accounts it is known that per capita hospital utilization and private health insurance purchases tend to be less in the West than in the rest of the United States.[25] For this reason, the expected signs of the included variables are positive.

The variable MEDPOP measures total Medicaid expenditures per person in the state in which the household head is located. Because Medicaid represents a substitute for private health insurance, its expected effect on the probability of being insured is negative. The expected effect on amount of insurance (once insurance is obtained) is less clear. There may be a slight tendency for some families to supplement Medicaid benefits with private purchases, in which case the impact would also be negative.

Mean hospital expense per adjusted patient-day in the household head's area is represented by EXPAPD. The areas are defined as SMSAs for urban-located heads and counties for rural residents. One expects fewer persons to self-insure as the expected costs of health service rise; yet utilization may fall. Phelps (1973) demonstrated (theoretically) that one cannot predict a priori whether the amount of insurance demanded will rise or fall as the price of health services rises. Newhouse (1976), in a review of empirical evidence on this issue, concluded that the relationship is likely to be positive, but with a low associated elasticity.

Means and standard deviations of dependent and independent variables are presented in table 4–3; insurance demand regressions (with standard errors in parentheses) are presented in table 4–4. From table 4–3, it is evident that the insured sample tends to have slightly fewer young, elderly, female, metropolitan, and nonwhite household heads than the total sample which includes uninsured members. In addition, insured sample members

Table 4–3
Private Health Insurance Regression Variable, Means and Standard Deviations, Sample of Household Heads, 1970

Variable[a]	Total Sample (Standard Deviation)		Insured Sample (Standard Deviation)	
INSURED	0.62	(—)	1.00	(—)
PREMIUM	—		250.2	(165.9)
TPREM	—		252.7	(150.0)
HPREM	—		174.5	(110.0)
AGE1	0.08	(—)	0.06	(—)
AGE3	0.31	(—)	0.33	(—)
AGE4	0.28	(—)	0.26	(—)
FEMALE	0.31	(—)	0.26	(—)
WHITE	0.74	(—)	0.82	(—)
EDUC	9.94	(3.74)	10.68	(3.48)
FAMINC (00)[b]	76.23	(101.82)	94.29	(120.96)
FAMSIZE	2.99	(2.02)	3.00	(1.93)
METRO	0.60	(—)	0.56	(—)
FARM	0.08	(—)	0.07	(—)
NEAST	0.19	(—)	0.21	(—)
MWEST	0.31	(—)	0.32	(—)
SOUTH	0.36	(—)	0.36	(—)
MCDPOP (00)	0.24	(0.17)	0.24	(0.16)
EXPAPD (00)	0.72	(0.13)	0.71	(0.13)

[a]Dependent variables are defined as follows: INSURED = 1 if the household head has some private health insurance coverage and 0 otherwise; PREMIUM is the total actual health insurance premium for insured heads; TPREM is the predicted total health insurance premium, based on regressions in table H-2; and HPREM is the predicted hospital-component health insurance premium, also based on regressions in table H-2. All premium and monetary independent variables were deflated by an area price index (1970 metropolitan area averge = 1.00). Independent variables are defined in the text.
[b]Variables FAMINC, MCDPOP, and EXPAPD are expressed in hundreds of dollars.

Table 4-4
Private Health Insurance Regression Results, Sample of Household Heads, 1970

	Total Sample		Insured Sample	
Variable	Insured/Uninsured (Standard Error)[a]	Total Premium (Standard Error)	Predicted Total Premium (Standard Error)	Predicted Hospital Premium (Standard Error)
AGE1	*−0.181 (0.036)	−18.4 (16.2)	−0.71 (12.8)	−2.5 (10.1)
AGE3	**0.057 (0.024)	−6.7 (9.2)	**−16.8 (7.3)	−8.2 (5.8)
AGE4	−0.011 (0.028)	*−125.1 (11.2)	*−165.8 (8.9)	*−106.5 (7.0)
FEMALE	*−0.099 (0.021)	*−69.7 (8.9)	*−72.4 (7.1)	*−49.6 (5.6)
WHITE	*0.216 (0.024)	*42.0 (10.5)	*25.7 (8.3)	*18.6 (6.5)
EDUC	*0.027 (0.003)	**2.3 (1.1)	1.5 (0.9)	0.44 (0.70)
FAMINC (00)[b]	*0.00054 (0.00009)	0.056 (0.031)	*0.067 (0.024)	**0.041 (0.019)
FAMSIZE	−0.005 (0.005)	*16.6 (2.2)	*15.7 (1.7)	*10.4 (1.4)
METRO	0.012 (0.024)	**−30.3 (9.6)	−8.3 (7.6)	**−12.3 (6.0)
FARM	*−0.074 (0.036)	−0.9 (14.9)	−30.3 (11.8)	−14.9 (9.3)
NEAST	*0.193 (0.033)	25.0 (13.8)	10.8 (10.9)	*44.8 (8.6)
MWEST	*0.158 (0.031)	*63.0 (13.0)	15.3 (10.3)	*22.3 (8.1)
SOUTH	*0.115 (0.032)	*61.7 (13.7)	**23.7 (10.9)	*28.8 (8.5)
MCDPOP (00)	−0.119 (0.075)	−6.65 (29.8)	−23.1 (23.6)	−16.5 (18.6)
EXPAPD (00)	**−0.233 (0.111)	*172.9 (42.6)	**83.0 (33.7)	*112.9 (26.5)
Constant	0.245	37.2	166.4	67.0
	$R^2 = 0.178$	$R^2 = 0.321$	$R^2 = 0.481$	$R^2 = 0.402$
	$*F(15, 2{,}429) = 35.1$	$*F(15, 1{,}493) = 47.1$	$*F(15, 1{,}493) = 92.3$	$*F(15, 1{,}493) = 66.9$

* = Significant at the 1% level (two-tail test).
** = Significant at the 5% level (two-tail test).
[a]Standard errors generated by OLS regressions on binary dependent variables are biased. Indications of statistical significance are therefore only approximate.
[b]Variables FAMINC, MCDPOP, and EXPAPD are expressed in hundreds of dollars.

tend to be more highly educated and have higher family incomes. Remaining characteristics show relatively little difference between the two samples.

On the whole, the parameter estimates tend to support the hypotheses presented above (when directions of effect can be determined in advance), with a few exceptions that are noted.[26] Judging by the Fs, all equations are statistically significant at conventional levels. Comparison of the actual total premium and predicted total premium regressions shows that, as anticipated, the latter equation obtained a better fit—a higher R^2 and generally lower standard errors of parameter estimates. However, there are no major qualitative differences between the two regressions.

As hypothesized, young household heads (AGE1) are less likely to purchase private health insurance than those aged twenty-five to forty-four, and the older age group, forty-five to sixty-four (AGE3), was slightly more likely to be insured. However, the latter group tended to have less coverage (lower premiums) than the reference group, perhaps reflecting the presence of greater amounts of supplementary coverage or subsidiary benefits available from other sources. The signs of the parameter estimates for these two age groups tend to be negative and statistically insignificant. Parameter estimates pertaining to the group over sixty-five (AGE4) showed virtually no lower likelihood to have private health insurance than the group twenty-five to forty-four. This supports the widely held view of the incompleteness of Medicare coverage and corroborates data on the extent of supplementary health insurance purchases. Negative parameter estimates on AGE4 in premium regressions are statistically significant and relatively large in absolute value. In the predicted total and hospital premium regressions, the coefficients are approximately two-thirds of the means of the dependent variables. Our prediction that the parameter estimate would be relatively greater (in absolute terms) in the hospital premium regression therefore is not supported.

The FEMALE coefficients imply that female household heads are less likely to have private coverage and, once covered, tend to purchase substantially less insurance. The results are similar with regard to the variable WHITE, showing that nonwhites are much less likely to have private coverage and less insurance once covered. In the case of women, this result may reflect availability of benefits from alternative sources. However, both results are likely to reflect differences in occupational characteristics between males and females and whites and nonwhites, a topic that is worthy of further investigation but beyond the scope of this book.

Results on the variable EDUC show that better-educated persons are more likely to insure. However, the effect of this variable is not great, and parameter estimates in the insurance regressions show near-zero effects. As suggested above, it is possible that educated persons are able to obtain lower prices for their insurance purchases and a higher level of health status, *ceteris paribus*, with a given outlay on health services, offsetting the positive effect on premiums of a preference for more insurance.

The effect of family income (FAMINC) on the probability of being insured is positive, as expected, in all regressions, but the magnitude of effect is not great relative to that of the demographic variables. The coefficient of FAMSIZE, the variable representing family size, is unexpectedly negative (but statistically insignificant) in the insured/uninsured regression and positive with low elasticities in the premium regressions. The latter result probably reflects the fact that family insurance premiums tend to be insensitive to family size. Positive coefficients in the premium regressions reflect the association between family size and the likelihood of purchasing individual or family insurance.

The variable METRO shows virtually no effect of metropolitan location on the probability of being insured and an unexpectedly negative impact on the amount of insurance. Estimated coefficients on the variable FARM, signifying a farming-related occupation of the household head, are also negative in the premium regressions. The variable FARM has a negative coefficient which is twice its standard error in the insured/uninsured regression.

The dummy variables signifying census areas are all positive and attain high levels of statistical significance. The reference group for these parameter estimates is the West. *Ceteris paribus*, the probability of having private health insurance is highest in the East, followed by the Midwest, South, and West; the largest difference is between the South and West. The census area dummies also have consistently positive signs in the premium regressions as well. Of interest is the difference in parameter estimates in the predicted total and hospital premium regressions. The coefficients tend to be much larger with lower standard errors in the latter regression, even though the mean of the predicted hospital premium is about 70 percent of the mean predicted total premium. These results suggest major interregional differences in the markets for private health insurance. There appears to be less emphasis on hospital services in the West and, by implication, relatively more emphasis on ambulatory services.

The variable measuring state per capita Medicaid expenditures (MEDPOP) has a negative but statistically insignificant coefficient in all regressions. Apparently, the availability of Medicaid health care benefits exerts very little influence on the demand for private health insurance. This suggests that the Medicaid program tends to provide coverage that would not otherwise be provided in the private sector.

Variable EXPAPD, which measures area hospital expense per adjusted patient-day, is negative in the insured/uninsured regression, but has a substantial positive impact in all premium regressions. Overall, if we combine the effects on the probability and the amount of insurance given coverage, the effect of EXPAPD is positive, a result that is clearly consistent with the growth in real (relative to the CPI) premiums over this decade.[27] Not surprisingly, the effect is more pronounced in the predicted hospital premium regression than in the predicted total premium regression. The elasticity in the former regression is 0.46 and in the latter is 0.23.

Stage Three: Depth of Coverage by County, 1970–1975

In the third stage, predicted values of depth of private coverage by county, calculated from stage-two parameter estimates and county data for the explanatory variables, have been constructed. The resulting variable is INS. Variants of the insurance demand equations, excluding EDUC and FARM and having age dummy variables for only the groups twenty-five to forty-four and over sixty-five, were used to form the county estimates. Data by county on the excluded variables are not available annually. Fortunately, omitting these variables from regressions has very little impact on the R^2s in stage two. For each county, the value of INS is the product of the estimated county proportion with private health insurance and the estimated depth-of-coverage value for insured persons in the county.

In constructing INS, we were faced with a choice of using parameter estimates from the estimated total premium regression or the estimated hospital-component premium regression. We chose the estimated total premium regression on grounds of goodness of fit. In addition, although a hospital-component insurance measure seemed more appropriate at first glance as an explanatory variable in hospital input and cost regressions, we contend that the joint-product nature of much of medical care mitigates this view. There is very little evidence of substitutions between hospital and other health services in response to private insurance programs under existing insurance configurations. Because there is a great deal of complementarity between different forms of health services, our view is that demand responses to variations in private insurance coverage are likely to be parallel for different types of providers. Therefore, we regard our use of a total health insurance measure in hospital performance regressions as appropriate.

As constructed, INS should reflect temporal as well as cross-sectional differences in depth of coverage. However, when we compared the growth in INS between 1970 and 1975 with the growth in actual real premiums, our series fell short. There have probably been intertemporal shifts in the insurance demand parameters that our cross-sectional regression analysis cannot capture. Changes in the levels of the explanatory variables do not fully explain the trend. Alternatively, a growth in the loading may be responsible for the discrepancy. We view the first explanation as much more likely and for this reason have adjusted our INS series so that its growth approximates the growth of actual real premiums per capita.

Clearly, INS, as constructed, is far from an ideal measure of depth of private insurance coverage. Its major advantages, compared to previously utilized state aggregate data, are that it is conceptually a "purer" measure of depth of coverage than actual enrollment, premium, or benefits data, in that it incorporates the multifaceted features of insurance in a single series, and it is measured on a small-area basis (the county). Health insurance is potentially an extremely important factor in hospital behavior, but large-area measures of coverage are too crude for investigating most important influences of insurance. Our construction of INS represents an attempt to develop a more refined measure that, we hope, will be improved on in future research via increased availability of insurance data for small geographic areas.

Summary and Conclusions

This chapter has presented a considerable amount of new information on private health insurance. Because our principal task has been to describe INS, this evidence does not receive further attention in later chapters. Therefore, in this section we provide a brief summary of some of the highlights of our investigation of depth of coverage under private health insurance and close with hypotheses regarding the effects of our insurance variables on hospital costs and input employment.

The chapter began with a description of primary characteristics of health insurance policies. Depth of coverage was shown to be a function of three factors: benefits covered, generosity of benefits, and patient copayment (deductibles and coinsurance). We further described aspects of private health insurance that are potentially related to depth of coverage. Of the three primary types of coverage—basic, major medical, and combined—the last is likely to provide the most thorough coverage, particularly for hospitalization episodes. However, the extent of coverage under any type depends largely on relationships among insurance policy parameters, patient utilization, and provider charge and reimbursement systems. We argued that coverage is also likely to be more thorough when service, as opposed to indemnity, benefits are provided. Service benefits are designed to minimize patient out-of-pocket expenditures for covered services. As shown in table 4–2, one of the major differences between Blue Cross and Blue Shield policies and commercial health insurance is that the Blues tend to market service benefits to a much greater extent than commercial firms.

A final factor related to coverage depth is the loading on health insurance policies. Loading was hypothesized to be related to whether the policy was sold on a group or individual basis, to whether it is Blue or commercial, and to the effects of state regulatory and taxation programs. Aggregate data clearly indicate that loading tends to be less on group policies and Blue policies, but parameter estimates pertaining to loading-related variables in premium regressions (Appendix H) yielded very little consistent evidence on how loading influences health insurance premiums. We found that the most consistent determinants of premiums pertain to benefits covered, particularly the generosity of coverage for inpatient hospital care.

From our private health insurance regressions based on a sample of household heads, we found that the probability of having private coverage tends to increase with age, up to age sixty-five. Despite the availability of Medicare coverage to the elderly, *ceteris paribus*, the probability of having private health insurance was virtually the same for those over sixty-five and between twenty-five and forty-four. Among demographic variables, race was the most important determinant of the probability of coverage, and sex, education, family income, and occupation were also influential. The low parameter estimates and statistical insignificance of variables measuring the availability of Medicaid benefits suggest that Medicaid tends to provide coverage that otherwise would not be provided in the private sector.

We found that the availability of Medicare benefits to the elderly has a substantial negative impact on premiums. Apart from this effect, age has very little influence on depth of coverage under private health insurance. Being a female head of household, however, has a strong negative impact. This result may reflect employment circumstances of female household heads and availability of health insurance benefits from other sources. Race, family size, and the area's average hospital expense per patient-day were also major determinants of private health insurance demand. The last variable was particularly important in the estimated hospital premium regression. The persistence of race as a determinant of private health insurance depth of coverage, when other demographic factors are held constant, may be viewed as a signal of financial barriers to access to health services of racial minority groups.

Our regional dummy-variable parameter estimates indicate substantial systematic differences among private health insurance markets in different parts of the country. In general, both the probability of having private coverage and the depth of coverage, once insured, are considerably less in the West than in other regions. Both the probability of coverage and the depth of coverage for hospital services are highest in the East; however, total depth of coverage is highest in the Midwest and South, with other factors held constant.

Three measures of health insurance coverage are defined for inclusion as independent variables in our analyses of hospital costs and input employment. Our Medicare variable, MCARE, measures over-sixty-five population proportions by county. Our Medicaid variable, MCAID, measures proportions of state populations eligible for Medicaid benefits, after eliminating the elderly Medicaid eligibles. Our private health insurance depth-of-coverage variable, INS, is estimated by county.

Although some studies have shown that insurance affects hospital costs and input use (Feldstein 1971b, 1977; Salkever 1972), there is room for new research on these issues, especially with refined measures. Past empirical research serves as a basis for the working hypothesis that health insurance in general raises cost and input employment. Its effects on the latter may not be uniformly positive since, for example, professional nurses may be preferred to licensed practical nurses in counties with high coverage depth.

Predicting the effects of MCARE and MCAID also involves some complexities. In particular, these variables may also act as proxies for patient demographic characteristics. For example, in areas where Medicare eligibility is relatively high, hospitals are likely to have a relatively high proportion of elderly patients. Patient age may exert an independent (of insurance coverage) effect on input employment and costs.[28] Similarly, Medicaid coverage is associated with demographic characteristics, including race, sex, and education. These factors may influence hospital input employment in unpredictable ways. Our specifications attempt to hold constant as many of these influences as data availability permits, but we may anticipate some residual effects to be manifested in our parameter estimates.[29]

Notes

1. Unless otherwise noted, data in this and the following paragraph are taken from Mueller (1977), The Health Insurance Association of America (HIAA) estimated that 87.2 percent of the under-sixty-five population had private hospitalization coverage at the end of 1975, somewhat higher than the federal estimate. Social Security Administration figures presented in Mueller are based on data from household surveys; HIAA figures are based on insurance company survey data presented in Health Insurance Institute (1977).

2. Blue Cross is typically the insurer for hospital services, but in some areas Blue Shield provides this insurance also. However, the latter, in the aggregate, accounts for only 3 percent of their combined hospitalization insurance enrolled populations. Blue Shield sells primarily insurance covering expenditures for physicians' services and some other forms of ambulatory health care.

3. Utilization varies substantially by state. See Feldstein (1971a).

4. Federal Medicaid regulations list services that state Medicaid programs may provide, eight of which are mandatory. The mandatory services include hospitalization and use of ambulatory hospital services. See Wendorf (1977) for a comprehensive presentation of characteristics of state Medicaid programs and relationships with hospitals.

5. Very little hard evidence exists to demonstrate that Medicaid reimbursement is significantly less generous than other forms for inpatient hospital services. However, see Sloan, Cromwell, and Mitchell (1978) for evidence that this is true for ambulatory services in general. Wendorf (1977) provides a sampling of hospital complaints regarding Medicaid reimbursement.

6. Variable construction is explained in more detail in Appendix J.

7. In the health economics literature, *coinsurance* also refers to the gross percentage of expenditures paid by the insured. In this context, however, the term refers to a specified percentage paid by the insured for expenses related to a covered benefit.

8. This includes both *comprehensive* major medical, which is designed to stand alone, and *supplemental*, which is designed to be combined with a basic plan.

9. It is also highly relevant to surgical coverage. For less expensive ambulatory care services, however, reimbursement under major medical coverage is more prevalent.

10. Health Insurance Institute (1976). Commercial figures include loss-of-income insurance. The "other hospital and medical plans" consist primarily of the independent plans mentioned earlier. The Blue Cross-Blue Shield *Fact Book, 1976*, reports an even higher payout ratio for Blue Cross in 1975—nearly 100 percent—but this is atypically high. The figures above are more representative of historical trends.

11. Blue plans, according to Frech and Ginsburg, desire to sell complete coverage because of ideological convictions and especially because complete coverage is in the interests of their sponsors, namely, physicians and hospitals. This theory is intuitively appealing and warrants future examination because of its welfare implications. For example, Feldstein (1973) estimates the welfare loss of excess health insurance to be on the order of several billion dollars annually. However, there are grounds for challenging some of the Frech-Ginsburg assumptions, particularly that health insurance regulation is generally harder on commercial companies than on the Blues.

12. See Lewin and Associates (1975a) for a description of characteristics of state health insurance regulatory programs and procedures.

13. Collusion may be too strong a term to describe Blue Cross-hospital relationships. However, this is implied by Frech and Ginsburg (1978) in their analysis of health insurance. See Law (1974) for an even more critical interpretation.

14. A full report of the findings from the CHAS-NORC survey is provided by Andersen, Lion, and Anderson (1976).

15. Family size averaged about 3.0 in the CHAS-NORC sample.

16. For information on this point, refer to discussions of the issue of

community versus experience rating [for example, Somers and Somers (1961, chap. 150].

17. Because premium and other data are for 1970, the time difference may be a source of measurement error.

18. We hypothesized that mandated utilization review (UR) programs, if effective, would tend to reduce hospital utilization, thereby reducing insurance claims and possibly premiums as well. A plausible *ex post* explanation is that UR programs tend to be instituted where utilization is relatively high, leading to a positive association with premiums. However, since one expects at least part of a premium tax to be passed on to consumers, we are unable to explain negative parameter estimates on the premium tax variable (TAX).

19. In a separate study using the CHAS-NORC data base, Hays (1978) attempted to gauge the impact of market conditions and regulatory programs on premiums paid by commercial health insurance policyholders. He found virtually no evidence of effect of regulatory programs or premium taxes on commercial premiums.

20. Based on data provided in Health Insurance Institute (1973), the proportion for 1970 was estimated to be 0.647.

21. The number of uninsured persons added to the insured-persons file was set such that the resulting proportion with private health insurance was equivalent to the corresponding insured proportion of CHAS-NORC respondents as a whole. The percentage of household-head respondents to the CHAS-NORC survey with some private health insurance was 61.7.

22. Some differences in effect of age between the insured/uninsured regression and premium regressions may be anticipated. The omitted category represents the prime child-rearing age group in which fewer additional health service benefits (say, from employed spouses or children) are likely to be available than in the other groups. This may influence the premiums in this group upward relative to other age groups represented in the regressions. In addition, because the Medicare program includes copayment provisions, there is substantial uncovered expense which constitutes fertile territory for insurance purveyors. Apart from the negative impact of Medicare, the positive effect of old age on the amount of the premium is likely to be greater in the hospital premium regression than in the total premium regression.

23. In a number of places we hypothesize that the availability of subsidies of health insurance purchases from employers will exert a positive influence on the probability of being insured and on the amount of actual or predicted premiums. Because this subsidy represents a form of income, it is not clear that employees would prefer the subsidy to higher wages. However, our hypothesis is based largely on the fact that group policies tend to be associated with lower insurance prices (holding benefits and other factors constant) than nonsubsidized policies. In addition, employees typically are

not given a choice of trading the subsidy for higher wages, and choices pertaining to the extent of coverage are infrequent.

24. Feldstein (1973) and Phelps (1973).

25. See, for example, National Center for Health Statistics (1976) and Health Insurance Institute (1973).

26. The insured/uninsured regression was estimated via ordinary least squares (OLS), even though the dependent variable is binary. Because the primary purpose of these regressions was to generate predicted values rather than precise estimates of causal relationships, we did not deem it necessary to engage in a more complex estimating process, such as probit or Tobit. Moreover, from our past experience and that of others (for example, Salkever and Seidman 1978) such alternative econometric techniques seldom yield results that are qualitatively much different from OLS. In any case, readers are cautioned that the parameter estimates in the insured/uninsured regression, and associated significance tests, can be regarded as only very approximate.

27. Recall that monetarily expressed variables have been deflated to eliminate the effect of area cost-of-living differences.

28. Based on data provided in Andersen, Kravits, and Anderson (1975) and Cooper, Worthington, and McGee (1976), hospital expenditures per patient-day were roughly 35 percent higher for the elderly than for all ages in 1970. This differential may be due, in part, to different health care needs of the elderly relative to the population at large. If the anticipated positive effect of Medicare coverage is obtained, it may not be due entirely to the insurance effect.

29. According to data presented in Andersen, Kravits, and Anderson (1975), the hospital discharge rate for nonwhites was approximately 16 percent lower than that of whites, but average length of stay was about 29 percent higher for nonwhites in 1970. These statistics are consistent with the view that nonwhites tend to be "sicker," on average, than whites, once hospitalized. This is suggestive of a demographically based, positive influence of Medicaid reimbursement on inputs and costs.

5

Hospital Regulation: Institutions, Empirical Evidence, and Research Issues

This chapter lays the groundwork for empirical analysis of the impact of regulation on hospital costs and inputs. We adopt a rather broad definition of regulation—it includes not only direct control of hospital behavior by government authorities, but also programs developed in the private sector. At the same time, the scope of this book is limited to regulations most relevant to current policy deliberations and suitable, in terms of data availability and hypothesis development, for the empirical analyses in ensuing chapters.

The years following enactment of Medicare and Medicaid in the mid-1960s have been a period of explosiveness in the formation and implementation of hospital regulations. Owing primarily to inflation in hospital costs and expenditures during this period, hospitals have become subject to a large and increasing number of controls which, according to many hospital spokespersons, often work at cross purposes without much anti-inflationary impact.[1] Existing evidence of the impact of major regulatory programs on hospital costs tends to be inconclusive. However, only recently have sufficient data become available to permit more thorough empirical tests than have been performed in the past.

The remainder of this chapter discusses capital and service expansion controls; rate, revenue, and reimbursement controls; and utilization and quality regulation. These constitute the major forms of hospital regulation enacted during the late 1960s and the 1970s. Each of the following three sections contains descriptions of background and current regulatory institutions, a review of empirical evidence on effects on hospital performance, and a discussion of research issues. The final section presents our specification of regulation variables.

Regulation of Hospital Capital and Service Expansion

Background and Current Regulatory Institutions

Current regulatory programs pertaining to hospital capital and service expansion largely grew out of the voluntary health planning movement in the United States (Anderson 1976; Havighurst 1973b). Health planning got its first legislative recognition in the Hill-Burton Act in 1946 which, among other things, required the states to develop plans for guiding hospital construction within their jurisdictions. However, up through the early 1960s, the planning movement was contained almost entirely in the private sector, primarily through the activities of areawide health planning agencies. Creation and growth of these organizations were encouraged through joint efforts by the American Hospital Association and the Public Health Service (May 1974a). When the Hill-Burton Act was extended in 1964 to make federal funds available for health planning, the number of agencies grew substantially, from 32 in 1964 to 75 in 1967 (Gottlieb 1974).[2]

Two laws that increased the federal government's role in health planning were passed in the mid-1960s: the Regional Medical Program (RMP) and the Comprehensive Health Planning (CHP) Act. The RMP was concerned primarily with the diffusion of medical technology; CHP created a framework for a two-tiered planning system whereby areawide (local) agencies would submit plans for approval and funding to state agencies which are statutorily required to be part of state government. Many existing agencies wished to maintain their focus on facility planning rather than broaden their scope of planning activities to become *comprehensive*, a term that was never explicitly defined by law (May 1974a). In any case, in excess of 150 agencies at the state and local levels were supported by the CHP program in 1972.

Policy developments at state and federal levels in the late 1960s and early 1970s made it clear that the "planning without teeth" concept embodied in the voluntary planning movement and fostered by CHP had been judged by the political process to be ineffective; yet the concept of planning per se garnered increased support. It became apparent to many policymakers that voluntary planning could do little to check hospital cost inflation. Consequently, during this period the boundary between voluntary and compulsory was emphatically crossed, and regulation of hospital expansion, largely based on the public-utility regulatory model, reached fruition.

At the state level, compulsory hospital capital-expansion regulation was initiated with enactment of the Metcalf-McCloskey Act in New York in 1964. This legislation contains most of the basic features of current certificate-of-need laws, including mandatory prior approval of changes in bed capacity and major equipment purchases (Curran 1974). The next states to adopt similar regulations were Maryland, Rhode Island, California, and Connecticut. The American Hospital Association endorsed this approach to facility regulation in 1968 (Havighurst 1973b).

At the federal level, two pieces of legislation, passed during the early 1970s, embody the current regulatory posture toward hospital capital and service expansion. First, Public Law 92-603, the Social Security Act amendments of 1972, contains section 1122, which authorizes state-designated planning agencies to review hospital plans for facility or service expansion. In principle, if a plan is judged to be inconsistent with community needs, the designated planning agency recommends disallowance of expenses (primarily interest and depreciation) related to the unapproved hospital capital investment in reimbursements to the hospital under the Medicare, Medicaid, and Maternal and Child Health programs. Designated planning agencies contract with the federal government and receive funding to perform this function.

Second, P.L. 93-641, the National Health Planning and Resources Development Act of 1974, created a system of health service areas and health systems agencies (HSAs) to guide the allocation of health resources within the states. It also mandated the development of certificate-of-need (CON) controls in all states by 1980.[3] To date, existing state CON laws have developed independently, and there are substantial differences among them. As CON develops further under the aegis of P.L. 93-641, interstate differences will likely lessen (Salkever and Bice 1976a, 1976b). However, variations in state laws in the 1970s provide an opportunity to empirically assess the effects of these differences on hospital costs and input employment.

The task of implementing "planning with teeth" mandated by these federal laws has been delegated, to a large extent, to existing comprehensive health planning agencies. These agencies were simply available to accept this task, although sometimes with reluctance (Curran 1974). However, some observers view CHP involvement in itself as a deterrent to effective health planning. Historically, these agencies have focused almost exclusively on hospital capacity expansion (Gottlieb 1974). It has been suggested that continued emphasis on controlling bed supply is more likely to shift the locus of inflation rather than reduce it (McClure 1976; Havighurst 1973a, 1973b). In addition, because areawide planning agencies supported under CHP were forced to raise one-half of their operating funds locally, many relied on local hospitals for financial support (Curran 1974). Thus it is feared that these agencies will be unable to sever their ties with hospitals, and as has been the case elsewhere in the economy, the regulators will serve the interests of the regulated industry to a greater extent than the public's interests are served.[4] The fact that the American Hospital Association was an early supporter of CON legislation gives credence to this suspicion (Curran 1974; Posner 1974).

Mandatory controls on hospital investment are emerging in direct and indirect forms. Direct controls are inherent in the certificate-of-need approach. Where CON programs are operative, a hospital desiring to expand its bed supply or purchase equipment in an amount that exceeds a specified threshold must obtain a certificate similar to the certificate of public convenience and necessity issued to public utilities. The authority for issuance of the certificate is usually vested in the state health department, which typically delegates local determination of need to areawide planning agencies (Curran 1974). As of January 31, 1978, thirty-six states had enacted CON laws (U.S. Department of Health, Education, and Welfare 1978).[5] In general, the emphasis of these laws is on controlling bed supply. However, several states also attempt to control equipment and service expansion.[6]

Indirect controls on hospital investment operate through public and private insurance and capital financing mechanisms. The major public initiative of this sort is the section 1122 program mentioned above, which uses Social Security Administration reimbursement as a regulatory tool. Approval by state-designated planning agencies of hospital capital expenditures exceeding $100,000, changes in bed capacity, and/or changes in services offered is required as a precondition for full reimbursement.[7] The major private program is operated by some Blue Cross plans, which link reimbursement for certain hospital capital expenditures to approval by health planning agencies.[8] By using an approach analogous to the section 1122 process, such plans may deny reimbursement for capital costs related to unapproved hospital investment projects. Also, the plans may deny participatory status to nonconforming hospitals. Usually the Blue Cross plan will accept the review determinations of agencies acting under the authority of certificate-of-need and section 1122 programs (Lewin and Associates 1975a).

Empirical Evidence

Despite the fact that many capital and service expansion regulatory programs are currently in existence, empirical evidence of their effects is limited. Moreover, isolating these effects is subject to considerable empirical complexity. One problem is that many hospital investment programs experience substantial time lags between the initial planning stage and the time when the program results in expanded capacity or services. In addition, "grandfathering" is common in this area of regulation. Consequently, it may take several years before the impact of an investment control program is observable. Other factors, such as the possibility that states with relatively high rates of hospital inflation and/or facility growth are most likely to implement investment controls, interactions between investment control and other regulatory programs, and the political environment of the state, add to the difficulty of evaluating these programs empirically (Blumstein and Sloan 1978).

Most studies of hospital investment control tend to be descriptive—either single-state case studies or national descriptions of program history, characteristics, and procedures. The following discussion focuses primarily on the

few multivariate analyses that have been performed in this area, followed by
an examination of descriptive evidence and indirect evidence from studies of
the impact of voluntary health planning on hospital behavior.

Hellinger (1976a) used regression analysis to investigate the impact of
hospital investment controls on state mean plant assets in short-term
hospitals in 1973. Several alternative specifications were estimated, all in
linear functional form. In half of the equations, a dummy variable indicating
the presence of CON programs by January 1, 1973, was included among the
explanatory variables. In the remaining half, a dummy variable indicating the
presence of CON program *or* a section 1122 contract by June 6, 1973, was
included. The impact of investment controls was inferred from parameter
estimates pertaining to these dummy variables.

Parameter estimates of the investment control variables were always
negative, as expected, but the magnitude of the coefficients was relatively
low, and *t* statistics did not exceed 1 in any one of the equations. Hellinger
appropriately concluded from these results that the evidence did not suggest
that CON and section 1122 regulation had reduced hospital investment
during the period investigated. However, in an effort to obtain further insight
into hospital response to investment control legislation, additional regressions were estimated with a dummy variable indicating states with CON laws
in effect for less than half a year. These parameter estimates were positive
and statistically significant, although not large in absolute terms, suggesting a
tendency for hospitals to anticipate CON legislation by increasing investment in the period immediately prior to the legislation taking effect.

Hellinger included lagged values of dependent variables in his equations
and used OLS rather than an econometric method more appropriate for his
time series of cross-sections specification. According to Hellinger (1976a, p.
190), "the large coefficients for the lag value of plant assets imply that the
rate of adjustment of plant assets toward the equilibrium level is slow."
While this would imply that any effect of CON would take a long time to be
fully realized, we doubt that this study offers reliable evidence on response
lags. Because parameter estimates of the lagged dependent variables are
biased in this specification, the speed of hospital response to CON and other
exogenous forces is almost certainly underestimated.

In a somewhat more comprehensive empirical analysis, Salkever and
Bice (1976a, 1976b) investigated the impact of CON laws, also using a
regression model, with cross-sectional data on short-term hospitals aggregated to the state level for 1969 through 1972. The Salkever and Bice
specification included demand factors, investment fund availability
measures, and other factors influencing investment as independent variables.
The CON variable included in the equations was the percentage of months
during the period that CON controls were in effect.

Three hospital investment measures were included as dependent variables in their regressions: change in plant assets, change in bed supply, and change in assets per bed. Two forms of the regression equations were estimated: linear in percentage changes and linear in logarithmic changes. Salkever and Bice also estimated the percentage change equations for non-CON states only and applied the estimated coefficients to data from CON states to see whether actual changes in hospital investment in these states differed substantially from those predicted. The two estimating approaches yielded very similar results.

In the total investment equations, parameter estimates of the CON variable were positive and generally statistically insignificant. However, the results indicated a negative impact of CON on bed supply and a positive impact on assets per bed. All parameter estimates were statistically significant in these equations, and the levels of effect were substantial. Retardation in bed supply expansion because of CON was estimated to fall between 5.4 and 9.0 percent and increase in assets per bed between 15.2 and 19.7 percent. Estimates corresponding to the second method were similar, but not as pronounced. The authors concluded, with appropriate caveats, that CON has controlled expansion in bed supply and stimulated other types of investment, resulting in negligible impact on total investment. Salkever and Bice expressed doubt that tightening investment controls would be a cost-effective solution to this compensatory effect of CON programs. According to the authors, CON treats the manifestations of the disease rather than its causes. Pressures to expand remain and are channeled into nonbed investments.

Descriptive studies of hospital investment control provide insight into the structure and processes employed by the regulatory agencies, but such studies can be misleading with regard to regulatory effects. The agencies have a natural tendency to evaluate their effectiveness in terms of number or percentage of applications for approval of capital expansion projects that are denied. For example, in a study of the certificate-of-need experience in Massachusetts, Bicknell and Walsh (1975) found that roughly 19 percent of proposed bed and facility improvement applications were disapproved. This percentage may underestimate the impact of CON because of hospital reluctance to submit applications for projects with a high probability of disapproval (Salkever and Bice 1976a, 1976b). However, disapproval rates cannot account for shifts of expenditures into areas not covered by CON laws, for example, physicians' offices, relatively low-expenditure projects not subject to CON review, or labor inputs. Nor do they capture capital expansion in anticipation of such programs.

In another single-state study, Rothenberg (1976) reported mixed results on the CON experience in New York during 1965–1970. She concluded that the introduction of CON during this period had a limited effect at best. Because single-state analyses cannot adequately control for non-CON factors that may have affected bed growth and other dependent variables of interest, it is difficult to isolate the effects of CON from such studies.

Lewin and Associates (1975a) examined the experience of several states with various forms of regulation including certificate-of-need and section 1122 programs. Some of this work involved interviews with hospital administrators which revealed a number of interesting points that really cannot be obtained from formal statistical analysis. First, not surprisingly, hospital administrators did not want to pursue projects that were likely to be rejected because of concern over both the impact a denial would have on hospital/regulatory agency relations and the costs involved in the application process. Second, CON seems to have increased intra-area planning and coordination among hospitals, including development of shared services and joint medical programs. Although desirable from the standpoint of the planner, coordination raises questions of an antitrust nature (Blumstein and Calvani 1978). Third, the threat of controls appears to have accelerated timetables for construction of facilities and the introduction of special services. Fourth, some hospital administrators commented that CON program reviewers favored existing providers to the detriment of new entrants.[9] In this sense, CON policies may serve to cartelize the hospital sector.

A MACRO Systems (1974) study of CON laws in existence in 1973 is similar to that of Lewin and Associates in terms of both its overall objectives and its methodology. These are among the major findings of this book. First, hospital associations have generally been among the most active supporters of CON, which again suggests that CON may serve as a vehicle for reducing competition among hospitals. Second, levels of funding of CON programs appeared to be inadequate. Agencies taking on the responsibility for CON often received little additional funding. Third, criteria used to determine the necessity for a capital item tended to be weak and poorly developed. Although the frequent lack of well-defined criteria is not unique to capital expenditures regulation, it does serve as a warning that decisions based on current criteria may not be well informed.

Indirect evidence regarding the possible impact of CON facility and service regulation can be inferred from studies of the effects of areawide planning agencies on local hospital expansion. While such agencies historically functioned without authority to impose strong sanctions on hospitals failing to comply, the goal of controlling hospital expansiveness was often stated. Moreover, these are largely the same agencies that are charged with the responsibility of implementing CON and section 1122 programs.

May (1974a) reported the findings of two previous studies of planning agency impact. In the earliest empirical study on this topic, May (1967) compared hospital growth in "matched" SMSAs, with and without established planning agencies. He found that bed supply per 1,000 population was virtually unchanged in the SMSAs with planning agencies, but decreased in unplanned areas. The market share of proprietary hospitals decreased substantially in the planned areas relative to the unplanned. Hospital cost increases showed no appreciable difference between planned and unplanned areas. In a more recent study, Palmiere (1970) examined decision making within forty-five planning agencies. This study found little evidence of effect of planning agencies on hospital behavior. However, Palmiere also found no evidence suggesting that planning agencies were controlled by hospitals.

In the most detailed study of the impact of planning on hospitals, May (1974b) examined planning effects via regression analysis of a cross section of 144 standard metropolitan statistical areas in 1970. Planning was defined as the existence of an areawide health planning agency for two or more years in mid-1970. According to this definition, roughly 60 percent of the SMSAs were planned areas. May found that planning agencies had a statistically significant positive impact on employees per bed, physical assets per bed, and financial assets (defined as endowments, short-term investments, and working capital) per bed. These measures were approximately 8, 9, and 16 percent higher in planned than in unplanned areas, respectively, with several exogenous influences held constant.

May recognized that his OLS regression estimates were subject to simultaneous-equations bias in that areas with relatively high levels of hospital staffing and capital investment may be more likely to form planning agencies than other areas. To correct for this potential bias, he reestimated the equations, using a two-stage process with predicted values for the planning variable. The results were similar to the OLS estimates, although levels of statistical significance were reduced. These findings must be interpreted with caution, for they are subject to the limitations of using aggregated cross-sectional data. However, they do support the view that, historically, planning agencies have been ineffective in controlling hospital capital and service expansion.

The net effect of this evidence is to create a climate of skepticism regarding the efficacy of hospital investment control legislation in controlling hospital growth. Direct evidence on this topic, limited as it is, does not show a tangible impact of CON or section 1122 programs on controlling total hospital investment. Indirect evidence suggests that these programs may have unintended side effects and reduce competition in the hospital care market.[10]

Empirical Issues

Empirical analyses in later chapters attempt to determine how hospital investment controls affect hospital costs and inputs. Hospital beds, the primary focus of this form of regulation, represent an obvious dependent variable. Yet it is clear from the above discussions that these controls may also have direct and indirect consequences for the allocation of other physical inputs and for the amount and types of labor inputs in the production of hospital services. Thus, our empirical analyses do not focus solely on fixed nonlabor inputs, but attempt to examine the full range of input decisions. The analysis considers the response of *individual* hospitals to investment controls. This has the advantage of examining regulatory effects at the micro level, but it also has the disadvantage of not addressing effects of regulation on community resource allocation, including entry and exit of hospitals from the marketplace and examination of such important factors as hospital expenditures per capita population. The latter topics must be left for future research.

Type of regulatory mechanism can be direct or indirect, as suggested above, with CON being the direct regulatory tool. There are many dimensions to certificate-of-need laws which cannot adequately be captured in empirical analysis. However, perhaps the most important dimension is the comprehensiveness of the law. We distinguish between CON laws restricted primarily to bed-supply regulation and those that also focus on equipment purchases and service expansion.

Indirect controls include section 1122 review and Blue Cross requirements for planning agency compliance. In assessing the impact of such controls, it is necessary to consider the size of the population within an area that falls within the program's purview. For example, the larger the market share of Blue Cross in an area, the greater the impact of compliance requirements on hospitals. Thus, our empirical specification weights these programs by the relative sizes of populations covered.

Although the main thrust of both direct and indirect investment controls is on fixed hospital plant and equipment, they may also affect the use of labor and other types of nonlabor inputs. Service regulations incorporated in some CON laws may have direct effects on noncapital inputs, and capital controls have two potentially offsetting indirect effects. To the extent that fixed capital and other inputs are substitutes, effective control of fixed plant and equipment will lead to greater use of the nonregulated inputs. However, in the hospital sector, it is more likely that the other inputs are complementary with fixed plant and equipment on the whole. In fact, the marginal operating costs associated with a hospital investment should generally exceed the costs of debt repayment and depreciation. Our empirical analysis attempts to determine the direction and magnitude of these indirect effects.

As discussed earlier, implementation of investment controls may be uneven with regard to different types of hospitals. This view derives in part from the possibility that the hospital industry, particularly the dominant community nonprofit sector, may be able to wield substantial influence, and in part from the consumer-oriented ideology of the planning agencies which administer these laws. We attempt to determine whether investment controls tend to be particularly stringent on proprietary hospitals and whether teaching hospitals are allowed greater input expansion than other hospitals.

A final issue relates to the timing of hospital response to investment controls. Research objectives related to timing include identifying the lag time between the point at which legislation becomes effective and a tangible impact (if any) on hospital behavior is realized and the passage of time before investment controls achieve their full effect. In addition, we attempt to determine the extent and locus of anticipatory response of hospitals to investment control legislation.

Rate, Revenue, and Reimbursement Regulation

Background and Current Regulatory Institutions

The current movement toward regulation of hospital service rates, revenues, and methods of reimbursement also can be traced to the inflationary period following enactment of Medicare and Medicaid in the late 1960s. Two trends affecting hospital reimbursement have materialized during this period. First, there has been a movement toward widespread adoption of prospective reimbursement systems in place of retrospective cost-based and charge-based reimbursement. This trend represents a partial culmination of experimentation with incentive reimbursement. Prospective reimbursement, described in depth below, has been seen by policymakers as the most promising method of installing efficiency incentives in third-party reimbursement.[11] Second, there has been a movement away from employment of voluntary cost-control incentives to imposition of mandatory controls. By 1974, three states had established overall authority to regulate hospital rates, and several others were engaged in regulation of rates pertaining to state purchases of hospital services (Lewin and Associates, 1975a). In the private sector, several Blue Cross plans have instituted controls on hospital payment rates as a condition for hospital participation in Blue Cross reimbursement programs. There is considerable overlap between the development of rate controls and prospective reimbursement systems.

At the federal level, the Carter administration's Hospital Cost Containment Act is the most recent manifestation of the trend toward mandatory cost controls. As of this writing, however, the only federal program in this area of regulation that was fully implemented was the Economic Stabilization Program (ESP).[12] Initially, beginning in August 1971, both wages and prices were controlled (although, inadvertently, not reimbursement of costs by third-party payers).[13] In December 1972, regulations specific to institutional health care providers were issued. These limited the growth in annual revenue resulting from price increases to 6 percent, and all price increases had to be cost-justified. Limitations on increases in specific costs—5.5 percent for wages, 2.5 percent for nonlabor costs, and 1.7 for "new" technology—could well have constrained many hospitals to service-charge increases below the 6 percent limitation. As ESP progressed, unanticipated administrative problems and political considerations led to exceptions. Probably for the latter reason, wages of low-paid employees were exempted from the 5.5 percent limitation. Furthermore, the hospital variant of ESP was patterned after the general ESP program, emphasizing limits on price increases rather than expenditure increases. Many health care experts would have preferred emphasis to have been placed on expenditures.

The debate over charge- versus cost-based reimbursement precedes the passage of Medicare.[14] The selection of the reimbursement base—costs or charges—may be regarded as an indirect form of regulation. As noted in chapter 2, under charge-based systems, the insuring organization pays the hospital according to its schedule of fees for various hospital services covered. Commercial insurance companies and some Blue Cross plans traditionally have used charge-based systems. This method presumes some degree of market restraint on hospital fee-setting practices. The restraint lies in the presence of uninsured patients and those with fixed-payment indemnity coverage in the market.[15] Proponents of this method maintain that it promotes efficiency because the hospital will fare best financially if it minimizes costs, given its charges. However, as the proportion of uninsured patients and those with fixed-payment indemnity coverage has shrunk, the restraining influence on charges imposed by such patients has diminished.

Under cost-based systems, the insuring organization pays the hospital its allowable costs, usually with an added factor to cover future capital replacement and expansion. This method is often termed *cost plus* because the added factor is usually computed as a percentage of allowable costs. Medicare, Medicaid, and some Blue Cross plans use this method of reimbursement. Its critics claim that this system provides an incentive to maximize costs in order to maximize the plus factor.[16] Cost-based systems contain provisions for disallowance of reimbursement of costs declared "unreasonable," which is typically defined as costs substantially in excess of those of a reference group of hospitals. This criterion has not been widely used by insuring organizations to deny reimbursement.[17] As seen in chapter 2, which of the two types is the more inflationary is an empirical question.

Prospective reimbursement (PR) represents a more recently instituted form of direct regulation of hospital reimbursement rates or revenues. Advocates of PR hope that under this type of system hospital cost inflation will be controlled. Yet, as seen below, empirical support for this position is currently lacking. Because many PR systems were instituted when pressure to contain the growth in outlays for hospital services was relatively high, it is difficult to separate the effects of PR per se from prevailing political climates. New York's and Rhode Island's PR systems, for example, were instituted as an alternative to more stringent government controls on hospitals in these states.

Dowling (1974) identified the following commonalities among all PR programs: rates of hospital reimbursement are set in advance for a future period, and hospitals are paid these rates regardless of costs actually incurred. Because PR systems shift part of the risk of cost increases from insurers to hospitals, proponents assert that hospitals reimbursed through PR have an incentive to be more cost-conscious and correspondingly more concerned with the cost implications of changes in quantity, quality, style of care, scope of services, and/or efficiency, since third-party payers under PR do not cover "overruns." If prospective rates are exceeded, the hospital suffers financial losses. If the hospital's unit costs are below the prospective rate, it keeps at least part of the savings.

Uniformity among PR programs in various states virtually ends with the above definition. Programs differ, *inter alia*, according to (1) whether they are mandatory or voluntary; (2) use of a formulary or budget review method for prospective rate setting; (3) payers covered (say, Medicaid, Blue Cross, private payers); (4) the payment unit, including patient-day, case, specific services, and total hospital or department budget; and (5) aspects of PR administration, including the locus of rate-setting authority.

Our PR variable includes only mandatory programs since voluntary PR programs are unlikely to show substantial effects and, for research purposes, are subject to substantial self-selection bias. By contrast, the formula-versus-budget-review distinction is an important one, and we develop separate PR variables in our empirical analysis for these two forms. Until the mid-1970s, the only formula PR system was New York's, and the New York experience, because of the number of years and hospitals covered, must dominate any current evaluation of formula PR, including ours. Under formula PR systems, the prospective rate is established by solving an equation consisting of variables pertaining to individual hospital characteristics (size, ownership, and teaching status), hospital performance (occupancy rate, prior cost experience), and factors external to the hospital (general inflation rate). The formula is recomputed periodically, usually yearly, to arrive at a new prospective rate. This method involves relatively little direct interaction between hospitals and the rate-setting authority and is therefore less costly to administer and, although possibly more arbitrary, less likely to be redirected to the hospital's advantage.

Under budget PR systems, the hospital develops a budget for the prospective year which is reviewed by the PR authority. Items in the budget deemed unecessary or excessive are eliminated or reduced. Hospitals are generally given the opportunity to negotiate and/or to appeal budget-reducing decisions. Once the final budget has been approved, a payment rate is established that covers the hospital's budgeted costs. Because this method permits maximum recognition of individual hospital characteristics, it tends to be preferred by hospitals over the formula method. In fact, when given the choice between being regulated by budget review or a formula, all New Jersey hospitals chose the former (Worthington 1976). This is indirect evidence that the formula method tends to be tougher on hospitals than the budget method.

Of course, a major difficulty in evaluating effects of tough versus weak regulatory programs of any sort is that one may expect the tough ones to be implemented in states in which there is political pressure on government to reduce inflation in hospital expenditures. The precise nature of the regulatory approach may be less important than the political atmosphere existing when regulatory programs are implemented. Unfortunately, there is really nothing one can do about this empirically.[18]

The extent to which patients in a hospital's market area have insurance covered by revenue-cost controls should bear a direct relationship to the influence of such controls on hospital behavior. This factor is incorporated into our analysis by defining our PR variables as proportions of patients in the market area covered by particular types of PR, either formulary or budget review.

The vast majority of PR programs use either per diem rates or payment rates based on specific services (Dowling 1974; Abt Associates 1978). All formula PR systems use the per diem method. The controls-on-specific-services method leaves open the possibility of generating output to boost hospital revenue, and hence programs using this kind of payment unit may be less effective in controlling growth in hospital costs and input use. The number of hospitals (weighted by the proportions of patients covered by PR) in our sample is too small to sustain a split between budget review–per diem and budget review–specific services. Given that the per diem method is likely, on balance, to be more stringent and the fact that formulary programs use it, one may infer that budget review PR programs tend to adopt the specific-services method of reimbursement in states less inclined toward hospital regulation (than formula states).[19]

During the early 1970s, several PR systems advanced from the experimental stage to large-scale systems encompassing the universe of hospitals in the catchment area of a rate-setting authority. However, most systems pertain to patients covered by a specific third-party payer—Blue Cross, Medicaid, or Medicare. Only a few statewide PR systems encompass all sources of payment for hospital services, but there may be a trend in this direction. Table I–2 presents information on the year instituted, population covered, and method of establishing rates (budget or formula) of large-scale

PR systems existing in 1975. Additional institutional details pertaining to existing PR systems are delineated in the discussion of past empirical findings below.

Empirical Findings

The discussion of empirical findings from past research begins with a review of studies of cost- versus charge-based reimbursement and of the impact of ESP on hospital costs. However, most of this section is devoted to empirical studies of prospective reimbursement.

Pauly and Drake (1970) examined data pertaining to four Blue Cross plans in the Midwest, focusing on the inflationary effects of cost-based reimbursement. Their data base consisted of accounting data pertaining to hospitals in the four states during the last six months of 1966. The four Blue Cross systems were differentiated as to their method of reimbursement (cost- or charge-based) and presence or absence of direct controls on hospital rates. To test the impact of the method of reimbursement and controls on hospital costs, regression equations were estimated on data from pairs of states. Dependent variables were cost per patient-day and cost per admission. The regression equations included a number of exogenous variables reflecting hospital and community characteristics and a dummy variable indicating the type of reimbursement scheme. In a pooled regression including all states, a continuous variable ranging from 0 to 1 was constructed to measure strictness of regulatory controls.

The regression results indicated no effect of reimbursement mechanism on cost per patient-day and a slight positive effect of cost-based reimbursement on cost per admission. Neither dependent variable was appreciably affected by the presence of direct controls on charges or allowable costs. As emphasized by Klarman (1970) and Davis (1973), this specification omits consideration of the proportion of patients in the hospital's market area covered by the reimbursement mechanism under study. Moreover, it may not be reasonable to assume, as Pauly and Drake implicitly did, that the hospital's demand schedule is unaffected by its level of costs. If some cost-increasing activities are devoted to enhancing quality, and this affects the hospital's demand function, one cannot deduce a priori that cost-based systems should be more inflationary than charge-based ones.

Davis (1973) estimated a regression model similar to the Pauly and Drake specification, but with several modifications. She performed both single-year cross-sectional estimates and pooled-time-series cross-sectional estimates using state data pertaining to 1965, 1967, and 1968. State average expense per hospital admission was the dependent variable, and the proportion of state hospital expenses covered by cost-based reimbursement was entered as an independent variable. Davis found that cost-based reimbursement exerted no statistically significant impact on hospital costs in the individual cross-sectional regressions, and a similar result was obtained from the pooled regression when dummy variables for time were included. Without the dummy variables for time, the cost-based proportion had a positive influence on hospital costs.

Davis' conclusion from these findings was that cost reimbursement has not had an appreciable impact on hospital costs within the range of cost reimbursement proportions observed. This conclusion was consistent with her theoretical argument that the proportion of patients covered by cost reimbursement would have to be extremely high (for example, 95 percent) for hospitals to have an incentive to increase costs.

Two additional studies provide further evidence on the impact of cost-based reimbursement on hospitals. Salkever (1972), in a time-series cross-sectional analysis of average cost per day in short-term hospitals in New York covering 1961 to 1967, included measures of the extent of coverage under major types of health insurance (Blue Cross, commercial, Medicare, and Medicaid) among the independent variables. Because Medicare, Medicaid, and (to a lesser extent) Blue Cross tend to use cost-based reimbursement systems, while commercial systems tend to be indemnity- or charge-based, parameter estimates pertaining to these variables can be used to infer relative inflationary effects. Salkever found generally small differences in cost impact, with an unexpected tendency for increases in commercial insurance to be the most inflationary of the four types.

Sloan and Elnicki (1978), in a cross-sectional analysis of nurse staffing in a national sample of short-term hospitals in 1973, included an estimate of the proportion of population with cost-based health insurance among the independent variables. They found that cost-based reimbursement exerts a positive influence on nurse staffing. In light of the fact that other studies have revealed no consistent impact of reimbursement type on hospital costs generally, the Sloan and Elnicki finding suggests that a full investigation of the cost- versus charge-based reimbursement issue requires examination of disaggregated components of hospital costs.

The evidence of the impact of the Economic Stabilization Program on hospital costs and inputs is somewhat mixed, but generally indicates a decline in input, cost, and price inflation rates during the period that ESP was in effect. Feldstein and Taylor (1977) reported that the increase in earnings per employee was 4.6 percent in 1972–1973 and 5.6 percent in 1973–1974, the years in which controls were entirely in effect, compared to an 8.1 percent increase in 1971–1972, and a 10.8 percent increase in 1974–1975. The increase in an index of inputs per patient-day during the 1972–1974 period was roughly half the increase of the 1971–1972 and 1974–1975 years. Altman and Eichenholz (1976) reported that the rate of increase in hospital room-and-board rates declined by over 50 percent from November 1971 to January 1973. The rates of increase in cost per patient-day and cost per admission declined by only about 25 percent, suggesting an overall reduction in hospital revenues per admission and per patient-day during this period.

Elnicki (1972) examined data from the 1960s pertaining to three hospitals in Connecticut to predict the effect of ESP on growth of hospital services. He found that, given the restrictions of ESP on increases in hospital revenues and plausible assumptions regarding input price and productivity increases, controls would permit less than half the historical growth rate in services. While no direct data on the effect of ESP on service growth were presented, the Elnicki study suggests a potentially negative effect on quality and diffusion of innovations if ESP-type controls were long-lasting.

In contrast to data indicating a decline in hospital cost and price increases during ESP, more recent studies suggest that ESP has had relatively little overall impact (Salkever 1978b). The most comprehensive work on this subject currently in the public domain is by Ginsburg (1976, 1978).[20] Ginsburg's empirical analysis began with an examination of time-series trends in hospital costs, revenues, and inputs. Based on these data, he did not concur with others, including the Council on Wage and Price Stability, which asserted that ESP controls had resulted in a reduction in hospital cost inflation. Ginsburg ascribed this discrepancy to the fact that other studies failed to express cost trends in real terms (thereby overstating declaration in rates of cost increase) and to the focus of other studies on charges rather than on costs or revenue per unit of output. From the second quarter of 1971 to the second quarter of 1973, semiprivate room charges increased at an annual rate of 5.8 percent while inpatient revenues per patient-day from reimbursement of costs increased at an annual rate of 9.3 percent.

Ginsburg also performed multivariate evaluations of the effects of ESP on hospitals. Using aggregate data for the nine U.S. Census divisions for forty-four quarters (1963–1973), he regressed a set of exogenous variables, including a dummy variable signifying the quarters that ESP was in effect, on a number of variables related to hospital costs. Both static and dynamic versions of his model showed no significant effect except on wages. In the static version, a decline in the ratio of labor to nonlabor inputs was attributable to ESP. Neither costs nor input intensity (gauged by the ratio of an index of input use to hospital outputs) appeared responsive to ESP. Ginsburg attributed the failure of ESP to have a major impact on costs to disincentives to control costs (for example, the 6 percent figure became a floor as well as a ceiling), ambiguous regulations, and expectations in the hospital community that ESP would be short-lived and hence not worth large-scale adjustments. The fact that Ginsburg's time series extended only through 1973 is unfortunate since the ESP variable may have picked up any trend In the terminal years of the 1963-1973 decade. More conclusive evidence could be obtained with a time series incorporating some post-ESP experience.

Much of the evidence on prospective reimbursement pertains to the formula PR system in New York State. We review three studies on this system.

Abt Associates, Inc., and Policy Analysis, Inc. (1976), performed a detailed analysis of the formula PR system in upstate New York.[21] In this system hospitals are grouped on the basis of size, ownership, and teaching status, and "routine" costs in excess of 110 percent of the peer group average for a rating year are disallowed. Routine costs are added to ancillary and education costs and are trended for inflation in input prices that are expected to occur between the base year and the rating year. Total projected costs for the rating year are divided by base-year patient-days to calculate the per diem reimbursement rate. If the hospital fails to meet occupancy minimums in the rating year (60 percent for obstetrics, 70 percent for pediatrics, 80 percent for medical-surgical units), patient-days are increased to the minimum level, reducing the per diem rate.

Until recently, the upstate New York PR system applied only to Medicaid and Blue Cross patients, accounting for approximately 55 percent of hospital revenues statewide. It was created under the authority of the Cost Control Act of 1969 and was implemented in 1970. Overall, the system is regarded as a tight one; it was instituted during a period of intense political pressure to control hospital costs when, for example, a Medicaid hospital payment rate freeze was a likely alternative.

The Abt-PAI evaluation design included development of a geographically "matched" comparison group of hospitals from most of Ohio and from the Milwaukee SMSA. American Hospital Association data were used to construct a time series of cross sections encompassing periods prior to and after institution of PR. The effect of PR was inferred from parameter estimates pertaining to a PR dummy variable in a series of regression equations.

The Abt-PAI study specified twenty-six dependent variables potentially influenced by PR in upstate New York. Overall, the impact of PR on hospital costs was consistently negative, but nearly all important estimates were statistically insignificant at conventional levels. The rates of increase in total cost per patient-day and per admission were, respectively, $0.88 and $11.00 lower than in the control group. Revenues per patient-day in upstate New York grew at a rate approximately $2 less per year than in the control group. Total losses resulting from the occupancy and group mean penalties and the per diem constraint were estimated to be, on average, about 5 percent of average total costs.

With regard to hospital inputs, the empirical results suggested that the impact of PR was primarily on ancillary (for example, laboratory and X-ray) and nonlabor costs. The authors suggested that this may be due to greater administrative control over equipment and facilities investment than other decisions influenced to a greater degree by the medical staff. The study found that PR had little impact on average hospital wages, but some evidence of reduced skill mix relative to that in control hospitals was obtained. In addition, there was evidence of a slower rate of increase in FTE employees per patient-day and in adoption of complexity-expanding services than in the control group.

The study found no impact of PR on hospital output, measured by either beds or admissions. However, evidence was obtained that PR had a positive impact on average length of stay. The authors speculated that this was probably due to the per diem reimbursement unit and the penalty for low occupancy.

From production function estimates, the authors found a statistically significant improvement in efficiency due to PR when bed size was used as the measure of capital. This result was regarded as evidence of reduced administrative slack in New York hospitals. There was no evidence that PR had any adverse impact on quality of care.

Dowling et al. (1976) analyzed the prospective reimbursement system in the seventeen-county Greater New York City Area–Downstate New York (DNY). In light of the similarity between upstate and downstate New York in key PR program characteristics (main differences pertain to Blue Cross reimbursement), the two systems may be regarded as nearly identical. Both have group mean restrictions and occupancy restrictions built into rate computations. Both project input price inflation from a base year to the prospective rating year to obtain the per diem prospective rate. Both were created in 1970 by the same (state) legislation under similar pressures to control hospital cost inflation in New York.

The approach employed by Dowling et al. to estimate the impact of PR in DNY is similar to the Abt-PAI approach in two major respects—creation of a geographically matched control group of hospitals for comparative purposes and use of time-series cross-sectional regression estimates to determine the impact of PR on a variety of hospital decision variables. The study period included two pre-PR years, 1968 and 1969, and four during-PR years, 1970 to 1974.

The control group selected for the empirical estimates consisted of hospitals in the Chicago, Cleveland, and Philadelphia SMSAs. These areas were deemed to be similar to DNY with respect to important hospital demand and supply factors, and measures were taken to enhance comparability. However, cost levels in the control group were considerably lower before and during the PR period, and it was determined statistically to be inappropriate to pool the DNY and control hospitals in estimating cost functions, which suggests a different structure of cost determination between DNY and control hospitals. The authors submitted that these factors limit comparability between study and control hospitals, but that this limitation is not substantial in light of the order of magnitude of the findings.

Dowling et al. compared cost trends of DNY and control hospitals and estimated cost functions to isolate the impact of PR. Both methods showed a negative impact of PR on cost per patient-day and a less substantial negative impact on cost per admission. Cost per day was affected more than cost per admission because PR had slowed the rate of decrease in average length of stay in DNY hospitals.

Mean cost per patient-day increased from $82 to $167 in DNY hospitals and from $69 to $142 in control hospitals over the seven-year period, but in comparing the periods before and during PR, the rate of cost inflation declined in DNY and rose slightly in control areas. Cost function estimates showed that PR had reduced the rate of increase in adjusted cost per day in DNY hospitals by 6.4 percent per year, a result that was statistically significant at the 1 percent level, and had reduced the rate of increase in adjusted cost per admission by 4.6 percent per year, a result that approached statistical significance at the 5 percent level. The authors noted that, because of different cost structures of DNY and control hospitals, these findings should be interpreted cautiously.

Dowling et al. obtained several other findings, mostly consistent with the view that PR restrained hospital costs in DNY. Most significant was the finding that PR had caused a substantial decline in the financial position of DNY hospitals relative to that of control hospitals. The average DNY hospital operating margin for the seven-year period was -0.07. Control hospitals suffered losses, but not nearly as great. To compensate, DNY hospitals reduced working-capital balances and unrestricted endowments. During the period 1973–1974, the ratio of unrestricted endowment funds to total assets in DNY nonprofit hospitals declined from 0.20 to 0.05, while this ratio remained steady at about 0.15 in control hospitals. The authors concluded that PR was not the only factor contributing to operating losses in DNY, but that it accounted for about half of the inpatient losses.

Berry (1976), in a less detailed analysis of prospective reimbursement in New York (upstate and downstate), ascribed great importance to the government programs introduced in the 1960s as chief sources of increases in hospital prices, net revenues, and input intensity in the 1970s. His explanation was intended to show how controls on hospital price increases would lead to a constraint on cost, the hoped-for result of the New York PR system.[22] Berry compared a variety of price, cost, and input measures pertaining to New York, New England, Ohio, and all hospitals nationally for 1965–1970, 1970–1973, and 1974. In the earliest period, New York compared unfavorably to the other areas with regard to inflation in hospital prices, costs, and inputs per unit of service. During 1970–1973, after New York had instituted its PR system and when, for much of the period, the entire United States was subject to ESP, New York compared much more favorably. Declines in rates of increase of price, cost, and input use were greater for New York than for other areas and for the entire United States in almost every instance. Berry tentatively credited this improvement in the relative position of New York to PR.

In the period following ESP, Berry's evidence shows that the constraints on prices and costs were eased in New England and Ohio, while rates of increase in these measures continued to decline in New York, which he again ascribed to PR. According to Berry, the major effect of formula PR in New York operated through the mechanism of reduced revenues. Price constraints arising from PR have produced deficits in New York, suggesting that revenues have been affected more than costs.

On the whole, these three studies suggest that formula prospective reimbursement in New York has reduced cost and revenue inflation, particularly the latter, but it is difficult to generalize from these findings. First, the empirical results are not so strong that they clearly signify a marked effect on costs attributable to PR. Second, the results pertain to a single state in which the political climate may have been the ultimate source of the negative impact on costs. Third, the concurrent existence of other regulatory programs, such as ESP, may have had a confounding effect. Comprehensive evaluations of formula PR covering more states, a longer period, and additional regulatory variables would be worthwhile.

Now we review evaluations of three budget-based prospective reimbursement programs. Geomet (1976) studied the budget review system in New Jersey over a six-year period, 1968 to 1973. In New Jersey, proposed hospital budgets are reviewed by an advisory committee to the insurance commissioner, and institutional comparisons are made to determine reasonableness of costs. Committee recommendations, which are negotiated with hospital administrators, are forwarded to the state commissioners of insurance and health whose offices establish the prospective per diem rate (final authority resides with the commissioner of health). If dissatisfied, hospitals can appeal to the commissioners and ultimately to the courts.

Hospitals that underspend budgeted prospective rates, based on cost data accumulated periodically, are compelled to return the difference to the insurer without sharing in the cost savings. Hospitals that overspend may apply for an interim cost review by the advisory committee and may receive recompense if the committee determines the additional costs to be reasonable. The New Jersey system covers Blue Cross and state hospital service purchase programs, including Medicaid. In 1973, these programs accounted for roughly 43 percent of total patient-days in the state.

The Geomet study was limited to nonfederal, short-term general hospitals that participated in the Medicare program from 1968 to 1973. Data consisting primarily of Medicare cost reports were obtained on eighty-nine such hospitals in New Jersey. A control group of twenty-eight hospitals from eastern Pennsylvania, matched on size, teaching status, and other factors with an equal number of hospitals from the New Jersey sample, was selected for comparative analysis. A time series of cross-sectional data was constructed. Overall study objectives were to assess the impact of PR on cost, productivity, and quality of care in New Jersey.

Analysis of the impact of PR on hospital costs consisted of descriptive evidence of cost trends and estimation of general cost functions by using regression methodology. A limitation of the analysis arises from the fact that hospitals entered the New Jersey PR system on a year-by-year basis, and there is a pronounced relationship between time of hospital entry into the program and cost experience (the more costly hospitals tended to enter the PR program earlier). Also, because the study period began in 1968 and hospitals began to enter the PR program in 1969, there was a very limited pretest period. The treatment of this problem in the cost regressions was to include as independent variables both a single dummy variable indicating whether the hospital was subject to PR and a vector of dummy variables signifying when the hospital became subject to PR (holding one year constant in the regressions). This approach was adopted to correct for the bias arising from the incremental entry. The year-of-entry dummy variable vector represents the correction, and the PR dummy variable is intended to represent the impact of PR on costs.

Average costs per patient-day and per admission were selected as dependent variables, and several variables representing exogenous influences on hospital costs were included. However, no evidence of an effect of PR on hospital costs in New Jersey was obtained.

The analysis of productivity also found that PR had had no significant impact on New Jersey hospitals. With regard to hospital inputs, regression estimates indicated that hospitals had not varied the labor/capital input mix or engaged in labor substitutions (that is, employed more lower-cost substitutes) in response to PR.

To a greater degree than other studies reviewed here, the Geomet study of New Jersey hospitals attempted to assess the impact of PR on quality. The primary technique employed was to derive quality-of-care scores through medical audit of three "tracer" diagnoses in each study and control hospital and to regress the score on a set of presumed quality-related variables with a PR dummy variable entered as an independent variable. This method showed no discernible impact of PR on quality of care in New Jersey hospitals.

Thornberry and Zimmerman (1976) and Zimmerman, Buechner, and Thornberry (1977) provide reviews of the Blue Cross budget-based prospective reimbursement system in Rhode Island during 1971 and 1972. As in other states, the system in Rhode Island was developed in response to rapid hospital cost inflation during the late 1960s. Blue Cross covers roughly 80 percent of Rhode Island's population, the largest Blue Cross plan enrollment proportion in the United States. When a rate-increase request for fiscal 1971 of 24.5 percent was cut to 18 percent, Blue Cross entered into a period of bargaining that ultimately resulted in the establishment of a negotiated budget-based PR system.[23] The system was in effect for Blue Cross reimbursement in 1971 and 1972 and terminated in 1973 owing to conflicts with ESP, but was reinstated in fiscal 1975, adding Medicare and Medicaid as participants.

The PR system instituted in 1971 required preparation of prospective budgets by hospitals and negotiation with Blue Cross until mutually acceptable budgets were obtained.[24] Hospitals agreed to adhere to prospective rates (obtained via standardized cost-finding techniques) provided that actual utilization did not deviate from that projected by more than specified amounts for different types of service, but per diem rates were renegotiated if actual utilization exceeded allowable variation. The system called for equal sharing of surpluses between hospitals and Blue Cross and total absorption of all losses by hospitals.[25]

Thornberry and Zimmerman (1976) constructed a comparison group of twelve hospitals in Massachusetts and assembled cost and other data pertaining to a pre-PR period (1966–1970) and a post-PR period (1971–1972). The study group consisted of the thirteen general hospitals in Rhode Island. The two hospital groups were comparable in most respects, except that on average the Rhode Island hospitals tended to be smaller. As with other PR studies, cost functions were estimated with cost per patient-day and cost per admission as dependent variables. This specification adjusted for interhospital variations in case mix to a greater degree than other PR analyses. The impact of PR was inferred from parameter estimates on a PR dummy variable included in the cost regressions.

Equations were estimated for Rhode Island hospitals for 1969–1972 and for Rhode Island and control hospitals for 1971–1972. Parameter estimates on the PR variable in the former equation were interpreted to signify the combined impact of PR and ESP; in the latter equations, of PR alone. The sign of the PR variable was consistently negative (seven regressions in all were reported), but the variable tended not to be statistically significant at conventional levels. The authors concluded that these findings are suggestive of potential cost savings from PR, but that the complicating influence of ESP, the short duration of the PR study period, and methodological limitations made it impossible to tell precisely from these data that PR had had an impact on hospital costs in Rhode Island in 1971 and 1972. No impact of PR was found on bed growth, admissions, patient-days, average length of stay, or occupancy level. Examination of revenue and expense data suggested that the financial position on Rhode Island hospitals did not deteriorate during the PR period.

An analysis of the combined formula and budget-review prospective reimbursement system of Blue Cross in western Pennsylvania was conducted by Applied Management Sciences (AMS) (1975). Although not the fault of the authors, this study suffers enormously from self-selection bias. During the study period of 1972–1974, the system was completely voluntary and only five predominantly rural hospitals participated.[26] Consequently, despite the authors' attempt to form valid experimental/control group comparisons, findings of this study regarding impact of PR cannot be accepted with a great deal of confidence.

Some evidence of reduced cost inflation in PR hospitals was detected, but (as the authors noted) this finding cannot reliably be attributed to PR per se. Poor financial positions of the study hospitals had influenced both the decision to participate in the PR experiment and subsequent actions to contain costs. Therefore, the AMS study does not receive further review. Moreover, we have excluded such voluntary programs from our empirical analyses.

Completed evaluations of budget-based prospective reimbursement cover more systems than evaluations of formula PR, but the former have yielded virtually no evidence of any cost-inhibiting influences on hospital behavior. The lack of such evidence may reflect the early stage in program development at which these evaluations took place, or they may indicate inherent weaknesses in this approach to hospital cost containment. The fact that hospitals and hospital associations have been supporters of budget-based PR in preference to more stringent forms of regulation again comes to mind. But we speculate no further—our empirical analyses attempt to generate more comprehensive evidence on effects of formula and budget-based PR on hospital behavior.

Empirical Issues

As seen in chapter 2, formal models advanced by economists tend not to produce unambiguous predictions of hospital response to reimbursement programs, and empirical studies also have not been able to identify consistent responses. As with the other regulatory program variables, no-effect null hypotheses are appropriate, yet the potential for perverse effects, especially in the analysis of hospital demand for inputs, cannot be disregarded.

Past research and theory on cost- versus charge-based reimbursement have not shown a tendency for either method to be more inflationary than the other. Our treatment of this issue is simply to provide further evidence of whether the two systems result in differences in hospital costs and/or input employment over time. There is little change in proportions of patients by cost- versus charge-based reimbursement over time, but changing proportions of patients covered by Blue Cross, Medicaid, and Medicare do permit limited examination of time-series response to reimbursement method.

Most studies of the Economic Stabilization Program indicate that ESP had a restraining influence on hospital prices and revenues during the period it was in effect. However, the behavioral response to ESP, including changes in the level and mix of inputs, has not been fully investigated. Our empirical analysis of ESP will benefit from having pre- and post-ESP years included in the time series.

Despite the enthusiasm of its proponents, neither theory nor the limited evidence available gives much cause to expect major cost savings from prospective reimbursement. Studies of budget-based PR systems are inconclusive with regard to effects on hospital costs and behavior.[27] Studies of formula PR in New York, taken as a whole, do suggest that the system had an effect, primarily through its constraining influence on hospital revenues. Of course, this evidence cannot be taken as indicative of relative efficacy of budget- and formula-based systems. As suggested earlier, the political and economic circumstances existing in New York during the period that PR was studied may have been the ultimate source of the constraint on hospital revenues, and the PR system can be viewed as one of several alternative vehicles for imposing tight controls on hospitals in the state. Nevertheless, hospital behavioral responses to the characteristics of the system are deserving of further empirical research. The possible tendency for hospitals to expand average length of stays, *ceteris paribus*, when reimbursement is on a per diem basis and when penalties for underutilized facilities are present, for example, has implications for both hospital cost performance and input employment. Incorporating information on all large-scale, mandatory PR programs existing in the first half of the 1970s, our empirical analysis investigates whether PR had an aggregate effect on cost inflation and levels and/or mix of hospital inputs in our hospital cohort.

Utilization and Quality Regulation

Background and Current Regulatory Institutions

The topic of utilization and quality regulation, although important from a public-policy standpoint, is accorded less attention in this book than other forms of regulation. First, although utilization and quality regulation has a much longer and diverse history than, say, investment control, the first half of the 1970s was not an active period in the implementation of mandatory utilization-quality controls. For example, the major national program, Professional Standards Review Organizations (PSRO), though part of the 1972 amendments to the Social Security Act, was not fully implemented during this period. Consequently, this program is not well suited for our empirical analysis. Nevertheless, an institutional overview of hospital regulation would not be complete without some description of utilization and quality regulation. More important, some data on utilization control programs are available for limited empirical testing. More detailed descriptions of this form of regulation are available elsewhere.[28]

As is the case with other forms of hospital regulation, the modern era of utilization and quality regulation in hospitals began with enactment of Medicare and Medicaid in 1965. These programs specified that, as a condition of participation, hospitals must have utilization review (UR) committees to analyze admissions, lengths of stay, and services delivered, and patients with extended stays must be recertified at periodic intervals to establish ongoing necessity of care (State of Michigan 1973). Both retrospective UR and extended-stay recertification were intended to be implemented with minimal intervention into provider and practitioner decision making. Emphasis was placed on extended-stay review because it was felt that this was the area of greatest abuse and greatest potential savings (Blum, Gertman, and Rabinow 1977). In general, the UR mechanisms mandated by Medicare and Medicaid have not been regarded as successful, nor have they been strictly enforced.

On the quality front, passage of Medicare required hospitals to obtain Joint Commission on Accreditation of Hospitals (JCAH) accreditation to be eligible for participation. This provision was included to ensure a minimum quality of services rendered to Medicare patients, but subsequently JCAH and the Social Security Administration (SSA) were criticized for laxity of the JCAH accreditation standards (Blum, Gertman, and Rabinow 1977; State of Michigan 1973). As a result, the 1972 Social Security amendments authorized HEW to withhold participatory status to JCAH-accredited hospitals with "significant deficiencies."

Trends in utilization and quality regulation have converged with the establishment of the Professional Standards Review Organization (PSRO) program (the so-called Bennett Amendment to P.L. 92-603, the 1972 Social Security Act amendments). The PSRO program was established to serve jointly the purposes of quality assurance and cost containment through utilization control (Blumstein 1976). Procedures were specified that must be followed by providers to obtain reimbursement for services delivered to Medicare and Medicaid patients. These procedures are designed to ensure that services conform to appropriate professional standards (quality), and payment is to be made only when services are medically necessary and economically provided (for example, inpatient service expenditures should not be reimbursed if the same services could have been effectively provided on an outpatient basis) (Blum, Gertman, and Rabinow 1977).

The impetus behind PSRO legislation was clearly cost containment, largely because experience with UR under Medicare had been regarded by Congress as a failure in this regard (Blum, Gertman, and Rabinow 1977). However, actual implementation of PSRO has been exceedingly slow. As of early 1977, five years after the program was created, 108 "conditional" and 58 "planning" PSROs had been established, but none were operationally fulfilling all requirements of the law (*Medical Care Review* 1977).[29]

The specific regulatory institutions governing control of hospital quality and utilization are diverse and complex. This discussion focuses on activities of third parties (insurers and government) that are primarily directed toward utilization control. Aside from PSROs, most quality regulation is vested in the licensure and certification procedures of state governments and professional associations.

Institutional UR and peer review have existed in hospitals for several decades, and both concepts are integrated into the current hospital regulatory movement. Hospital UR generally involves review of both concurrent and after-treatment care by physician-controlled UR committees. Peer review functions overlap with UR; however, the main emphasis of the former is on professional competence of professionals, especially physicians. Thus, the focus of peer review has traditionally been on professional quality, which potentially includes, to some extent, detection of instances of over- or underutilization of hospital services (State of Michigan 1973).

Claims-review activites are carried out by third-party payers for hospital services. Much of claims review is simply to determine whether a patient is entitled to reimbursement for services and, if so, to what extent, However, an increasing amount of attention is being paid to whether services rendered are necessary, and in some cases payment is denied if services are deemed unnecessary. While it would appear to be in the best interests of insurers to reduce utilization whenever possible, potential conflicts with hospitals, doctors, and patients, all of whom may become responsible for payment of a denied claim, have limited the aggressiveness with which insurers pursue utilization-reduction claims-review activities. Consequently, most insurers rely heavily on hospital UR committee judgments.[30] Many Blue Cross plans require participating hospitals to have functioning UR programs meeting specific criteria.

In contrast to programs that review utilization, quality, and costs of services already delivered, other utilization controls seek to monitor hospital services prospectively. Among the latter, preadmission screening and recertification measures are the most germane to current regulatory trends.[31] These forms of regulation were initiated with the Medicare program and expanded with PSRO legislation. Considerable federal money has been made available to support the development of organizations and functions within organizations to monitor utilization and quality of health services. In recent years, most of this money has been devoted to the development of PSROs.

The chief review activities undertaken by PSROs are precertification of institutional services, periodic sample reviews by diagnosis or condition, and regular review of patient and provider profiles; PSROs are also responsible for monitoring the certification requirements of SSA, physician education regarding the program, and reporting violations (Decker and Bonner 1973). Preadmission screening and retrospective review are permitted, but not required; but concurrent review to determine necessity and appropriateness of utilization is required (Blum, Gertman, and Rabinow 1977). And PSROs are authorized to delegate UR functions to hospitals in their catchment areas.[32]

Empirical Evidence

In contrast to other major regulatory programs of the 1970s, including CON and PR, the chief utilization and quality control program, PSRO, has been initiated as a nationwide program without incremental enactment of laws at the state level. Consequently, there is little evidence on early programs from which to generalize. In addition, there are no comprehensive longitudinal studies of Medicare and Medicaid utilization control mechanisms. Consequently, this review is confined to a few isolated studies of the impact of specific utilization control mechanisms on hospital use.

In general, studies of preadmission certification and recertification programs have produced few concrete findings of utilization reduction. Exceptions are found in studies of the preadmission certification program operated by the Medi-Cal program in the early 1970s (Brian 1972, 1973) and a study of the Hospital Admission Surveillance Program (HASP) in Illinois (Flashner et al. 1973). Brian (1972) compared utilization trends before and after implementation of the preadmission certification program which consisted primarily of prior authorization for hospital admission by a state-employed or consultant physician. While this is a relatively uncontrolled experimental design (probably the only available under nonexperimental circumstances), Brian observed an immediate decline in the Medi-Cal hospital admission rate during a period when non-Medi-Cal hospital admissions rates were increasing. The admission rate declined from 17.4 per 1,000 eligible persons in 1969 to 16.1 in 1970, the first year of operation of the program. Brian (1973) compared the Medi-Cal program to the Certified Hospital Admission Program (CHAP) operated by the Sacramento Foundation for Medical Care and found that both programs resulted in reduced admission rates and average lengths of stay.

In a preliminary study, Flashner et al. (1973) compared length-of-stay data on hospitals covered by the HASP program before and after program implementation. He found that average length of stay declined from 7.2 to 6.2 days, but because of the uncontrolled nature of this study, it would not be warranted to ascribe the change entirely to the implementation of HASP.

In a more recent study, Dumbaugh and Neuhauser (1976) examined the impact of preadmission testing in selected hospitals in Massachusetts in 1973–1974. Preadmission testing, in which patients undergo diagnostic testing on an outpatient basis prior to hospital admission, is intended to reduce unnecessary admissions and lengths of stay, primarily of patients scheduled for elective surgery. Dumbaugh and Neuhauser focused on the latter objective by examining randomly selected cases pertaining to two common diagnoses and constructing experimental/control group comparisons of patients with and without preadmission testing. That study found no impact of preadmission testing on average length of stay, which the authors ascribed primarily to a lack of financial incentive of physicians to modify admitting practices to take advantage of the stay-reducing potential of the program. While preadmission testing is not a mandated part of the PSRO program, it has many advocates. Perhaps the most relevant aspect of that study in the present context is the implicit support of the view that utilization control measures cannot be expected to be highly successful without generating incentives for physicians to comply with regulatory objectives.

Recertification of appropriateness of hospital stay is designed to reduce average lengths of stay by curtailing unnecessary use of hospital beds. Blue Cross has found that recertification programs operated by member plans generally have had little or no impact on hospital length of stay (Blue Cross Association 1966). This finding is supported by the conclusion of the General Accounting Office that the recertification procedures required by the Medicare program have not been as successful as hoped in reducing the length of stay (State of Michigan 1973). Bailey and Reidel (1968) studied the New Jersey Blue Cross Approval by Individual Diagnosis (AID) program to determine impact on length of stay in New Jersey hospitals. Immediately following introduction of AID the average length of stay decreased markedly, but returned to prior levels by the end of the first year.

Most studies of hospital utilization have found that excessive use of hospital services is prevalent, but empirical evidence, albeit limited, does not indicate worthwhile reductions in hospital use from recertification programs and UR generally. Findings of a study of Medicare-mandated UR in Connecticut (Berman 1969) and a study of Medicare recertification at Massachusetts General Hospital (Kolb and Sidel 1968) found no substantial impact on hospital bed use. However, two studies of the impact of hospital UR on length of stay in Pennsylvania hospitals (Marcom 1965; Grimes 1970) did find a negative impact of hospital UR procedures on average length of stay. These findings appear to be an exception; moreover, the level of empirical investigation of this issue must be regarded as very rudimentary.[33]

Two more recent studies have questioned the PSRO emphasis on reducing hospital bed utilization through concurrent certification of length of stay. Goldberg and Holloway (1975) pointed out that this type of review is based on the premise that most unnecessary utilization occurs in the latter part of a hospital stay, but that this premise is contradicted by some recent evidence suggesting that much inappropriate hospital usage occurs in relatively short stays and in early days of the hospital stay. Averill and McMahon (1977), using plausible assumptions regarding the incidence of detection of inappropriate utilization and the timing of detection and remedial action, concluded that it is very unlikely that continued-stay certification under the PSRO program will be cost-effective. Overall, these two studies support the generally negative impression from review of past studies on the impact of UR procedures on curbing hospital use and extend this skepticism to the PSRO program. However, assessment of this impact cannot be definitive until controlled studies of operational PSROs are performed.

Empirical Issues

One form of reasoning pertaining to hospital utilization and quality regulation recognizes that there is considerable uncertainty surrounding much of medical practice and that, for most illnesses, a range of treatments can be viewed as acceptable on purely medical grounds. With this view as a premise, it seems logical to some observers that government should promote, through regulation, delivery of the least expensive service package in the acceptable range in publicly financed medical care programs. Quality regulation can be performed to ensure that minimum standards are met, and utilization regulation can be used to control expenditures beyond the minimum acceptable point.

Albeit simplistic, this line of thinking is at least as reasonable as the rationales underlying most public-policy development. However, there is substantial doubt that current regulatory policy reflects this point of view with much vigor. Havighurst and Blumstein (1975) pointed out that historically very little attention has been paid to quality-cost-trade-offs in the delivery of medical care and that the incentives of the prevalent modes of practice have promoted adherence to a "quality imperative" in health care delivery. Furthermore, to the degree that independent physicians retain considerable control in quality and utilization regulatory decisions, as is presently the case with PSRO, there is little likelihood that regulatory activities will be successful in controlling hospital expenditures. Thus, to some observers, the potential for utilization regulation to curb hospital expenditure inflation is in part a matter of reducing physician control or altering their incentives.[34]

Empirical investigation of the impact of utilization controls on hospital behavior is extremely limited in this book, and assessment of the effects of quality controls is virtually nonexistent. Existing state information on utilization controls is confined to cross-sectional data pertaining to utilization review programs operated by Blue Cross and Medicaid in 1974. These data are presented in table J-3.

A detailed examination of the multifaceted effects of utilization review, such as on occupancy, inpatient/outpatient service mix, frequency of elective surgery, and use of long-term-care beds, is beyond the scope of this book. However, to the extent that these effects are reflected in hospital costs or inputs, our empirical analysis considers them indirectly.

Variable Specification

Eleven regulation variables have been constructed for the empirical analyses of hospital costs and inputs. These variables are described below, and concise definitions are presented in Appendix A.

Five binary variables represent certification of need in our empirical analyses. The variable PRECON is 1 for hospitals located in a state in the year immediately preceding the introduction of CON. Thus PRECON can be 1 for, at most, one of the six years. This variable is designed to account for anticipatory behavior. An operating CON program is classified as either comprehensive or noncomprehensive. As defined, comprehensive programs include service expansion review *and* have a threshold less than $100,000. These programs presumably leave less room for the kind of compensatory impacts reported by Salkever and Bice (1976a, 1976b), such as on growth in assets per bed and/or in hospital demand for labor. We make a further distinction between *new* (the first or second year of operation) and *mature* programs (greater than two years of operation). It is possible that CON becomes more effective through a form of learning by doing. Several states changed from new to mature status during 1970–1975. Hence, in a limited way, we are able to gauge changes in CON impact as the program matures. Prefixes "C" and "N" in front of CON designate comprehensive and noncomprehensive programs, respectively; suffixes 1 and 2 identify new and mature programs, respectively.

Most of our remaining regulatory variables operate in conjunction with third-party reimbursement. To construct the variable, a binary variable indicating that the regulatory program exists is multiplied by the proportion of the population in the hospital's area with the kind of insurance for which the regulation in questions applies. The variable S1122 is the product of a binary variable indicating whether the program exists in the hospital's state and the sum of Medicare and Medicaid population proportions, since section 1122 applies to these programs. The variables BCPPA is a product of (1) a binary variable, which equals 1 if the Blue Cross plan in the hospital's area requires local planning agency approval for capital expenditures, and (2) Blue Cross' market share in the (Blue Cross plan catchment) area. As noted previously, neither section 1122 nor the Blue Cross program forbids the hospital from undertaking capital expansion and/or modernization; however, current expenditures associated with these capital purchases can be disallowed.

To discern the effects of cost- versus charge-based reimbursement on hospital costs and input use, we have constructed the variable COSTB. This variable is the sum of Medicaid and Medicare population proportions, since these are always cost-based, and the Blue Cross plan area population proportion when the plan uses a cost-based payment method.

The Economic Stabilization Program variable (ESP) is the fraction of the year that ESP was in effect, ranging from 0.25 to 1.00. Formula (FPR) and budget review (BPR) prospective reimbursement programs are defined as the products of binary variables identifying that the program was in effect and the proportions of the relevant populations covered. Since PR may apply to virtually any type of insurer (and there is substantial interstate variation on this score), we have devoted considerable effort to computing the relevant population proportions.

Our measure of utilization review (UR) is the proportion of patients in the hospital's market area covered by Blue Cross and Medicaid utilization review programs. Because data for UR are available for 1974 only, the only reason for intertemporal variation in UR is a change in the proportions of the population with various forms of third-party reimbursement.

Notes

1. A good example of this view is Kinzer (1976), who provides an illustration of the complexity of controls facing hospitals in Massachusetts.

2. May (1974a) reported an even more rapid rate of increase in growth of health planning agencies.

3. See Blumstein and Sloan (1978) for a thorough description of this act and its relationship with certificate-of-need laws.

4. May (1974b) provides evidence, cited later in this section, supporting this viewpoint.

5. In one additional state, North Carolina, a CON law had been

enacted and subsequently repealed prior to 1978, only to be reenacted in 1978 to bring the state in conformance with P.L. 93-641.

6. Table I–1 shows which states had CON in effect during 1970–1975. Additional descriptive data and information on indirect control programs are also provided in this table.

7. Table I–1 identifies the thirty-nine states having section 1122 review programs in 1976. Only one state, West Virginia, had neither a CON nor a section 1122 review program. Some states may have decided not to enter into a section 1122 agreement with DHEW because they did not wish to create competing and/or overlapping bureaucracies to achieve essentially the same goals.

8. Very little information on Blue Cross planning agency compliance requirements exists in the public domain. Table I–1 identifies plans having such requirements in 1976.

9. In a separate analysis of data collected for Lewin and Associates (1975a, 1975b), Harmon (1977) noted that CON disapproval rates were higher for proprietary hospitals and that many CON agency representatives expressed a bias against proprietary hospitals and multifacility chains. Because proprietaries represent a major competitive threat to nonprofit hospitals in several areas of the country, agency implementation of CON laws may have the effect of reduced competition in the hospital sector. Harmon also identified evidence of agency hindrance of innovative services, such as ambulatory surgical facilities, in some states.

10. The hospital investment control debate is intimately related to the controversy over whether hospitals should be regarded as public utilities for regulatory purposes. This issue has been addressed several times in the literature, both pro (McClure 1976; Priest 1970; Somers 1969) and con (Drake 1973; Noll 1975; and Havighurst 1973a).

11. This is evidenced by the enormous amount of funding made available in recent years by HEW to perform demonstrations and evaluations of prospective reimbursement systems. Findings from completed evaluation are reviewed in this chapter.

12. See Altman and Eichenholz (1976) and Ginsburg (1978) for more complete descriptions of the ESP program and its specific control.

13. Ginsburg (1976) has argued that it is likely that few hospitals took advantage of this loophole because, at the time, hospitals believed the controls would be short-lived and were uncertain whether cost increases realized during this period would be included in subsequent rate bases.

14. For example, see Tekolste (1963) and Sigmond (1963). See Weiner (1977) for a concise legal history of reimbursement trends.

15. Under fixed-payment indemnity coverage, the patient is covered for

a fixed amount per day hospitalized. When the hospital's charge is above this amount, the indemnified patient, like the uninsured, must pay 100 percent of the marginal dollar charged. See chapter 4 for more details.

16. The same criticism has been levied against public utilities that are paid on an "allowable rate-of-return" basis.

17. See Evans (1970) and Weiner (1977) for discussions of reimbursement criteria and Law (1974) for a critique. There has been some variation among private reimbursement programs in the extent to which the insuring organizations have attempted to limit hospital cost inflation through application of charge- and cost-based reimbursement criteria. There is considerable variation among Blue Cross plans in specific items regarded as allowable. Items exhibiting the most variation are bad debts, charity care, educational expenses, and treatment of depreciation and debt expenses. In plans where such provisions tend to be most restrictive, the percentage of billed charges reimbursed under charge-based systems and the amount of the plus factor in cost-based systems tend to be highest. See American Hospital Association (1971, 1974, 1977) and table I–2.

18. Even a social experiment would not be adequate if, in fact, the effect of a particular regulatory approach depended on the political environment.

19. Gaus and Hellinger (1976), Hellinger (1976b), and Worthington (1976) address this and related issues.

20. There are several other studies on ESP effects. For example, there is descriptive evidence that hospital profits fell during ESP. See Furst and Dunkelberg (1978) for evidence on North and South Carolina hospitals and a review of evidence on profits nationally during ESP. See also additional work by Ginsburg (1974, 1976) and Taylor (1977).

21. Hereafter cited as Abt-PAI (1976). Upstate New York includes non–New York City counties in the state.

22. This argument represents the "demand pull" view of inflation in the hospital industry. For evidence that at least part of the inflation is the "cost push" variety, see chapter 7.

23. Dowling (1974) and others have identified budget negotiation and budget review and approval as distinct models of PR. However, because budget review systems generally include negotiation with hospitals (as in New Jersey) and negotiation systems involve review and approval by the insurer and/or rate-setting agency (as in Rhode Island), these methods are regarded as essentially the same in this chapter and in subsequent empirical specifications.

24. The negotiation process was somewhat more detailed in fiscal 1972. A peer review committee was appointed by the Hospital Association of Rhode Island to review prospective budgets prior to submission to Blue

Cross, and Blue Cross review procedures were formalized. According to Zimmerman, Buechner, and Thornberry (1977), the entire process showed "little resemblance" between the first and second years.

25. In 1975, the system was altered such that hospitals were permitted to keep 100 percent of surpluses.

26. While it is true that the hospitals studied in the New Jersey PR system reported in Geomet (1976) participated voluntarily, the fact that all New Jersey hospitals were eventual participants permits viewing the New Jersey system as de facto mandatory.

27. These studies systematically provided information on PR program implementation and acceptance and a variety of attitudinal responses which may be useful to policymakers. However, as a foundation for empirical assessment of the impact of PR, their usefulness is limited.

28. See, for example, Blum, Gertman, and Rabinow (1977), O'Donoghue (1974), Donabedian (1966), and State of Michigan (1973).

29. *Conditional* and *planning* are HEW administrative terms designating PSROs in early stages of development. With federal financial support, PSROs are initiated as planning organizations and begin functioning on conditional terms before they become operationally qualified to satisfy the provisions of the law.

30. Insurers have been criticized for failing to take a more active role in controlling hospital utilization and costs. See chapter 4 for a discussion.

31. However, an important underlying rationale for copayment provisions of Medicare is to restrain utilization of health services, and HEW has spent considerable sums to discover how consumers respond to varying arrangements involving patient sharing of insured health service expenditures. Such controls differ substantially in nature from the more direct restraints imposed by programs whose intent is to verify necessity of service prior to delivery.

32. While these details describe the primary features of the PSRO program, considerably more could be written, unwarranted in the present context, but necessary to achieve a full understanding of the PSRO law, procedures, and relationships among government agencies, providers, and other parties. A good recent text on the subject is that of Blum, Gertman, and Rabinow (1977).

33. Study findings reported in the previous two paragraphs were abstracted from State of Michigan (1973) and O'Donoghue (1974).

34. Havighurst and Blumstein (1975) and Enthoven (1978a, 1978b), among others, feel that the altered physician incentives embodied in HMO-type medical care organizations offer the best potential for injecting cost consciousness into utilization and quality control decisions.

6 Descriptive Evidence

This chapter presents an overview of the variables we have constructed for our analysis of hospital costs and input employment. In the early stages of our research, we devoted considerable time to collecting data from numerous published and unpublished sources. Most researchers would readily agree that data reconnaisance is an extremely tedious process but one absolutely crucial to the thoroughness and ultimate policy value of the research effort. Our user file pertaining to the cohort of 1,228 short-term, general hospitals from 1970 to 1975 is one of the most comprehensive data bases ever constructed for analysis of hospitals. Tables interspersed throughout this chapter present variable means and rates of change of dependent and independent variables. The discussion of individual tables is preceded by a brief summary of national trends and characteristics of the hospital industry.

Annual expenditures in the hospital industry are currently well above the $50 billion mark.[1] At this level of expenditure, relatively minute changes in factors affecting the hospital market may have major consequences on the number of dollars spent for hospital care. Because of the degree of government involvement in financing these expenditures, such changes have potentially large effects on government budgets and on the availability of tax dollars for alternative uses. Annual increases in hospital expenditures were double-digit from 1967 through the mid-1970s, and the percentage of gross national product devoted to hospital care has been consistently increasing for the past decade and longer.

Trends in physical hospital outputs during the 1970s seem trivial in comparison to those on expenditures. For example, the 1974–1975 growth in hospital expenditures was 17.6 percent, while the corresponding percentage increases in inpatient admissions and outpatient visits were only 1.8 percent and 1.7 percent, respectively. The number of beds in community hospitals increased 1.7 percent while decreases in long-term-care beds caused beds in all hospitals to decline 3.1 percent.[2]

Increases in hospital inputs fall in between outputs and expenditures in order of magnitude. Hospitals are a major employer, having surpassed 3 million full-time-equivalent (FTE) employees in 1975. The increase in FTE community hospital employees in 1974–1975 was 4.8 percent. Total community hospital assets per bed increased 11.1 percent, and total assets of all U.S. hospitals increased 10.8 percent in 1974–1975.

Thus, a simple profile of hospital performance in the 1970s is one of rather modest increases in output with substantial increases in gross inputs and alarming increases in costs. This is admittedly an oversimplified profile since it ignores the problem of defining and measuring changes in the hospital product, an issue that has been discussed previously and receives further treatment in ensuing chapters.

Hospital Costs

Trends in hospital costs per adjusted patient-day and per admission are presented in tables 6–1 and 6–2. Time series of undeflated and deflated total and labor costs are contained in table 6–1.[3] In general, costs per admission increased less than costs per adjusted patient-day, reflecting a secular decline in average length of stay during the period. In addition, labor costs have increased more slowly than total costs, which largely reflects a rapid increase in prices of nonlabor inputs utilized by hospitals. Labor costs, including fringe benefits, were approximately 64 percent of total costs in 1970, declining to about 59 percent in 1975.[4]

The first differences in both undeflated and deflated cost measures were U-shaped during the 1970–1975 period. For our cohort, only in 1974 was the rate of inflation in hospital costs less than that of economywide prices in general. The reduction in hospital cost inflation during 1973 and 1974 has been attributed to the Economic Stabilization Program. The implied impact of ESP on costs is much more evident from these tables than from the cost regressions presented in chapter 7 and is generally consistent with other descriptive evidence on hospital costs during ESP.[5] The largest cost increases occurred in 1970–1971 and 1974–1975. The deflated series shows quite clearly that hospital cost inflation has been considerably greater, on the whole, than price inflation in general during the 1970–1975 period.

Table 6–2 presents cost per adjusted patient-day and per admission tabulations by census division. Averages (means) for the entire six-year period are shown in the table. The deflated series have been adjusted so that the means across all census divisions equal their undeflated counterparts to facilitate comparisons of deflated and undeflated means within census divisions. For example, general price levels are relatively high in New England; deflation lowers average hospital costs from well above to well below the national average. With two exceptions, the mid-Atlantic and Pacific census divisions, deflating causes census division means of these variables to be closer to the national means.

Interarea variations in average length of stay are also indicated in table 6–2. For example, average costs in mid-Atlantic hospitals move from lower to higher than the national average in changing from adjusted patient-day to admission denominators because stays tend to be relatively long in this

Table 6-1
Cost per Adjusted Patient-Day and per Admission, 1970–1975

Cost	1970	1971	1972	1973	1974	1975	Percentage Change 1970–1975
Cost per Adjusted Patient-Day ($)							
Total cost, undeflated	79.40	91.40	102.60	111.40	122.70	144.40	—
Growth rate	—	15.1	12.2	8.6	10.2	17.6	81.9
Total cost, deflated[a]	85.56	94.42	102.60	104.90	104.07	112.20	—
Growth rate	—	10.4	8.7	2.2	-0.8	7.8	31.3
Labor cost, undeflated	50.69	57.30	63.86	68.27	73.51	84.56	—
Growth rate	—	13.0	11.5	6.9	8.1	15.0	66.8
Labor cost, deflated[a]	54.62	59.19	63.86	64.28	62.35	65.70	—
Growth rate	—	8.4	7.9	0.7	-3.0	5.4	20.3
Cost per Admission ($)							
Total cost, undeflated	736.90	823.64	919.57	1,001.49	1,110.95	1,296.40	—
Growth rate	—	11.8	11.7	8.9	10.9	16.7	75.9
Total cost, deflated[a]	794.07	850.87	919.57	943.02	942.28	1,007.30	—
Growth rate	—	7.2	8.1	2.6	-0.1	6.9	26.9
Labor cost, undeflated	468.93	521.50	578.23	616.28	671.86	767.80	—
Growth rate	—	11.2	10.9	6.6	9.0	14.3	64.7
Labor cost, deflated[a]	505.31	538.74	578.23	580.30	569.86	596.58	—
Growth rate	—	6.6	7.3	0.4	-1.8	4.7	18.1

[a]Divided by an area price index (1972 mean for metropolitan areas = 1.00). See Appendix B.

Table 6-2
Cost per Adjusted Patient-Day and per Admission by Census Division, 1970–1975

Cost	New England	Mid-Atlantic	East North Central	West North Central	South Atlantic	East South Central	West South Central	Mountain	Pacific	All
Cost per Adjusted Patient-Day[a] ($)										
Total cost, undeflated	117.1	101.2	103.2	101.9	83.8	93.3	92.8	103.8	136.6	107.7
Total cost, deflated[b]	101.4	97.1	110.1	102.0	94.0	94.7	104.7	111.1	137.1	107.7
Labor cost, undeflated	75.1	67.1	62.4	65.1	49.6	59.1	51.3	61.4	79.7	66.8
Labor cost, deflated[b]	65.3	64.4	66.7	65.5	55.8	60.2	58.1	66.0	80.2	66.8
Cost per Admission[a] ($)										
Total cost, undeflated	1,105	1,086	915	964	714	905	675	816	1,027	972
Total cost, deflated[b]	962	1,046	976	971	806	928	765	877	1,034	972
Labor cost, undeflated	711	725	558	619	426	575	377	484	604	611
Labor cost, deflated[b]	621	698	597	625	483	591	430	522	610	611

[a]Cost figures are averages for 1970–1975.

[b]Divided by an area price index (1972 mean for metropolitan areas = 1.00) and adjusted so that deflated and undeflated means for all the United States are equal. See Appendix B.

region. By contrast, relatively short stays on the West Coast bring average costs per admission much closer to the national mean than per diem costs, and labor costs per admission are actually lower in the West than the national average in sample hospitals.

Deflating clearly reduces interarea and interhospital variation in average hospital costs, but considerable variation remains. On an area-by-area basis, the difference between the lowest and highest average cost per adjusted patient-day (South Atlantic versus Pacific) is 46 percent and between the lowest and highest average cost per admission (West South Central versus mid-Atlantic) is 37 percent. Some caution is warranted in comparing these statistics across census divisions—our data base is representative nationally in ways indicated in chapter 3, but it is not designed to be truly representative regionally. This, of course, applies to the input and explanatory variables as well.

Hospital Input Use

Hospital labor and nonlabor input trends are presented in tables 6–3 and 6–4. All inputs increased during 1970–1975, but, unlike the cost averages, there appears to be little pattern in these changes over time. Only the growth rate of current nonlabor expenses exhibits the same U-shaped pattern as the cost growth data. Despite the level of inflation during the period, RN employment increased at a much faster rate than that of LPNs, indicating some substitution toward higher quality or more expensive inputs. Unfortunately, AHA data do not permit more comparisons of this sort.

By far the fastest growing input was current nonlabor expense. Like assets, this input is necessarily measured in (deflated) dollar terms rather than in physical units, and, as suggested earlier (chapters 1 and 3), our price index may understate the rate of growth in hospital-specific nonlabor input prices, especially during 1974–1975. Our current nonlabor expense measure excludes expenses linked to capital formation, such as interest and depreciation, but includes items that hospital spokespersons claim are the source of much of the inflation in hospital prices, such as food, fuel, insurance, and so on.

Table 6–4, which presents the input variables by census division in 1975, displays important interarea variations in input combinations. For example, New England, which has the highest number of FTE employees per bed, is lowest of the nine census divisions in deflated plant assets per bed. The South Atlantic and West South Central census divisions are lowest in RNs per bed, but the former is highest in LPNs per bed. Mountain census division hospitals are relatively low on FTE employees, but have the highest deflated plant assets per bed. The Pacific census division is relatively low in

Table 6-3
Trends in Labor and Nonlabor Input Variables, 1970–1975

	1970	1971	1972	1973	1974	1975	Percentage Change 1970–1975
RNs							
Per hospital	116	123	125	131	140	146	—
Per bed	0.44	0.46	0.45	0.47	0.48	0.50	—
Growth rate (%)[a]	—	2.7	−0.4	3.1	2.3	3.7	12.6
LPNs							
Per hospital	49	52	51	52	54	55	—
Per bed	0.20	0.20	0.20	0.20	0.20	0.21	—
Growth rate (%)[a]	—	3.6	−2.5	−1.0	2.0	0.5	2.5
Other Employees							
Per hospital	463	478	484	504	531	538	—
Per bed	1.64	1.65	1.65	1.70	1.75	1.77	—
Growth rate (%)[a]	—	0.8	0.0	2.7	2.7	1.7	8.1
Net Plant Assets, Deflated ($)[b]							
Per bed	30,711	31,509	31,397	31,939	32,437	32,433	—
Growth rate (%)[a]	—	2.6	−0.4	1.7	1.6	−0.0	5.6
Current Nonlabor Expense, Deflated ($)[b]							
Per bed	6,821	7,460	7,914	8,240	8,548	9,658	—
Growth rate (%)[a]	—	9.4	6.1	4.1	3.8	13.0	41.6
Beds							
Per hospital	250	254	258	261	265	268	—
Growth rate (%)	—	1.9	1.3	1.3	1.5	0.9	7.2

[a]Input growth rates are on a per bed basis and were calculated from more precise (that is, more significant decimal places) input estimates than those shown in the table.

[b]Divided by an area price index (1972 mean for metropolitan areas = 1.00). See Appendix B.

Table 6-4
Labor and Nonlabor Inputs by Census Division, 1975

Input	New England	Mid-Atlantic	East North Central	West North Central	South Atlantic	East South Central	West South Central	Mountain	Pacific	All
RNs per bed	0.66	0.55	0.49	0.47	0.35	0.45	0.35	0.57	0.51	0.50
LPNs per bed	0.21	0.20	0.19	0.18	0.32	0.18	0.27	0.15	0.19	0.21
Other employees per bed	1.93	1.80	1.90	1.86	1.72	1.60	1.62	1.72	1.66	1.77
Plant assets per bed, deflated ($)[a]	29,104	31,912	35,272	34,332	34,429	32,971	30,597	37,335	30,844	32,433
Current nonlabor expenses per bed, deflated ($)[a]	9,067	8,931	10,965	9,063	8,899	8,538	9,865	9,873	11,001	9,658
Beds	224	320	305	304	256	287	225	262	190	268

[a]Divided by an area price index (1972 mean for metropolitan areas = 1.00). See Appendix B.

employees, assets, and beds, but has the highest current deflated nonlabor expenses per bed. These figures, in part, reflect geographic differences in styles of care and clearly indicate the presence of several types of input substitution possibilities in hospitals.

Explanatory Variables

Table 6–5 presents annual means of the explanatory variables and percentage changes from 1970 to 1975. Variable construction is described in chapters 3 through 5 and in the appendixes. As noted above, all monetary variables are deflated by an index to correct for intertemporal and geographic variations in price levels. The table excludes variables that, as defined, have no intertemporal variation, including hospital characteristics and size classes. Information on such factors and on our method of classifying variables is presented in chapter 3.

Seven product demand variables have been defined, three of which pertain to extent of coverage under different health insurance programs. Real per capita income increased during the period, but all the increase occurred during 1970–1973. Surprisingly, mean population density declined, most likely because of suburban emigration. Declines in population per physician and in the general-practitioner proportion reflect the trends toward rapidly expanding medical school capacity and increased medical specialization. The increase in population per "other" hospital bed is a reflection of a slowdown in bed expansion relative to population during the period.

Increases were registered in each of the three reimbursement demand variables. The modest growth in the Medicare proportion is a reflection of population aging, while the relatively large growth in the young Medicaid proportion is probably due in large part to rising unemployment over the half decade. Probably the most important increase in health insurance coverage over 1970–1975 was in the area of major medical protection—the number of persons with major medical coverage rose by 30.1 percent during these years (Carroll 1978). Also, according to Health Insurance Institute (1977, 1978), the proportion of expenses covered by commercial health insurance increased for most types of claims from 1967 to 1977.

Real factor prices all increased during 1970–1975, but the nonlabor increases were much greater than the labor increases.[6] Mean real wages paid to RNs, LPNs, and other hospital employees actually declined during 1973–1975. By contrast, the price of capital and cost-of-living measures increased the most during these years. Because our cost-of-living measure is the same variable used to deflate all monetary dependent and independent variables, including wages, an inverse relationship between first differences in cost-of-living and some of the deflated variables is expected.

The time series of the unionization varibles is largely dependent on the limited data that were available to construct these variables and the method of defining them (see Appendix K); therefore, these data should be interpreted with caution. Nevertheless, the series does indicate a substantial increase in unionization activity during 1970–1975.[7] This is especially true of requests for recognition as a collective-bargaining agent, which presumably tend to precede formal collective-bargaining agreements and job actions. Based on these data and on the 1974 modifications of the Taft-Hartley Act, one may infer that union activity will have become an increasingly prevalent force in hospitals throughout the 1970s and into the 1980s.[8]

The regulation/reimbursement measures consist of five variables pertaining to certificate-of-need (CON) programs and seven variables whose common denominator is that each pertains to a program which uses hospital reimbursement as a regulatory tool. With regard to certificate of need, the method of variable definition makes the time series appear somewhat curious because programs shift from young to mature. However, these data do indicate a fairly steady growth in such programs over 1970–1975. (The growth pattern is evident in the variable PRECON which indicates the year immediately prior to program inception.) The peak year for establishment of new CON programs, in terms of proportion of sample hospitals affected, was 1972, followed by 1973. As defined, the preponderance of CON programs are noncomprehensive—they focus primarily on limiting growth in hospital beds (see Appendix I). In 1975, roughly 60 percent of sample hospitals were under the jurisdiction of noncomprehensive CON programs, while about 11 percent were subject to comprehensive programs. According to legislative mandate, all states were to have instituted CON programs by 1980.

With regard to the reimbursement variables, yearly values reflect a combination of program presence *and* estimates of proportions of area population affected by such programs.[9] Thus, time series of these variables are measures of program additions and expansion of populations covered, which is why some yearly changes shown in table 6–5 are abrupt and others are gradual. In addition, the time series are also affected to varying degrees by limitations on data availability. This is especially true of the Blue Cross planning agency approval and utilization review variables.

On the whole, the regulation and reimbursement trends shown in table 6–5 indicate a steady growth in regulatory programs affecting hospitals during 1970–1975, and it is likely that this trend will continue. Hospitals least affected by regulation are those located in areas without certificate of need or prospective reimbursement, where private commercial insurance covers a relatively large fraction of patients and where Blue Cross and Medicaid

Table 6–5
Trends in Explanatory Variables, 1970–1975

Variable	1970	1971	1972	1973	1974	1975	Percentage Change 1970–1975
Demand Variables							
County per capita income (PERCAP)[a]	3,861	3,991	4,110	4,268	4,253	4,266	10.5
County population per square mile (DENS)	4,736	4,657	4,608	4,560	4,512	4,491	−5.2
County population per nonfederal office-based physician (POPMD)	1,034	1,000	980	985	982	960	−7.2
County general-practitioner proportion (GPPROP)	0.263	0.249	0.240	0.229	0.221	0.210	−20.2
County population per "other" hospital bed (POPBD)	2,133	2,164	2,234	2,577	2,582	2,609	22.3
County population proportion age 65 and over (MCARE)	0.097	0.098	0.098	0.101	0.102	0.102	5.2
State population proportion under 65 and eligible for Medicaid (MCAID)	0.074	0.077	0.081	0.082	0.092	0.096	29.7
County depth of coverage under private health insurance (INS)[a]	205	217	238	250	248	256	24.3
Factor Price Variables							
Hourly wage for RNs (RNWG)[a]	4.32	4.47	4.62	4.68	4.54	4.48	3.7
Hourly wage for LPNs (LPNWG)[a]	3.17	3.31	3.45	3.53	3.45	3.41	7.6
Hourly wage for "other" hospital employees (OTHWG)[a]	3.17	3.33	3.40	3.31	3.18	3.21	1.3
Price of capital index (CAP)[a]	95.9	94.9	100.0	111.3	140.6	162.3	69.2
Cost-of-living index (CPI)	0.943	0.982	1.015	1.079	1.194	1.292	37.0
Unionization Variables							
Hospital has received collective-bargaining request (COLREQ)	0.134	0.160	0.187	0.213	0.309	0.405	b
Hospital has signed collective-bargaining agreement (UNION)	0.204	0.221	0.237	0.253	0.272	0.292	b

							b
Hospital has had strike or other work stoppage (STRIKE)	0.036	0.036	0.051	0.059	0.059	0.059	
Regulation/Reimbursement Variables							
Proportion of hospitals in states with:							
Year prior to certificate-of-need program taking effect (PRECON)	0.048	0.160	0.110	0.017	0.078	0.071	47.9
Noncomprehensive, young certificate-of-need programs (NCON1)	0.181	0.225	0.125	0.191	0.112	0.080	−55.8
Noncomprehensive, mature certificate-of-need programs (NCON2)	0.104	0.104	0.285	0.326	0.047	0.517	397.1
Comprehensive, young certificate-of-need programs (CCON1)	0.013	0.017	0.082	0.078	0.015	0.015	15.4
Comprehensive, mature certificate-of-need programs (CCON2)	0.000	0.000	0.013	0.017	0.096	0.096	—
Proportion of population in areas where hospitals are subject to:							
Section 1122 regulation of capital expansion (S1122)	0.000	0.000	0.000	0.041	0.102	0.105	—
Blue Cross requirements for planning agency approval of capital expansion (BCPAA)	0.149	0.149	0.150	0.219	0.224	0.226	51.7
Formula prospective reimbursement program (FPR)	0.088	0.089	0.090	0.092	0.096	0.109	23.9
Budget prospective reimbursement program (BPR)	0.029	0.030	0.048	0.061	0.086	0.087	200.0
Utilization review (UR)	0.351	0.357	0.359	0.364	0.380	0.384	9.4
Cost-based reimbursement (COSTB)	0.479	0.485	0.489	0.502	0.521	0.529	10.4
Proportion of months the Economic Stabilization Program in effect (ESP)	0.000	0.250	1.000	1.000	0.250	0.000	—

[a] Deflated by an area price index (1972 mean for metropolitan areas = 1.00). See Appendix B.

[b] Percentage changes are not meaningful for unionization variables.

programs tend to be relatively "loose" with respect to requirements of participating hospitals. Clearly, very few hospitals, if any, are not affected by several of the regulatory programs examined in this book, and many hospitals will have been affected by most of them. Our empirical estimates in chapters 7 and 8 should shed some light on the consequences of this movement.

Notes

1. Data for this section were taken from American Hospital Association (1976).

2. Community hospitals are defined by the AHA as "short-term general and other special hospitals," which excludes federal, tuberculosis, psychiatric, and all hospitals where the average stay is more than thirty days. This definition differs slightly from our cohort in that we have excluded the "other special" hospitals, which provide ophthalmic, obstetric, orthopedic, and other specialized services.

3. See Appendix B for a description of the deflating process, which converts all monetary variables to 1972 dollars, adjusting for interarea differences in price levels.

4. In published American Hospital Association reports, fringe benefits are included as a nonlabor expense. Throughout our analysis they have been recomputed as a labor expense.

5. See, for example, Altman and Eichenholz (1976) and U.S. Council on Wage and Price Stability (1977).

6. Our wage variables do not include the monetary value of fringe benefits. Because fringe benefits increased markedly during the 1970s, wage variables incorporating the monetary value of fringe benefits would probably have displayed greater increases than the wage variables in table 6–5.

7. All unionization variables are cumulative; that is, the value in year t is the value in $t - 1$ plus any measured activity taking place in the period between $t - 1$ and t.

8. Considerably more information on union activity and its effects on hospitals is contained in our companion book, Sloan and Steinwald (1980).

9. In the case of the Economic Stabilization Program, the population proportion can be set at 100 percent during all months that ESP was in effect.

7

Analysis of
Hospital Costs

This chapter presents and evaluates empirical results of our multivariate analysis of cost measures—total and labor expenses per admission and per adjusted patient-day. Although the discussion emphasizes total expense measures, the analysis of labor expense also merits attention, particularly for what it reveals about the effect of alternative regulation and reimbursement methods on the labor/nonlabor mix of expenses in hospitals. As indicated in chapter 6, labor, inclusive of wages and fringe benefits, constituted approximately 60 percent of total hospital expenses during the first half of the 1970s.

Measures of expense per adjusted patient-day recognize contributions to hospital expenses from provision of outpatient services.[1] This is not true of expense per admission, which is simply total hospital expenses divided by total admissions. The primary advantage of an admission-based measure is that it reflects cost savings realized by early discharge of inpatients whereas expenses per patient-day may be relatively high because procedures are spread over fewer days. Because expense per adjusted patient-day rose even faster than expense per admission during 1970–1975, one can infer that hospitals on the whole have devoted extra resources to getting patients out of hospitals sooner.[2] Thus, both admission- and day-based cost measures have advantages and disadvantages, and it is clearly sensible to evaluate determinants of hospital costs with each of these measures.

The theoretical analysis in chapter 2 considered hospital behavior in unregulated and regulated environments separately. Predicted effects of selected exogenous variables sometimes differ depending on which of the two environments applies. However, in the empirical work it is not practical to maintain the regulated-unregulated distinction by, say, stratifying hospitals according to regulatory intensity of the states where they are located. Similarly, the theoretical discussion of inputs in chapter 2 is limited to two general aggregate input categories, which is an analytical convenience but is unduly restrictive for empirical analysis. Thus, in several respects, there is only limited correspondence between the chapter 2 models and the regressions presented in this and the following chapter. In both chapters we (conservatively) use two-tailed tests of statistical significance because of ambiguities in predicted effects of several exogenous variables.

Regression results are presented in table 7–1. The majority of coefficients are statistically significant at conventional levels. A higher percentage of ordinary-least-squares (OLS) coefficients are statistically significant, but this is not surprising, given the large number of transformations involved in the time-series cross-sectional (TSCS) methodology. Although theoretical ambiguities limit the formulation of specific hypotheses, the signs of the coefficients are mostly plausible in the sense that they agree with past research results and/or are readily interpreted. The R^2s, ranging from 0.31 to 0.61, are high for cross-sectional analysis with several thousand degrees of freedom. The coefficients on the lagged dependent variables (LDEP) are 0.39 and 0.42 in the total expense regressions and 0.14 and 0.35 in the labor expense regressions. From the Koyck lag structure, these coefficients imply that over 60 percent of the difference in the logarithms of actual average expense and desired or equilibrium average expense is made up within a year. In other words, the effect of changes in the exogenous variables is realized rather quickly.[3]

The dependent variables, lagged dependent variables, demand variables, factor price (OTHWG), and asset index (ASSETB) are in logarithmic form. Thus, the associated parameter estimates are elasticities. The remaining explanatory variables, which are either binary or proportions, enter linearly. Our discussion of parameter estimates is divided into explanatory variable categories: product demand, wage rate and union, hospital characteristics, and regulation/reimbursement variables. A brief concluding section ends the chapter.

Product Demand Variables

As seen in chapter 2, using a simple model of the unregulated hospital with composite output and profits as arguments in the utility function, one can show that outward shifts in the hospital's product demand curve raise hospital costs. Regressions presented in this and the next chapter contain a number of demand shift variables which are defined in chapter 3.

Our measure of per capita income of patients in the hospital's market area (PERCAP) has no clear effect on hospital costs. This variable was eliminated from our TSCS regressions for reasons of multicollinearity; the PERCAP variable is closely related to our wage measure (OTHWG), and it does not appear possible to distinguish separate effects of the two variables. As noted in chapter 6, personal per capita income has been rising very slowly in real terms during the 1970s. In fact, between 1970 and 1975, median real family income rose only 0.3 percent.[4]

Population per square mile in the county in which the hospital is located is represented by DENS. Although the effects of density on demand for hospital care are ambiguous because of offsetting influences reviewed in chapter 3, density has been included in past hospital demand and cost studies (for example, Bentkover and Sanders 1977; Davis 1974; Feldstein 1971b,

1977; Salkever 1972). The parameter estimates on DENS in table 7–1 are uniformly positive and statistically significant, implying that costs are higher in densely populated areas. Since monetarily expressed variables have been deflated by an area price index, it is doubtful that the positive coefficients reflect differences in cost of living, which do indeed vary directly with density. Rather, the positive signs most likely reflect a combination of case-mix factors and density-dependent differences in the style of hospital care. The fact that the estimated elasticities are higher in total expense per admission regressions than in their adjusted patient-day counterparts lends support to the view that DENS accounts for the relatively complex case mix in hospitals located in populous communities.

In recent years, the physician-population ratio has increased dramatically, as has the number of specialists as a proportion of all U.S. physicians. Over the 1970–1975 period alone, the ratio of nonfederal patient-care physicians to the civilian U.S. population rose 8 percent (American Medical Association 1976, p. 153). During the same period, general practitioners as a proportion of all U.S. physicians declined from 17.3 percent to 13.9 percent (U.S. Bureau of the Census 1977). Projections for further growth place the number of active physicians per 100,000 population between 190 and 200 by the year 1980 and between 220 and 225 by 1990 (U.S. Department of Health, Education, and Welfare 1974; Reinhardt 1975). The comparable ratio in 1970 was 155.

Considering that the demand for hospital care may be linked to both physician availability and the generalist-specialist proportion, these trends have definite policy implications. We argued in chapter 3 that the expected effect of physician availability on demand for hospital services is uncertain; yet, because specialists' services tend to be hospital-intensive, the generalist proportion should exert a negative influence on hospital demand.[5]

Our physician variables, POPMD (population per nonfederal office-based patient-care physician, by county) and GPPROP (proportion of these physicians in general practice, by county), measure the impact of physician availability on costs through the influence of availability on demand for hospital services. With the exception of the total expense TSCS regressions, in which POPMD shows essentially no effect, our results support the view that doctor availability and specialization positively affect hospital costs. Given current trends described above, one may expect further inflation from this source. In general, these results are consistent with past research on this subject (Salkever 1972; Davis 1974). On the whole, we find the impact of GPPROP on hospital costs to be the stronger of the two influences, gauged in terms of both statistical significance and elasticities.

Although there has been very little "hard" research on the topic, most competition in the hospital sector is widely believed to be of a nonprice nature.[6] Hospitals allegedly compete for patients and their doctors by

Table 7-1
Average Cost Regressions

Variable[a]	Total Expense per Adjusted Patient-Day		Total Expense per Admission		Labor Expense per Adjusted Patient-Day		Labor Expense per Admission	
	TSCS (1)	OLS (2)	TSCS (3)	OLS (4)	TSCS (5)	OLS (6)	TSCS (7)	OLS (8)
PERCAP	—	0.18* (0.023)[b]	—	-0.012 (0.27)	—	0.12* (0.024)	—	-0.074* (0.029)
DENS	0.0072*** (0.0042)	0.020* (0.0022)	0.010* (0.0040)	0.048* (0.0026)	0.018* (0.0044)	0.027* (0.0023)	0.013* (0.0041)	0.055* (0.0028)
POPMD	0.0048 (0.0087)	-0.030* (0.0030)	0.0070 (0.0082)	-0.052* (0.012)	-0.013 (0.0095)	-0.048* (0.011)	-0.0053 (0.0086)	-0.070* (0.013)
GPPROP	-0.097* (0.015)	-0.065* (0.0090)	-0.097* (0.014)	-0.058* (0.011)	-0.10* (0.016)	-0.043* (0.0095)	-0.079* (0.014)	-0.035* (0.011)
POPBD	0.0076** (0.0032)	-0.00042 (0.0028)	0.0022 (0.0030)	-0.015* (0.0033)	0.0072* (0.0035)	0.0016 (0.0029)	0.00042 (0.0031)	-0.013* (0.0035)
MCARE	0.053** (0.025)	0.0046 (0.014)	0.087* (0.023)	0.14* (0.016)	0.023 (0.026)	-0.0048 (0.014)	0.068* (0.025)	0.13* (0.017)
MCAID	0.035* (0.0060)	0.052* (0.0053)	0.014 (0.0056)	0.059* (0.0064)	0.034* (0.0064)	0.040* (0.0057)	0.0062 (0.0060)	0.048* (0.0068)
INS	0.20* (0.021)	0.017 (0.020)	0.17* (0.020)	0.12* (0.024)	0.15* (0.022)	-0.056** (0.0057)	0.10* (0.021)	0.045** (0.025)
ASSETB	0.0051 (0.0034)	0.050* (0.0039)	-0.0011 (0.0032)	0.028* (0.0047)	0.0066*** (0.0036)	0.030* (0.0041)	-0.0014 (0.0034)	0.0077 (0.0049)
OTHWG	0.064* (0.016)	0.63* (0.046)	0.056* (0.015)	0.56* (0.055)	0.074* (0.017)	0.51* (0.048)	0.060* (0.015)	0.43* (0.058)
COLREQ	0.025* (0.0057)	0.030* (0.0066)	0.030* (0.0054)	0.027* (0.0079)	0.023* (0.0062)	0.022* (0.0069)	0.028* (0.0057)	0.019* (0.0083)
UNION	0.033* (0.0090)	0.047* (0.0067)	0.021* (0.0085)	0.044* (0.0081)	0.047* (0.0097)	0.086* (0.0071)	0.026* (0.0090)	0.083* (0.0085)
STRIKE	0.039** (0.018)	0.042* (0.012)	0.027 (0.017)	0.045* (0.014)	0.068* (0.019)	0.066* (0.013)	0.026 (0.017)	0.069* (0.015)

	(1)	(2)	(3)	(4)	(5)	(6)	(7)	(8)
PRECON	0.0099** (0.0050)	0.031* (0.0094)	0.0043 (0.0047)	0.014 (0.011)	0.017* (0.0054)	0.033* (0.0099)	0.0026 (0.0049)	0.015 (0.012)
NCON1	0.024* (0.0054)	0.075* (0.0081)	0.0087*** (0.0051)	0.047* (0.0097)	0.024* (0.0059)	0.072* (0.0086)	0.00042 (0.0054)	0.044* (0.010)
NCON2	0.047* (0.0069)	0.19* (0.0086)	0.035* (0.0064)	0.14* (0.010)	0.054* (0.0073)	0.16* (0.0091)	0.022* (0.0068)	0.11* (0.011)
CCON1	-0.00054 (0.0085)	0.075* (0.014)	0.015*** (0.0080)	-0.0018 (0.017)	-0.0061 (0.0092)	0.063* (0.015)	0.0097 (0.0085)	-0.014 (0.018)
CCON2	-0.0082 (0.0098)	0.15* (0.015)	0.0060 (0.0092)	0.033*** (0.018)	-0.015 (0.011)	0.13* (0.016)	0.00042 (0.0098)	0.0097 (0.019)
S1122	0.0018 (0.020)	0.21* (0.037)	-0.014 (0.019)	0.16* (0.044)	0.050** (0.022)	0.098** (0.039)	-0.018 (0.020)	0.050 (0.046)
BCPAA	-0.0066 (0.073)	-0.019 (0.014)	-0.014** (0.0069)	0.027*** (0.016)	-0.0038 (0.0079)	0.0081 (0.014)	-0.015** (0.0072)	0.054* (0.017)
FPR	0.017 (0.031)	-0.26* (0.017)	0.076* (0.029)	-0.14* (0.020)	0.055*** (0.033)	-0.17* (0.018)	0.11* (0.031)	-0.059* (0.021)
BPR	-0.030* (0.011)	-0.035* (0.016)	-0.0083 (0.010)	0.069* (0.019)	-0.015 (0.012)	-0.022 (0.017)	0.0056 (0.011)	0.082* (0.020)
UR	0.017 (0.052)	-0.17* (0.018)	-0.063 (0.049)	-0.076* (0.022)	0.017 (0.052)	-0.17* (0.019)	-0.084 (0.053)	0.013 (0.023)
COSTB	-0.13* (0.050)	-0.11* (0.017)	-0.0037 (0.048)	0.029 (0.021)	-0.0087 (0.051)	0.059* (0.018)	0.049 (0.052)	0.075* (0.022)
ESP	-0.0055*** (0.0032)	0.0085 (0.0066)	-0.0067** (0.0030)	0.00081 (0.0080)	0.031* (0.0035)	0.032* (0.0070)	0.011* (0.0032)	0.024* (0.0084)
GOVT	0.036 (0.033)	0.069* (0.0076)	0.039 (0.032)	0.10* (0.0092)	0.080* (0.032)	0.092* (0.0081)	0.056 (0.035)	0.13* (0.0097)
PROP	0.053 (0.043)	0.10* (0.011)	-0.041 (0.040)	-0.0069 (0.013)	-0.25* (0.042)	-0.044* (0.011)	-0.16* (0.045)	-0.15* (0.013)
MEDSCH	0.13* (0.028)	0.15* (0.0074)	0.14* (0.027)	0.19* (0.0089)	0.26* (0.027)	0.16* (0.0078)	0.21* (0.029)	0.20* (0.0094)
NURSCH	-0.022 (0.031)	0.0025 (0.0072)	0.016 (0.030)	0.014 (0.0086)	0.067** (0.030)	0.027 (0.0076)	0.054*** (0.032)	0.039* (0.0091)
SIZE1	0.047* (0.015)	-0.0021 (0.011)	-0.046* (0.014)	-0.18* (0.013)	0.089* (0.016)	-0.071* (0.011)	-0.010 (0.015)	-0.25* (0.014)
SIZE2	0.013 (0.012)	-0.033* (0.0088)	-0.034* (0.011)	-0.14* (0.011)	0.028** (0.012)	-0.064* (0.0093)	-0.020*** (0.012)	-0.17* (0.011)

Table 7–1 *(continued)*

Variable[a]	Total Expense per Adjusted Patient-Day		Total Expense per Admission		Labor Expense per Adjusted Patient-Day		Labor Expense per Admission	
	TSCS (1)	OLS (2)	TSCS (3)	OLS (4)	TSCS (5)	OLS (6)	TSCS (7)	OLS (8)
SIZE3	0.014	−0.042*	−0.013	−0.12*	0.027*	−0.053*	0.00033	−0.12*
	(0.0088)	(0.0079)	(0.0083)	(0.0094)	(0.0095)	(0.0083)	(0.0088)	(0.010)
LDEP	0.39*	—	0.42*	—	0.14*	—	0.35*	—
	(0.011)		(0.011)		(0.010)		(0.011)	
CONST	0.62	1.79	1.19	5.72	0.72	2.57	1.45	6.50
	$R^2 = 0.50$	$R^2 = 0.54$	$R^2 = 0.51$	$R^2 = 0.56$	$R^2 = 0.31$	$R^2 = 0.52$	$R^2 = 0.38$	$R^2 = 0.61$
	$F(32, 6110)$	$F(32, 6,110)$	$F(32, 6,110)$	$F(32, 6,110)$	$F(32, 6,098)$	$F(32, 6,110)$	$F(32, 5,917)$	$F(32, 6,110)$
	$= 188.4*$	$= 219.1*$	$= 200.2*$	$= 240.7*$	$= 86.1*$	$= 203.9*$	$= 110.1*$	$= 293.1*$

*Significant at the 1% level (two-tailed test).
**Significant at the 5% level (two-tailed test).
***Significant at the 10% level (two-tailed test).
[a]Variables are defined in Appendix A.
[b]Figures in parentheses are standard errors.

offering sophisticated equipment, amenities, and the like. For this reason, it is plausible to expect that hospitals in a monopoly position in their communities might have lower costs. Our measure POPBD (population divided by the number of beds in *other* hospitals in the county) gauges the impact of competition from other hospitals.[7] Contrary to our expectations, parameter estimates on POPBD are positive and over twice their standard errors in the TSCS regressions for total and labor expense per adjusted patient-day. However, the signs are not consistently positive in remaining regressions, and levels of statistical significance are low. The estimated POPBD coefficients do not support the notion that hospital costs are higher in densely bedded communities.

The remaining demand variables pertain to the extent of third-party reimbursement in the hospital's market area. With one exception, the private health insurance (INS) coefficients are positive and much larger than their respective standard errors. For the TSCS coefficients, the implied short-run elasticities are as high as 0.2. The long-run elasticity is as high as 0.3 [from the regression in column 1 of table 7–1: $0.20/(1 - 0.39)$, where 0.39 is the coefficient of the lagged dependent variable]. In comparing the total expense TSCS regressions with their labor expense counterparts, INS has a greater impact on total than on labor expense, suggesting that private insurance has a more pronounced effect on nonlabor expenses. Furthermore, INS shows a greater effect on expense per adjusted patient-day than on expense per admission, implying that private insurance influences service intensity more than the number of days of care.

The OLS coefficients on INS are smaller (less positive) than their TSCS counterparts. We are unable to explain the difference. But, when viewed as a whole, the regressions clearly suggest that increased depth of health insurance coverage has boosted both labor and nonlabor costs.[8]

Public-subsidy third-party reimbursement variables in our regressions are MCARE, the county proportion of population age sixty-five and over, and MCAID, the proportion of state population under sixty-five and eligible for Medicaid. As seen in chapter 6, the growth rates of these variables from 1970 to 1975 were 5.2 percent for MCARE and 29.7 percent for MCAID (the former is a demographic trend, and the latter is a reflection of rising unemployment). With one exception, the MCARE and MCAID coefficients are positive in table 7–1, and the vast majority of coefficients are statistically significant at the 1 percent level. The highest elasticities correspond to MCARE in the TSCS regressions for total expense and labor expense per admission (0.15 and 0.10, respectively, for the long run).

Although the MCARE results are not surprising, the positive MCAID coefficients are somewhat unexpected because of Medicaid's reputation for being a less than generous reimbursement program. Yet the results from table 7–1 are largely confirmed by our analysis of inputs, discussed in chapter 8.

The positive MCAID coefficients probably reflect, in part, the relative complexity of Medicaid cases.[9] There is insufficient information from other sources to allow us to attribute the observed relationships between MCAID and the cost dependent variables to Medicaid reimbursement practices alone.

Wage Rate and Union Variables

In chapter 2 we considered potential effects of variables shifting the hospital's cost curve. In no case was it possible to conclude unambiguously that an upward shift in the cost function, reflecting, for example, an increased real wage, would raise hospital costs. The source of the ambiguity is the indirect effect from a reduction in output (which, as defined, might not be reflected in adjusted patient-days or admissions) and/or amenities. Much of the recent empirical literature on hospital costs has attempted to distinguish between the effects of developments on the product demand side and on the factor supply side (for example, Davis 1973, 1974). As we have said, demand and supply influences are somewhat difficult to distinguish because of collinearity between area per capita income and wages.

Our wage variable OTHWG is a measure of average real hourly wage for hospital personnel other than RNs, LPNs, employed physicians, and all trainees. As described in chapter 3 and Appendix E, values of OTHWG were predicted from a wage-generating equation. If we had not used an instrumental-variable approach, we might have introduced an important source of bias into our multivariate cost analysis. It would have been inappropriate to specify an average wage variable with actual payroll data because these data enter the numerators of the total expense and labor expense dependent variables.

The OTHWG parameter estimates are uniformly statistically significant, but the implied elasticities vary from 0.10, the long-run OTHWG elasticity from the first regression in table 7–1, to 0.63 in the second regression, based on OLS. We would have hoped for more stability in these parameter estimates; the instability is partly attributable to multicollinearity with PERCAP. Further, one would expect OTHWG to have a larger impact on labor than on total expenses, but the implied effects are about the same in the two types of regressions. Hence, although it is clear from table 7–1 that real growth in wages has an impact on hospital costs, the level of precision in these estimates is less than desired. In any event, as seen in chapter 6, the growth in OTHWG nationally over 1970–1975 was modest.

Unionization is represented by three binary explanatory variables: COLREQ (hospital has received a request by an organization for recognition as a collective bargaining agent), UNION (hospital has at least one signed collective bargaining agreement), and STRIKE (hospital has experienced a strike or other work stoppage in its recent past). As specified, COLREQ represents a threat effect and STRIKE represents the intensity of union activity. Besides affecting wages, unions may reduce turnover and absenteeism and improve productivity and job satisfaction, which in turn should lower hospital costs. Unions would argue that efficiency gains offset wage gains, at least in part, thus mitigating the effect of union activity on inflation in this sector.[10]

With two exceptions, the coefficients on the binary union variables are statistically significant, and the parameters are uniformly positive. As anticipated, the union coefficients tend to be somewhat higher in the labor expense regressions. In fact, the TSCS regression for labor expense per adjusted patient-day (see column 5 in table 7–1) implies that a nonunionized hospital acquiring an active union (UNION = 1 and STRIKE = 1) would experience an almost 12 percent short-run increase in real labor cost per adjusted patient-day. The long-run equilibrium response in this case is 14 percent. The corresponding effects on labor expenses per admission are 5 percent in the short run and 8 percent in the long run. The COLREQ coefficients imply that unionization threats do affect hospital costs, although not as much as collective bargaining per se. For example, the effect on cost of a request implied by the first and third total expense regressions is about 3 percent in the short run. In conjunction with the influence of real wage changes, it must be concluded that developments on the factor supply side have contributed to increases in hospital costs during the first half of the 1970s.

Hospital Characteristics Variables

Hospital characteristics variables measure factors that are virtually fixed during the period under study. These include ownership (GOVT, PROP), affiliation with teaching programs (MEDSCH, NURSCH), and bed-size class (SIZE1, SIZE2, SIZE3). An exception is ASSETB, our continuous measure of plant assets per bed, which is subject to some intertemporal variation. As described in chapter 3 and Appendix C, variable ASSETB is predicted from a generating regression with explanatory variables representing hospital facilities, service programs, and other input and output characteristics. According to our method, facilities and services requiring greater amounts of fixed capital will have a comparatively large influence on predicted assets per bed. Since hospital facilities and services are probably related to case mix, ASSETB represents both the influence of variations in the sophistication of hospital plant and interhospital differences in case-mix complexity. However, this variable proves to be uniformly insignificant in the TSCS regressions, and although it is statistically significant in three out of four OLS regressions, the associated elasticities are low.[11] Empirical analysis of variations in ASSETB as a dependent variable are presented in chapter 8.

The labor cost regressions show that, as expected, (nonfederal) government hospitals (GOVT) tend to have relatively high, and proprietary hospitals (PROP) relatively low, labor costs, *ceteris paribus*. However, both government *and* proprietary hospitals appear to have higher total expense per adjusted patient-day, once the numerous other factors in the cost equations are held constant. Overall, cost differences by ownership are more evident in the labor expense than in the total expense regressions, implying that a large part of these differences are due to variations in hospital staffing practices.

Also intuitively plausible are the parameter estimates on the medical education (MEDSCH) and nursing education (NURSCH) variables. Average costs, especially labor, are substantially higher in hospitals with medical school affiliations. This may be due to case-mix differences and/or costs associated with teaching that are reflected in patient-care expenses. The nursing school affiliation coefficients are positive and statistically significant in the labor cost regressions; but judging from the essentially zero coefficients in the total expense regressions, extra labor expense is offset to a considerable extent by lower nonlabor expense.

Hospital cost studies throughout the 1960s emphasized the economies-of-scale issue,[12] which is a less important aspect of more recent research on hospitals, including this book. The SIZE variables represent bed size of less than 100 (SIZE1), of 100 to 249 (SIZE2), of 250 to 399 (SIZE3), and of 400 and over (the omitted bed-size category). The TSCS regression for total expense per adjusted patient-day shows economies of scale; its counterpart, total expense per admission, shows the opposite. These results, taken together, imply that length of stay is longest in the 400-plus size category of hospitals. Since the first days of hospitalization tend to be comparatively expensive, a longer length of stay means, *ceteris paribus*, a lower cost per adjusted patient-day.

Regulation and Reimbursement Method Variables

As discussed earlier, the main thrust of regulatory programs in the 1970s has been to curb the rate of hospital cost inflation. Regulatory emphasis has been placed on constraining the growth of hospital capital through state certificate-of-need legislation (PRECON, CCON1, CCON2, NCON1, NCON2); Public Law 92-603, section 1122, controls on Medicare and Medicaid reimbursement for capital expenditures (S1122); and Blue Cross reimbursement requirements for planning agency approval of capital expansion projects (BCPAA). Remaining programs addressed in this book include formula- and budget-based prospective reimbursement (FPR, BPR); utilization-review programs operated by Blue Cross and Medicaid (UR); federal revenue/price controls (ESP); and cost-based reimbursement under Blue Cross, Medicare, and Medicaid (COSTB). Our comments in this section focus on empirical results presented in table 7–1, but a complete verdict is inappropriate before we have examined results from the input analysis.

Even though chapter 2 contains very cautious statements about predicted hospital responses to regulatory programs, from the standpoint of a policy-maker the intended effects are unambiguously negative. At first glance (and with later glances as well), the regression results in table 7–1 are not very encouraging about the success of current efforts at direct regulation of hospitals, at least gauged in terms of hospital costs. The majority of the parameter estimates of the regulation variable are positive, not negative as proponents of regulatory strategies would desire.[13] One possible reason for positive parameter estimates is that states and/or areas in greatest need of regulation adopt it; that is, the regulation variables pick up omitted state effects. This argument has some merit with regard to the OLS regressions, but the combination of the lagged dependent variables and our approach to pooling should have eliminated this problem in the TSCS regressions. In fact, there are a few more negative signs in the TSCS than in the OLS regressions, but sign reversals are infrequent, and the resulting negative coefficients are often insignificant. For methodological reasons, the TSCS regressions merit emphasis in our discussion of empirical results.[14]

Five of our twelve regulation/reimbursement variables pertain to state certificate-of-need regulations. Although, according to the intent of this legislation, CON should have a negative effect on costs, there are conceptual reasons enumerated in previous chapters to doubt that this is so. Referring to the parameter estimates of PRECON in the regressions for total and labor expense per patient-day, we find a slight, but statistically significant, positive anticipatory response of costs to CON.[15] The parameter estimates in table 7–1 also suggest that comprehensive programs (CCON1 and CCON2) have essentially no impact on hospital costs, while noncomprehensive programs (NCON1 and NCON2), especially the more mature ones (NCON2), tend to have positive impacts. The short-run effect of a mature noncomprehensive CON program is to raise total expense per adjusted patient-day by nearly 5 percent; the long-run equilibrium effect is over twice this. To the extent that compensatory actions are taken in response to certificate of need, it is not at all surprising that such responses are more pronounced in states with noncomprehensive programs.[16]

Although one TSCS coefficient pertaining to S1122 is positive and statistically significant at the 10 percent level, two of the remaining three coefficients are negative with relatively high standard errors. These results, taken together, imply that section 1122 reimbursement regulation of capital expansion has had no impact on hospital costs. The TSCS coefficients for BCPAA are negative in the cost per admission regressions and statistically significant but with small implied long-run effects.[17] Of the capital-facilities regulation programs, Blue Cross planning agency approval requirements appear in the most favorable light. We are at a loss to explain why they should be more effective than other programs included in our analysis.

As indicated in chapter 5, several evaluations of state efforts to control hospital costs via prospective reimbursement (PR) were conducted during the mid-1970s.[18] Probably the best inference that can be drawn from past research is that PR may have had a small moderating influence on hospital costs, but the estimates of PR impact were often statistically insignificant and the methodologies frequently raised more questions than were answered. We reemphasize that we measured only a few of several potential effects of PR. For example, tabular evidence strongly suggests that the primary effect of PR in New York State has been to reduce hospital net revenues (Berry 1976). Our methodology is not designed to capture this type of effect.

At least in principle, the stronger form of prospective reimbursement is formula PR, which, compared to budget-based systems, gives much less discretionary power to program administrators. Unfortunately, our empirical analysis of this program is dominated by New York State. New York had formula PR for all years, and Colorado and Massachusetts instituted formula systems covering only Medicaid reimbursement in 1974 and 1975, respectively. Thus, our evaluation of formula PR is essentially a tale of regulation in one state. It is possible that Nerlove's TSCS pooling methodology, which is designed to eliminate time-invariant hospital or area effects, may in instances such as this "throw out the baby with the bath water," that is, discard information on the effect of New York formula PR as well as other unspecified New York effects. For this reason, our formula PR results (FPR) should be considered tentative.

The TSCS parameter estimates associated with FPR in table 7–1 are difficult to interpret. These estimates are all positive, and, in contrast to the general statement made above about TSCS versus OLS parameters, OLS estimates are negative, statistically significant, and implausibly large in absolute value. It is best to defer any judgment until we have examined the input regression results.

The TSCS budget-based prospective reimbursement estimates (BPR), based on hospitals located in several states, are more plausible. The coefficient in the total expense per adjusted patient-day regression is negative and statistically significant at the 1 percent level, implying that if *all* a hospital's patients were to obtain coverage under insurance programs using budget-based PR, the short-run (first-year) impact would be to reduce costs per patient-day by 3 percent. The implied long-run equilibrium effect is 4.8

percent. Of course, few, if any, hospitals currently have all patients with insurance covered by budget-review PR. The BPR parameter estimate in the TSCS total expense per admission regression is essentially zero. The labor cost regression coefficients imply that budget prospective reimbursement does not reduce labor costs; by inference, all the cost-reducing effects of budget PR are on the nonlabor side.

It seems plausible that budget PR is more effective than formula PR. We have cited evidence in chapter 5 that hospitals tend to prefer budget-based systems to formula systems, at least in New Jersey, where hospitals were permitted to chose between the two. This type of evidence, while not conclusive, suggests that formula PR should be more constraining. Again we find it advisable to defer conclusions until we have examined the input regression results.

Between the last quarter of 1971 and the end of the first quarter of 1974, the Economic Stabilization Program (ESP) was in effect. The TSCS total expense regressions imply that ESP did, in fact, reduce the rate of hospital cost inflation during the years it was in effect. According to the TSCS estimates presented in table 7–1, having ESP in effect for an entire year reduced hospital cost inflation by 0.5 to 1 percent, far less than the descriptive evidence presented in chapter 6 implies. The program had the opposite and much larger (in absolute terms) impact on average labor costs. Hence, if we judge from the cost regressions, it appears that nonlabor inputs bore the brunt of ESP. This result is consistent with our finding that *real* wages of hospital employees actually reached their peak during the ESP period (Sloan and Steinwald 1980). Ginsburg (1978) reported the ESP reduced hospital wages, but his specification differs from ours. We deflate all monetarily expressed variables; he entered the consumer price index as a separate explanatory variable. Thus, the wage dependent variable in Ginsburg's regressions is in nominal rather than real terms. Further discussions of effects of ESP is deferred to the next chapter.

The final direct regulation variable represents utilization review (UR). As we noted earlier, we are able to measure the effects of only Blue Cross and Medicaid efforts at utilization review and have no evidence on the PSRO program established under the 1972 amendments to the Social Security Act. Also, it is worth reemphasizing that since utilization measures are the denominators of our cost dependent variables, some effects of utilization review may be missed. Yet, it is possible that utilization review has a negative effect on the provision of certain expensive and sometimes unnecessary services. Our UR measure should capture at least part of this type of influence.

The TSCS estimates imply that UR has no impact on total expense per adjusted patient-day, but the corresponding coefficient in the total expense per admission regression is negative and larger than its standard error. If UR reduces length of stay, it should have a greater impact when an average-cost measure with an admissions denominator is used. As noted in chapter 5, data on utilization review are available for 1974 only, and therefore the only source of interyear variation in UR is changes in the proportions of patients with types of insurance covered by utilization review programs. Since these proportions change slowly over time, most of the variation by far in this variable is cross-sectional. The pooling methodology may be unduly hard on UR, forcing UR parameter estimates toward zero. Thus, the OLS coefficients of -0.17 in the regressions for total and labor expense per adjusted patient-day, both significant at the 1 percent level, merit some interest. If the UR coefficients were picking up an omitted state effect, it is more likely that the coefficient would have been positive rather than negative.

Policy discussions of hospital costs often assert that cost-based reimbursement (COSTB) is a relatively inflationary way to pay hospitals. If we judge from Davis (1973) and our theoretical work in chapter 2, it is clear that one should be cautious about making such statements without reference to empirical evidence. Past empirical tests of the comparative effect of cost-based versus other forms of reimbursement (charge-based and direct patient payment) have not shown the cost-based payment method to be relatively inflationary (Pauly and Drake 1970; Salkever 1972; Davis 1973).

Our results, using COSTB to measure the proportion of patients with cost-based insurance, are consistent with the findings of past research. With regard to total expense per adjusted patient-day, significantly negative coefficients were obtained in both TSCS and OLS regressions. In comparing the coefficients of total expense to those of labor expense, the main difference (that is, savings) appears to be in nonlabor costs. In fact, in one labor-cost regression (column 8 of table 7–1) the parameter estimate of COSTB is significantly positive. Thus, while we find no evidence that cost-based reimbursement is more inflationary on the whole, the results suggest that this method may have stimulated the growth of labor costs.

Summary

This chapter has assessed determinants of variation in total and labor expenses per admission and per adjusted patient-day based on a cohort of 1,228 U.S. hospitals observed over 1969–1975. Both static and dynamic cost equations have been estimated. The static equations were estimated via OLS, and the dynamic estimates, which merit more confidence, used a TSCS pooling technique developed by Nerlove.

Explanatory variables fall into four general categories: product demand shift, cost function shift, hospital characteristics, and regulation and reimbursement methods. Parameter estimates from the cost regressions are largely plausible and consistent with findings of past research. Three general findings are noteworthy.

First, as a group, the regulatory programs did not succeed in constraining the growth in hospital costs during the first half of the 1970s. In fact, we obtained evidence that some programs had perverse effects—they raised hospital costs above what they might otherwise have been. A more complete evaluation of regulatory strategies should await an examination of the input results in chapter 8.

Second, most of the product demand shift variables show substantial effects on hospital costs. Particularly relevant from the standpoint of policy are results on the insurance and physician availability variables. Both private health insurance and public programs demonstrate positive effects on hospital costs. In the case of Medicare and Medicaid parameter estimates, case-mix and reimbursement effects are probably mingled. The regressions also indicate that costs tend to be higher in geographic areas where specialists are dominant numerically. The unexpectedly poor performance of per capita income in the cost regressions is more likely due to relatively slow growth in this variable during the study period and to collinearity with the wage variable rather than to the absence of an effect of income on hospital costs.

Third, a substantial portion of the rise in hospital costs over the first half of the 1970s is attributable to cost-push factors. In particular, we found strong union influences in both total cost and labor cost regressions. The combination of acquiring a union and having a strike or other job action was estimated to raise our cost measures from 12 to 18 percent in the long run. Just having a union generates long-run effects on costs about half this large.

Notes

1. Adjusted patient-days are the sum of inpatient days and weighted outpatient visits. The weight is the proportion of average revenue per outpatient visit to average revenue per inpatient-day. See Greenfield (1973) for a critique of this method of combining inpatient and outpatient services.

2. Average length of stay in nonfederal, short-term general U.S. hospitals declined from 8.08 days in 1970 to 7.53 days in 1975.

3. Our estimates of the speed of the cost response to changes in exogenous variables are considerably faster than those reported in a hospital cost study by Salkever (1972). We suspect the difference lies in the econometric techniques employed. Salkever used an instrumental-variable approach based on the rank order of the lagged dependent variable. In previous work by Sloan (1977), it was determined that the estimated speed of response was particularly sensitive to the number of categories used in the

ranking procedure. That is, if one used deciles, one would obtain a quicker response than if one used quintiles. Because this procedure seems quite sensitive to the method of ranking, more confidence should be placed on the table 7–1 results, based on Nerlove's (1971) TSCS pooling technique. In his study of hospitals, Feldstein (1977) obtained rapid adjustment speeds for 1966–1973 versus slow speeds for 1959–1966.

4. U.S. Bureau of the Census (1977). Our PERCAP measure rose 10.5 percent over these years (see table 6–5). Personal per capita income variables have not performed very well in previous hospital cost studies. For example, Salkever (1972) found that per capita income had no effect on hospital costs. Salkever attributed this finding to increases in income, bringing about improvements in health status, and time costs of consuming hospital care increasing with income. Both influences might result in a negative association between per capita income and the demand for hospital care.

5. As discussed in chapter 2, the importance of the physician in determining who is admitted, lengths of stay, and ordering of tests is widely accepted. Recent research (for example, Pauly 1978) has begun to establish specific links between physician characteristics and hospital costs. Our data unfortunately are not sufficiently detailed to permit further examination of these relationships.

6. See Salkever (1978a) for a summary of existing literature on competition among hospitals.

7. If there were no other nonfederal, short-term general hospitals in the observational hospital's county, the number of other beds was set equal to 1 and thus POPBD equals county population in such cases.

8. As discussed in chapter 4, INS is predicted from a set of instrumental variables, defined for the hospital's county. For this reason, it is unlikely that the INS parameter estimates reflect a simultaneous relationship between hospital costs and private insurance.

9. See chapter 4, note 29.

10. Previous studies on the effects of hospital unions on wages include Davis (1973), Feldman and Scheffler (1977), Fottler (1977), Link and Landon (1975), and Sloan and Elnicki (1978). The consensus of this research is that unions have raised hospital wages, but not dramatically. These studies are reviewed in detail by Sloan and Steinwald (1980) who also present new information on union impacts on hospital wages.

11. For this reason, we are not concerned about the possible criticism that ASSETB should be considered endogenous in table 7–1.

12. For a comprehensive review, see Hefty (1969).

13. Strictly speaking, COSTB does not measure the impact of regulation; rather this variable is intended to measure the effects of alternative reimbursement methods. All other variables discussed in this section fit our definition of direct regulation.

14. Variable ASSETB and bed-size dummy variables, which have been entered separately in the cost regressions, may themselves be affected by capital-facilities regulation. However, because ASSETB demonstrates a negligible impact on costs in the TSCS regressions and the bed-size categories are quite large, we are not concerned about potential indirect effects of the regulatory programs on costs. Given our parameter estimates pertaining to ASSETB and BDTOT and dependent variables, such indirect effects appear to be slight. Much more detail on indirect effects is presented in chapter 8.

15. This result is supported by findings of Hellinger (1976a). Parameter estimates of PRECON in input regressions, reported in chapter 8, are possibly more illuminating.

16. Although the nature of their sample is different and they do not distinguish between comprehensive and noncomprehensive, and new and mature, programs, our results are consistent with those of Salkever and Bice (1976a, 1976b). If anything, Salkever and Bice's estimates of certificate-of-need effects on hospital costs are *slightly* more favorable toward CON than ours.

17. Responsiveness of hospital costs to BCPAA is far less than the (absolute) maximum coefficient of −0.015 suggests since, unlike the binary certificate-of-need variables, BCPAA is the proportion of area population with Blue Cross coverage where a Blue Cross planning agency approval requirement exists; otherwise BCPAA is zero.

18. For a summary of these programs and a synopsis of the empirical results of the studies, see Gaus and Hellinger (1976) in addition to our descriptions in chapter 5.

8 Empirical Findings on Hospital Demand for Inputs

In this chapter, we present our multivariate empirical findings on determinants of hospital employment of labor inputs (RNs, LPNs, and other employees) and nonlabor inputs (assets, current nonlabor purchases, and beds). As before, for the sake of convenience, we have divided the explanatory variables into four categories: product demand, factor price, hospital characteristics, and regulation and reimbursement method. Results pertaining to these variable classes are discussed separately in the next four sections. A fifth section is devoted to evaluation of dynamic properties of the input model. Finally, we summarize this chapter's most important findings.

Our empirical results are contained in eight tables. Tables 8–1 and 8–2 contain the time-series cross-sectional (TSCS) and ordinary-least-squares (OLS) parameter estimates of structural equations for labor and nonlabor inputs. In general, we emphasize the TSCS results.[1] Tables 8–3 through 8–5 present short-run (one-year) impact multipliers, depicting reduced-form effects of the explanatory variables on input use. The method for calculating the impact multipliers was explained in chapter 3. The impact multipliers measure the total effect of explanatory variables on the dependent variables, taking account of indirect effects on beds and assets. Instead of giving estimates of effects on inputs per bed, as in tables 8–1 and 8–2, the impact multipliers are "per hospital" measures.

Table 8–6 provides structural-equation estimates of interactions among regulation variables and two of the binary hospital characteristics variables measuring proprietary ownership and medical school affiliation. These empirical tests are intended to ascertain whether nonneutralities exist in the application of hospital regulatory programs. Table 8–7 presents information on dynamic interrelationships among the inputs, showing the effects of a shortage or surplus of one input on employment of the other inputs. Longer-run effects of explanatory variables on inputs are presented in tables 8–8 through 8–11.

Because this chapter contains considerable material, we concentrate on what we view to be the more important findings, rather than bombard readers with minutiae. We refer to the cost findings in chapter 7 where such comparisons are enlightening. Although the input results are a bit more difficult to interpret in some cases than the cost results, findings on hospital input use provide considerably more insight into hospital behavior than can be derived from the cost results alone.

Product Demand Variables

The first set of explanatory variables in tables 8–1 and 8–2 relates to demand for the hospital's product: PERCAP, DENS, POPMD, GPPROP, POPBD, MCARE, MCAID, and INS. In comparing input and cost regressions, directions of impact, with a few exceptions, tend to be the same. As in the cost regressions, more of the OLS coefficients are statistically significant than their TSCS counterparts, and the OLS coefficients tend to be larger. The OLS regressions are based on a static structure. By contrast, the TSCS estimates in the two tables represent first-year responses in a dynamic framework.

Table 8–3 presents the short-run (one-year) impact multipliers pertaining to the demand variables, based on the TSCS structural estimates in tables 8–1 and 8–2. Because the impact of the demand variables on assets per bed and on beds is usually positive, the multiplier coefficients tend to be larger than their TSCS structural counterparts. However, there are very few qualitative differences between the TSCS structural estimates in tables 8–1 and 8–2 and the multipliers.

Parameter estimates pertaining to PERCAP, county per capita real income, are generally positive, but tend to be statistically insignificant. An exception is assets per bed, where the elasticity of PERCAP is 0.58 and the TSCS regression and the impact multiplier in table 8–3 is 0.61. This finding suggests that growth in facilities and services, in both numbers and degree of sophistication, is responsive to community income growth. The poor performance of PERCAP in the TSCS regression for RNs per bed is surprising in view of the strongly positive effects gotten by using the same dependent variable reported in past research.[2] However, the corresponding impact multiplier, 0.085, is more than double the structural parameter estimate.

Most of the parameter estimates pertaining to DENS, county population per square mile, are positive and significant at the 1 percent level. An exception is the LPNs per bed regression, where the impact of DENS is definitely negative. This is the first of several findings suggesting that employment of LPNs often responds to demand variables in a manner opposite to the other labor inputs. This is not surprising in view of the fact that LPNs have a higher "quality" substitute, namely, RNs. On the whole, however, the elasticities depicting the influence of DENS on input employment are low, as was the case in the cost regressions.

Of the two area physician variables, POPMD and GPPROP, results pertaining to the latter are more interesting. Variable POPMD, which measures county population per nonfederal office-based physician, has unstable and generally insignificant parameter estimates. By contrast, most coefficients pertaining to GPPROP, the county proportion of physicians in general practice, are significantly negative, suggesting that hospital employ-

Table 8-1
Labor Input Regressions

Variable	RNs per Bed		LPNs per Bed		Other Employees per Bed	
	TSCS (1)	OLS (2)	TSCS (3)	OLS (4)	TSCS (5)	OLS (6)
PERCAP	0.039	0.14*	0.059	−0.058	0.0037	−0.0039
	(0.048)[a]	(0.044)	(0.091)	(0.081)	(0.037)	(0.031)
DENS	0.0016	0.032*	−0.039*	−0.050*	0.013*	0.029*
	(0.0071)	(0.0037)	(0.013)	(0.0068)	(0.0054)	(0.0026)
POPMD	−0.0075	−0.13*	0.013	0.13*	0.0033	0.023***
	(0.018)	(0.018)	(0.034)	(0.034)	(0.014)	(0.013)
GPPROP	−0.049***	0.018	−0.090**	−0.16*	−0.032	−0.11*
	(0.028)	(0.016)	(0.050)	(0.029)	(0.021)	(0.011)
POPBD	0.0012	0.024*	−0.0013	−0.0098	0.0058	0.013*
	(0.0067)	(0.0049)	(0.013)	(0.0090)	(0.0052)	(0.0034)
MCARE	−0.16*	−0.24*	0.029	−0.072	0.0085	−0.015
	(0.044)	(0.024)	(0.079)	(0.045)	(0.033)	(0.017)
MCAID	0.036*	0.14*	−0.040***	−0.13*	0.013	0.018*
	(0.012)	(0.0099)	(0.023)	(0.018)	(0.0095)	(0.0070)
INS	−0.16*	0.12*	0.15***	−0.37*	0.046	0.13*
	(0.049)	(0.042)	(0.091)	(0.078)	(0.037)	(0.030)
RNWG	−0.40***	−0.82*	—	—	—	—
	(0.22)	(0.24)				
LPNWG	—	—	−0.72	−3.16*	—	—
			(0.40)	(0.44)		
OTHWG	—	—	—	—	0.31***	0.64*
					(0.17)	(0.17)
RELRN	—	—	0.36	0.65*	0.23**	0.082
			(0.26)	(0.18)	(0.11)	(0.070)
RELLPN	0.083	0.22*	—	—	−0.022	0.15**
	(0.10)	(0.086)			(0.078)	(0.061)
RELOTH	0.041	−0.19**	−0.039	−0.13	—	—
	(0.10)	(0.087)	(0.19)	(0.16)		

Table 8–1 (continued)

Variable	RNs per Bed		LPNs per Bed		Other Employees per Bed	
	TSCS (1)	OLS (2)	TSCS (3)	OLS (4)	TSCS (5)	OLS (6)
RELCAP	-0.15 (0.12)	-0.33*** (0.20)	-0.48*** (0.22)	-1.25* (0.37)	0.073 (0.090)	0.20 (0.14)
ASSETB	0.028* (0.0070)	0.091* (0.0061)	0.0037 (0.013)	0.026** (0.011)	0.027* (0.0055)	0.053* (0.0043)
GOVT	-0.055 (0.037)	-0.0098 (0.013)	0.026 (0.063)	0.13* (0.024)	0.033 (0.027)	0.028* (0.0094)
PROP	-0.24* (0.049)	-0.27* (0.018)	-0.027 (0.085)	0.064** (0.032)	-0.12* (0.036)	-0.16* (0.012)
MEDSCH	0.044 (0.032)	0.065* (0.011)	0.048 (0.056)	0.072* (0.020)	0.12* (0.024)	0.20* (0.0079)
NURSCH	-0.012 (0.035)	0.067* (0.012)	-0.13** (0.059)	-0.19* (0.023)	-0.011 (0.025)	0.063* (0.0089)
PRECON	-0.0088 (0.011)	0.034** (0.017)	-0.0094 (0.020)	-0.015 (0.031)	-0.0037 (0.0082)	-0.024** (0.012)
NCON1	0.0071 (0.011)	0.094* (0.015)	0.014 (0.021)	0.047*** (0.028)	0.022* (0.0087)	0.026* (0.011)
NCON2	0.011 (0.015)	0.17* (0.019)	0.014 (0.029)	0.072** (0.035)	0.023*** (0.012)	0.0059 (0.014)
CCON1	-0.0030 (0.018)	0.15* (0.025)	0.032 (0.035)	-0.20* (0.047)	-0.016 (0.014)	-0.061* (0.018)
CCON2	0.0018 (0.012)	0.17* (0.028)	0.083** (0.039)	-0.16* (0.052)	-0.011 (0.016)	-0.037*** (0.020)
S1122	0.079*** (0.047)	0.18** (0.078)	0.17*** (0.091)	0.28*** (0.14)	0.045 (0.037)	-0.14* (0.055)
BCPAA	-0.0030 (0.015)	0.012 (0.024)	-0.014 (0.029)	0.0038 (0.044)	0.032* (0.012)	0.014 (0.017)
FPR	-0.056 (0.052)	-0.33* (0.031)	0.19** (0.095)	0.092 (0.057)	-0.023 (0.040)	-0.025 (0.022)
BPR	0.030 (0.023)	-0.0036 (0.030)	0.023 (0.044)	0.0035 (0.055)	0.019 (0.018)	0.037 (0.021)
UR	-0.089 (0.070)	-0.20* (0.033)	0.075 (0.12)	0.43* (0.062)	-0.069 (0.052)	-0.18* (0.024)

	(1)	(2)	(3)	(4)	(5)	(6)
COSTB	0.11*** (0.068)	0.27* (0.032)	-0.16 (0.12)	-0.025 (0.058)	-0.055 (0.051)	0.018 (0.022)
ESP	-0.010 (0.013)	-0.047** (0.022)	-0.039 (0.025)	0.018 (0.041)	-0.025** (0.010)	-0.037** (0.016)
LAGRN	0.28* (0.012)	—	-0.099* (0.023)	—	0.11* (0.0094)	—
LAGLPN	-0.032* (0.0061)	—	0.30** (0.012)	—	-0.0042 (0.0047)	—
LAGOTH	0.13* (0.013)	—	0.16* (0.025)	—	0.22** (0.010)	—
LAGASS	-0.0084 (0.0068)	—	-0.018 (0.013)	—	-0.0027 (0.0053)	—
LAGEXP	-0.027** (0.012)	—	-0.029 (0.023)	—	0.0033 (0.0093)	—
LAGBED	0.032** (0.014)	—	-0.033 (0.026)	—	0.050* (0.011)	—
TIME	0.023* (0.0066)	-0.0024 (0.010)	0.018 (0.013)	0.084* (0.018)	-0.0031 (0.0051)	-0.0046 (0.0071)
CONST	0.213	-1.07	0.172	6.74	-0.491	-2.76
	$R^2 = 0.18$ $F(36, 5,980)$ $= 35.6*$	$R^2 = 0.34$ $F(30, 6,443)$ $= 108.7*$	$R^2 = 0.12$ $F(36, 5,980)$ $= 23.6*$	$R^2 = 0.09$ $F(30, 6,443)$ $= 20.8*$	$R^2 = 0.18$ $F(36, 5,980)$ $= 36.9*$	$R^2 = 0.35$ $F(30, 6,443)$ $= 113.8*$

*Significant at the 1% level (two-tailed test).
**Significant at the 5% level (two-tailed test).
***Significant at the 10% level (two-tailed test).
[a]Figures in parentheses are standard errors.

Table 8–2
Nonlabor Input Regressions

Variable	Assets per Bed		Current Nonlabor Expenses per Bed		Total Beds	
	TSCS (1)	OLS (2)	TSCS (3)	OLS (4)	TSCS (5)	TSCS (6)
PERCAP	0.58*	0.67*	−0.017	0.085**	0.030	0.018
	(0.092)[a]	(0.089)	(0.052)	(0.041)	(0.030)	(0.028)
DENS	−0.016	0.0020	0.017**	0.033*	0.014*	0.013**
	(0.015)	(0.0076)	(0.0080)	(0.0042)	(0.0055)	(0.0051)
POPMD	0.043	−0.045	−0.029	−0.058*	−0.012	−0.014
	(0.033)	(0.038)	(0.020)	(0.017)	(0.011)	(0.0099)
GPPROP	0.063	−0.049	−0.061**	−0.11*	−0.013	0.00028
	(0.058)	(0.033)	(0.030)	(0.017)	(0.011)	(0.018)
POPBD	−0.043*	0.032*	0.0057	0.013*	0.0067***	0.0037
	(0.012)	(0.010)	(0.0073)	(0.0046)	(0.0039)	(0.0036)
MCARE	−0.11	−0.23*	−0.048	−0.084*	0.085*	0.10*
	(0.094)	(0.050)	(0.046)	(0.023)	(0.033)	(0.030)
MCAID	0.042***	0.066*	0.0016	0.039*	0.0031	−0.0013
	(0.024)	(0.020)	(0.013)	(0.0095)	(0.0078)	(0.0072)
INS	0.088*	−0.096	0.014	0.090**	0.083**	0.059***
	(0.010)	(0.087)	(0.054)	(0.039)	(0.033)	(0.033)
CAP	0.44	−0.033	—	—	−0.076	−0.030**
	(0.44)	(0.49)			(0.10)	(0.14)
CPI	—	—	0.20	0.18	—	—
			(0.31)	(0.18)		
RELRN	0.36	−0.085	0.10	0.20**	−0.14	−0.22**
	(0.28)	(0.20)	(0.16)	(0.10)	(0.093)	(0.089)
RELLPN	−0.22	−0.18	0.0053	−0.048	0.10	0.10***
	(0.19)	(0.18)	(0.11)	(0.085)	(0.063)	(0.058)
RELOTH	0.32	0.46**	0.30*	0.42*	−0.092	−0.11***
	(0.20)	(0.18)	(0.10)	(0.084)	(0.064)	(0.064)
ASSETB	—	—	0.011	0.093*	—	—
			(0.0078)	(0.0056)		

GOVT	-0.10	-0.17*	-0.0042	-0.0051	-0.052	-0.0027
	(0.11)	(0.027)	(0.037)	(0.012)	(0.063)	(0.058)
PROP	-1.22*	-1.31*	0.11**	0.13*	-0.32*	-0.29*
	(0.14)	(0.032)	(0.050)	(0.016)	(0.080)	(0.075)
MEDSCH	0.096	0.25*	0.15*	0.21*	0.35*	0.39*
	(0.092)	(0.023)	(0.033)	(0.010)	(0.053)	(0.049)
NURSCH	0.015	0.086*	-0.012	-0.013	0.20*	0.26*
	(0.10)	(0.026)	(0.035)	(0.012)	(0.060)	(0.055)
PRECON	-0.013	-0.0029	-0.012	-0.0086	0.014**	0.0081
	(0.020)	(0.035)	(0.012)	(0.016)	(0.0062)	(0.0058)
NCON1	-0.023	0.0033	0.013	0.066*	-0.000076	-0.0028
	(0.021)	(0.031)	(0.012)	(0.014)	(0.0069)	(0.0065)
NCON2	-0.033	0.034	0.0088	0.082*	0.00037	-0.0018
	(0.028)	(0.039)	(0.017)	(0.019)	(0.0090)	(0.0086)
CCON1	-0.019	-0.0026	-0.023	-0.017	0.023**	0.019***
	(0.034)	(0.052)	(0.020)	(0.024)	(0.011)	(0.010)
CCON2	-0.024	0.0037	-0.023	0.035	0.012	0.0082
	(0.039)	(0.058)	(0.023)	(0.027)	(0.013)	(0.012)
S1122	-0.033	0.28**	-0.0012	-0.077	-0.040	-0.058**
	(0.087)	(0.16)	(0.052)	(0.073)	(0.028)	(0.026)
BCPAA	0.079*	0.025	-0.013	-0.048***	-0.020**	-0.016***
	(0.028)	(0.049)	(0.017)	(0.022)	(0.0092)	(0.0085)
FPR	0.046	0.070	-0.037	-0.13*	0.042	0.053
	(0.11)	(0.064)	(0.055)	(0.030)	(0.041)	(0.038)
BPR	0.022	-0.014	-0.025	0.036	0.0054	0.0045
	(0.043)	(0.062)	(0.025)	(0.028)	(0.014)	(0.013)
UR	-0.11	0.18*	-0.086	-0.25*	-0.047	0.034
	(0.18)	(0.068)	(0.073)	(0.031)	(0.085)	(0.079)
COSTB	-0.081	-0.27*	0.0065	0.0082	-0.000086	0.0089
	(0.18)	(0.065)	(0.077)	(0.033)	(0.084)	(0.078)
ESP	-0.069*	-0.048	-0.029**	-0.056*	0.0080	-0.0039
	(0.024)	(0.046)	(0.012)	(0.012)	(0.0076)	(0.0072)
LAGRN	0.014	—	0.031**	—	—	0.025*
	(0.023)		(0.013)			(0.0068)
LAGLPN	-0.012	—	0.021*	—	—	0.013*
	(0.011)		(0.0067)			(0.0032)

Table 8–2 *(continued)*

Variable	Assets per Bed		Current Nonlabor Expenses per Bed		Total Beds	
	TSCS (1)	OLS (2)	TSCS (3)	OLS (4)	TSCS (5)	TSCS (6)
LAGOTH	0.016 (0.024)	—	0.34* (0.14)	—	—	−0.21* (0.0068)
LAGASS	0.40* (0.011)	—	0.016* (0.0075)	—	—	0.0052 (0.0034)
LAGEXP	0.0078 (0.022)	—	0.17* (0.013)	—	—	0.084* (0.0067)
LAGBED	0.069** (0.030)	—	0.014 (0.015)	—	0.54* (0.0097)	0.57* (0.0098)
TIME	−0.025** (0.012)	0.016 (0.021)	0.057* (0.014)	0.068* (0.0076)	—	0.0062 (0.0038)
CONST	0.037	5.79	2.73	5.70	0.705	0.713
	$R^2 = 0.23$	$R^2 = 0.28$	$R^2 = 0.34$	$R^2 = 0.35$	$R^2 = 0.44$	$R^2 = 0.53$
	$F(35, 5,981)$ $= 51.5*$	$F(29, 6,444)$ $= 87.5*$	$F(36, 5,980)$ $= 84.5*$	$F(30, 6,443)$ $= 117.9*$	$F(29, 6,032)$ $= 161.7*$	$F(35, 6,026)$ $= 190.7*$

*Significant at the 1% level (two-tailed test).
**Significant at the 5% level (two-tailed test).
***Significant at the 10% level (two-tailed test).
[a]Figures in parentheses are standard errors.

Table 8-3
Short-Run (One-Year) Impact Multipliers of Product Demand Variables

Variable[a]	RNs	LPNs	Other Employees	Current Nonlabor Expenses	Assets	Beds
PERCAP	0.085	0.091	0.049	0.007	0.610	0.030
DENS	0.015	−0.025	0.027	0.031	−0.002	0.014
POPMD	−0.010	0.001	−0.008	−0.037	0.031	−0.012
GPPROP	−0.060	−0.103	−0.043	−0.073	0.050	−0.013
POPBD	0.007	0.006	0.011	−0.000	−0.036	0.007
MCARE	−0.078	0.114	0.091	0.027	−0.025	0.085
MCAID	0.040	−0.037	0.017	0.005	0.045	0.003
INS	−0.070	0.101	0.131	0.098	0.171	0.083

[a]Based on the TSCS regressions. Parameter estimates for beds come from table 8-1, regression no. 5.

ment of nonphysician inputs tends to increase as medical specialization in the hospital's area increases. The coefficient of GPPROP is unexpectedly positive, although not statistically significant, in the TSCS regression for assets per bed. Relative to the corresponding structural estimates, the impact multipliers in table 8-3 show a slightly increased negative effect of GPPROP on input employment with a reduced positive impact on assets per bed.

Three variables, MCARE, MCAID, and INS, measure the extent of third-party reimbursement in the hospital's market. As seen in chapter 7, each variable exhibited a positive impact on costs, but we find some variability in the input regressions. Also, as stated previously, these variables are related to hospital case mix and patient demographics, which, in turn, may exert an influence on resource employment independent of the effects of reimbursement per se.

Parameter estimates of MCARE, our Medicare variable, are unstable. In the TSCS regressions, the MCARE coefficient is significantly negative in the RNs per bed regression and significantly positive in the beds regression, while all other coefficients are statistically insignificant. It may be true that elderly hospitalized patients require less skilled nursing care, so that, *ceteris paribus*, less input intensity is required for such patients. However, the TSCS coefficient of our Medicaid variable (MCAID) is positive in the RNs per bed and assets per bed regressions but negative in the LPNs per bed regression. The elasticities are not high, but these results suggest a higher level of input intensity associated with caring for the typical Medicaid patient, who probably is more likely to be acutely ill than most Medicare patients. This finding is generally supported by the impact multipliers in table 8-3, although the table suggests that Medicare has the greater impact on other employees, nonlabor expenses, and beds.

Parameter estimates in tables 8–1 and 8–2 pertaining to INS, our private health insurance depth-of-coverage variable, resemble the MCARE coefficients more than those for MCAID, especially in the RNs per bed and beds regressions. However, unlike MCARE, INS shows an insignificantly positive effect in the assets per bed regression. The negative sign in the RNs regression is very difficult to explain; this is the only negative sign on INS in the TSCS regressions. Table 8–3 tends to show a larger impact of INS on hospital resource employment. The positive elasticities on LPNs, other employees, and assets are all greater than 0.1, and the current nonlabor expense elasticity approaches this level. Given the results from chapter 7, and the finding with regard to RNs notwithstanding, it is clear that private insurance depth of coverage has positive effects on hospital costs and input employment.

Factor Price Effects

Most economic studies of demand for labor have emphasized the role of factor prices, both own and cross, as determinants of factor demand.[3] From parameter estimates on factor price variables, it is possible to determine the degree to which various inputs are substitutes. These relationships also have some policy interest. For example, with an estimate of the effect of input prices on demand for various types of labor, one can calculate the impact of a wage subsidy on the quantity of labor demanded. In the mid- and late 1970s, wage subsidies, using tax rebates, were proposed as a means of stimulating employment. Likewise, payroll taxes, such as Social Security, potentially affect input demand, and estimates of factor price effects may be useful for gauging the employment effects of raising payroll taxes.

In the hospital sector, interest in factor price effects has been twofold. First, given the predominance of hospitals organized on a not-for-profit basis, there is a fundamental issue of whether hospitals are cost minimizers. Hospital responsiveness to factor prices may provide one clue.[4] Second, for purposes of health workforce policy, it is useful to know the degree to which various types of labor are substitutes in hospital production.[5] Our data base is somewhat limited, especially for the latter purpose, because several of our input categories are general, and measurement of factor prices in this context is unavoidably imprecise. As seen in chapter 2, comparative statics analysis generally shows negative own-price effects. Cross effects may take either sign.

To calculate own-price effects from tables 8–1 and 8–2, one must consider that own prices enter the input regressions in two places: in absolute terms, such as RNWG in the RNs per bed equation, and in the denominators of the REL price terms. Since all factor prices are expressed in logarithms, the own-price effect is calculated by subtracting the REL coefficients from the term expressing own prices. Thus, for RNs per bed, the structural own-price elasticity from the TSCS regression is -0.37 [$= -0.40$ (on RNWG) $- 0.083$ (on RELLPN) $- 0.041$ (on RELOTH) $+ 0.15$ (on RELCAP)]. Structural own-price elasticities, based on tables 8–1 and 8–2, are presented in table 8–4. This table also shows reduced-form own-price effects on input levels (as above, obtained by substituting parameter estimates for ASSETB and beds from table 8–2 according to the method outlined in chapter 3).

The vast majority of both TSCS and OLS own-price elasticities are negative; those for RNs and LPNs are largest in absolute value. The results suggest that hospitals are sensitive to factor prices, confirming the predictions in chapter 2. We are reluctant to emphasize the implied magnitudes of response (that is, the elasticities) because the price measures used for estimation are unavoidably crude.

The number of cross-factor price terms in tables 8–1 and 8–2 is too numerous to discuss individually. Given the accuracy of the price data, we would not push these particular findings too far. Estimates of dynamic interrelationships among inputs, based on much more accurate data, merit far greater scrutiny.

Hospital Characteristics

Hospital characteristics are represented by one continuous variable, ASSETB, and four unchanging binary variables, GOVT, PROP, MEDSCH, and NURSCH. As noted earlier, ASSETB is predicted from a set of instruments which predominantly relate to the hospital's facilities and

Table 8–4
Own-Factor-Price Effects (Elasticities)

Equation	Structural		Reduced Form	
	TSCS	*OLS*	*TSCS*	*OLS*
RNs per bed	−0.37	−0.52	−0.50	−0.58
LPNs per bed	−0.56	−2.43	−0.46	−0.46
Other employees per bed	−0.03	0.21	−0.11	−0.13
Current nonlabor expense per bed	−0.21	−0.39	−0.21	−0.21
Assets per bed	−0.02	−0.16	0.04	−0.09
Beds[a]	0.06	−0.07	0.06	−0.07

[a]All beds estimates are based on TSCS. The second column of each pair of estimates is based on the second TSCS regression in table 8–2.

services mix. As an explanatory variable, it is intended to capture effects of variations in the hospital's scope of services, in both number and sophistication, on decisions to employ other inputs. Each of the binary variables is defined as of 1970 and, as constructed, is not permitted to change over the six-year period. Thus, the *very* few instances in which, for example, a hospital may have changed ownership status or closed a nursing school during the period are ignored. Nongovernmental, nonprofit hospitals without medical or nursing school affiliations represent the reference hospital group.

The asset variable is included as an explanatory variable in all labor input and in the current nonlabor expense regressions. Parameter estimates in both the TSCS and OLS regressions indicate that there is complementarity between hospitals' asset bases and other inputs. All coefficients are positive; however, in the TSCS regressions, ASSETB is statistically significant only in the regressions for RNs per bed and other employees per bed. These parameter estimates suggest that new or expanded facilities and services tend to generate additional staffing, but not across the board (for example, there is virtually zero impact of ASSETB on LPN staffing).

Because they enter linearly, coefficients pertaining to the four binary hospital characteristics variables indicate percentage differences in the dependent variable between hospitals with and without the referenced attribute. In general, directions of effect are the same in TSCS and OLS regressions, but orders of magnitude tend to be lower in the TSCS regressions and standard errors higher. Therefore, fewer of the TSCS results are statistically significant.

The variable indicating state and local government ownership, GOVT, shows relatively little impact on hospital inputs. The parameter estimates suggest that, compared to the voluntary hospital reference group, such hospitals tend to employ less expensive inputs (for example, the negative sign in the RNs per bed regression and positive sign in the LPNs per bed regression), but few of the coefficients were statistically significant at conventional levels. Parameter estimates on PROP, the variable indicating for-profit ownership, show marked differences between such hospitals and the reference group. Proprietary hospitals tend to employ significantly lower levels of all inputs except current nonlabor purchases. Parameter estimates on PROP in both OLS and TSCS assets per bed regressions were below -1.0, implying that assets per bed in proprietary hospitals are over 100 percent below voluntaries—an impossibility. Positive parameters estimates in the current nonlabor expense regressions are much lower (in absolute value), but still statistically significant at conventional levels. Taken as a whole, these results suggest that production in proprietary hospitals tends to be less input-intensive, *ceteris paribus*, than in other short-term general hospitals.

Results pertaining to the medical school and nursing school variables, MEDSCH and NURSCH, show that production in hospitals with medical school affiliations tends to be more input-intensive than in hospitals without such affiliations. In part, this pattern reflects joint production of teaching, research, and patient care in teaching hospitals. To a lesser extent, the same argument might be applied to nursing school–affiliated hospitals, but the NURSCH parameter estimates imply much lower input intensity than those for MEDSCH. An offsetting argument is that hospitals typically receive in-kind returns (that is, services compensated at less than a theoretical market rate) from students and trainees, who substitute, to some extent, for fully paid inputs.

The OLS regressions show that both medical and nursing education is associated with higher input levels, but these associations are weakened considerably in the TSCS regressions. The negative NURSCH parameter estimates in the LPNs per bed regressions are certainly plausible because one expects RN substitutes to be more readily available to hospitals with professional nursing schools. However, for the same reason, the negative NURSCH coefficient in the TSCS regression for RNs per bed is unexpected. If we view the two affiliation variables together, the most consistent results are in the total beds regressions, where the parameter estimates were positive and statistically significant in both OLS and TSCS regressions.

Regulation and Reimbursement Methods

A major objective of this book is to evaluate effects of various forms of regulation on hospital costs and input employment. Representing certificate of need in the empirical analysis are variables PRECON, NCON1, NCON2, CCON1, and CCON2. Since certificate of need is always implemented statewide, all these variables are binaries. Other facility and services regulation variables in our analysis are S1122 for the P.L. 92–603, section 1122, review program and BCPAA for Blue Cross planning agency approval programs. These programs use hospital reimbursement as a device to influence capital expansion. Revenue-cost regulation is measured by FPR and BPR for formula and budget-review prospective reimbursement and ESP for the Economic Stabilization Program. Utilization review effects are gauged by UR, which measures Blue Cross and Medicaid utilization review efforts at the local level. Strictly speaking, COSTB is not a regulation variable, but because it describes a reimbursement method and is measured similarly to most of the other variables in this group, it is appropriate to consider it here. As defined, all the reimbursement-related variables are bounded by 0 and 1 and depend on the extent to which reimbursement programs cover the populations served by sample hospitals. Structural parameter estimates of the regulation variables are presented, as before, in tables 8–1 and 8–2, and short-run impact multipliers are found in table 8–5.

Table 8–5
Short-Run (One-Year) Impact Multipliers of Regulation Variables

Regulation Variable[a]	Input					
	RNs	LPNs	Other Employees	Current Nonlabor	Assets	Beds
Capital-Facilities Regulation						
PRECON	0.005	0.005	0.010	0.002	0.001	0.014
NCON1	0.007	0.014	0.022	0.013	−0.023	−0.000
NCON2	0.011	0.014	0.023	0.009	−0.033	0.000
CCON1	0.020	0.055	0.007	0.000	0.004	0.023
CCON2	0.014	0.095	0.001	−0.011	−0.012	0.012
S1122	0.039	0.130	0.005	−0.041	−0.073	−0.040
BCPAA	−0.023	−0.034	0.012	−0.033	0.059	−0.020
Revenue-Cost Regulation						
ESP	−0.002	−0.031	−0.017	−0.021	−0.061	0.008
FPR	−0.014	0.250	0.019	0.005	0.088	0.042
BPR	0.035	0.027	0.028	−0.020	0.027	0.005
Utilization Review						
UR	−0.160	0.028	−0.120	−0.130	−0.160	−0.047

[a]Based on the TSCS regressions in table 8–1 and 8–2. Beds parameter estimates come from table 8–2, regression 5.

From the standpoint of cost containment, negative effects of the regulation variables on input levels are the desired result. However, 64 percent of the impact multipliers in table 8–5 are positive. By coincidence, this is precisely the same percentage of positive signs as in the TSCS cost regressions in chapter 7. There is certainly nothing magic about this figure, but it serves to emphasize our overall result—by and large, regulatory programs implemented throughout the late 1960s and 1970s have not been effective cost containment tools. First we review results depicting the overall effects of regulation on inputs. Then we assess findings describing effects of regulatory interventions on specific types of hospitals.

Effects of Regulation on Inputs

Our certificate-of-need findings are discussed in light of results obtained in two previous studies reviewed in chapter 5, those by Salkever and Bice (1976a, 1976b) and by Hellinger (1976a). Salkever and Bice found that over the years 1968–1972 CON retarded growth in hospital beds but stimulated investment in services and equipment. The latter result was interpreted by the authors as a compensatory response to this form of regulation. Expansionary pressures, according to Salkever and Bice, were channeled into other forms of investment in the face of restrictions on bed supply growth. Hellinger found that CON had not significantly reduced hospital investment over 1972–1973, but he did find some evidence of increased investment in anticipation of implementation of CON laws by the states.

As noted in chapter 5, our empirical analysis differs from the above studies. First, it covers a more recent period. Many states adopted CON during the 1970s. Second, our research encompasses a greater number of inputs, both labor and nonlabor, while the two previous studies focused on nonlabor inputs. Third, we explicitly assess a larger number of regulatory programs concurrently, thereby reducing the problem of separating CON effects from those of other regulatory programs. Last, we distinguish between types of CON programs with regard to age and comprehensiveness. This permits an assessment of whether variations in CON program characteristics are associated with different degrees of effectiveness.

With regard to beds, we find evidence of anticipatory response to certificate of need. If we judge from the PRECON parameter estimate in the first beds equation in table 8–2, there is (on average) a 1.4 percent increase in bed growth during the year preceding introduction of certificate of need. The corresponding parameter estimate in the second beds regression is somewhat smaller, but still positive. This result is quite robust—in preliminary regressions with fewer explanatory variables, the magnitude of this coefficient was considerably higher than 0.014. The noncomprehensive programs, which presumably emphasize controls on bed supply, have no impact on beds whatsoever. By contrast, the comprehensive programs, which have more general aims, have a positive impact, especially during the first two years (CCON1). It is possible that the CCON1 coefficient and even that of CCON2 reflect some anticipatory effects not captured by PRECON. In any event, there is no way to conclude from table 8–2 that CON has reduced the growth in beds in our cohort of 1,228 hospitals. In fact, these programs seem, through anticipatory effects and other forces, to have actually stimulated bed growth in some instances.

Although the coefficients of the CON variables in the assets per bed regression are statistically insignificant at conventional levels, they are indeed uniformly negative, as are the impact multipliers with two exceptions (in which the positive coefficients are very small). In terms of both assets per bed and assets per hospital (see table 8–5), the noncomprehensive programs show a slightly more negative effect than their comprehensive counterparts. We are unable to explain why. For both comprehensive and noncomprehensive programs, the mature programs (designated with the suffix "2") have somewhat more strongly negative effects than their younger counterparts.

Current nonlabor and labor inputs are not directly controlled by any certificate-of-need program. According to the simple two-input model presented in chapter 2, binding restraints on one input will tend to reduce the use of the nonregulated input. However, compensatory responses, as argued by Salkever and Bice, are potentially important in the context of CON regulations. For example, funds not permitted to be used for one form of investment may be used to improve staffing and/or purchase other (noncovered) types of equipment. Their line of reasoning, which was applied to investments in facilities and services, has even greater applicability to inputs that are not subject to any control by CON.[6]

Although there are some negative signs on the CON variables in the labor input regressions reported in table 8–1, all labor impact multipliers in table 8–5 are positive. The largest positive effect is on the demand for LPNs in states with comprehensive programs. The positive signs in the LPN and the other labor input regressions suggest a definite compensatory response. The CON coefficients are often negative in the TSCS regressions for current nonlabor expense per bed in table 8–2, but the corresponding impact multipliers are essentially zero.

In sum, our results on certificate of need are consistent with Salkever and Bice's notion of compensatory responses, but we find them on the labor rather than the nonlabor side. Since Salkever and Bice did not assess CON impacts on labor use, there is no way to ascertain whether this form of compensatory response would have been evident in the earlier period covered by their study. Our finding of a (slight) negative effect of CON on assets is more consistent with Hellinger's results than with those of Salkever and Bice. Like Hellinger, we also obtained evidence of an anticipatory response by hospitals to impending implementation of CON controls. On the whole, results from our analysis of inputs are broadly consistent with our results on costs, but the compensatory effect of CON on hospital use of labor inputs is more evident in the input analysis.

In chapter 7, we found that section 1122 programs had essentially zero effects in the TSCS total expense regressions; however, the programs had a significantly positive effect on labor expense per adjusted patient-day. These results are confirmed in tables 8–1, 8–2, and 8–5, even though not all S1122 parameter estimates are statistically significant. Section 1122 program impacts on nonlabor inputs tend to be negative, but these negative impacts are offset by positive S1122 coefficients in the labor demand regressions. Basically the same arguments apply to section 1122 as to certificate of need. If third-party payers do not want to pay for nonlabor inputs, hospitals will find other ways to spend money. This finding, coupled with the certificate-of-need results, suggests that projections of savings resulting from reducing excess bed capacity may seriously miss the mark because pressing in one place (nonlabor inputs) may create a bulge elsewhere (labor inputs).[7]

The Blue Cross planning agency approval variable (BCPAA) demonstrated negative and significant effects on both total expense and labor
expense per admission and negative but insigifnicant effects on average costs
per adjusted patient-day. The results on inputs are mixed: BCPAA has a
significantly negative impact on bed expansion, but not on assets (or assets
per bed). These programs seem to have reduced hospital demand for RNs
and LPNs but stimulated demand for other employees. We frankly do not
know what to make of this pattern.

Although states' experiences with prospective reimbursement have been
studied at length, there is little evidence on PR effects on input use per se.[8]
Berry (1976) stressed that New York's formula PR system allows for general
inflation in the cost of certain inputs purchased by hospitals, but excludes
capital costs from the inflation allowances. Tables presented by Berry
showing trends in capital/labor and planned assets/payroll costs ratios
suggest that New York hospitals, as might be expected, have substituted
labor for capital in response to PR. Although the TSCS parameter estimates
for FPR are positive in our total cost regressions in table 7–1, they are, in
fact, more positive in the labor cost regressions, which also implies a shift
among New York hospitals from nonlabor to labor inputs.[9]

Overall, the results presented in tables 8–1, 8–2, and 8–5 confirm the
TSCS cost regressions in that formula PR does not have a negative impact on
most inputs. An exception is RNs, where a substitution of LPNs (which may
have occurred for cost reasons) is evident.[10] The OLS labor input estimates
show this RN-LPN substitution in much more dramatic terms than the TSCS
regressions. We find no support whatsoever for the view that formula PR
lowered the capital/labor ratio. Both assets per bed and beds rise rather than
fall in response to FPR.[11]

The BPR coefficients do not indicate as much stimulation of internal
hospital growth as was suggested by the FPR coefficients; nor is the implied
reduced-form positive impact on assets as great (see table 8–5). On the
whole, however, the input analysis is less favorable to budget PR than is our
cost analysis. Of the six BPR impact multipliers reported in table 8–5, only
the current nonlabor expense estimate is negative. The TSCS and OLS
parameter estimates in tables 8–1 and 8–2 are mostly positive, yet none is
statistically significant at conventional levels. These results do not suggest
any firm conclusions regarding the effects of budget PR on hospital input
employment.

Of all the regulation variables considered, ESP has the most definite
negative effects on input use. Although ESP, not surprisingly, had no effect
on beds because of its temporary nature, the ESP variable shows significantly negative impact on assets per bed and current nonlabor expenses per
bed. Signs on the ESP coefficients in all three labor regressions are also
negative, albeit insignificant, in two of the three labor regressions. With the

exception of beds, all impact multipliers relating ESP to levels of input use are negative. Multipliers are as high as −0.06, the multiplier on assets, suggesting that ESP had a substantial effect on expansion of facilities and services. For purposes of comparison, one should recall that ESP had negative effects in the total expense regressions but positive effects in the labor expense regressions. The total expense results are certainly consistent with our input results. Our findings with respect to labor expense would appear to be inconsistent, but there is a missing link—real wages of hospital personnel, which Sloan and Steinwald (1980) show, based on two independent data sources, reached an all-time high during the ESP years.[12] Thus, ESP may have influenced real labor expense positively while exerting a negative influence on physical units of labor.

Our final direct regulation variable relates to utilization review (UR). Most of the TSCS parameter estimates for UR are negative in the input regressions, although never statistically significant. The implied savings on inputs, however, are substantial, almost too high to be believed. The negative UR impact multipliers receive some support in the expense regressions, especially total and labor expense per admission. We are reluctant to stress these results more, because conceptually and institutionally this type of program would be expected to be comparatively weak and our UR variable is not well-measured. Nevertheless, these results suggest that further investigation of utilization review, including the UR component of the PSRO program, would be worthwhile.

The final reimbursement variable is COSTB, which measures the proportion of area insured persons with insurance that reimburses hospitals on a cost basis. On the basis of the theoretical discussion in chapter 2 and our review of past evidence of cost-based reimbursement in chapter 5, we concluded that there is little evidence to support the view that this form of reimbursement is either more or less inflationary than the alternative forms. This conclusion was supported by parameter estimates in cost regressions presented in chapter 7 and further reinforced by the input regression results in tables 8–1 and 8–2. Our nonlabor regressions indicate no impact whatsoever. On the labor side, we have a positive and statistically significant parameter estimate in the TSCS regression for RNs per bed, as did Sloan and Elnicki (1978), and insignificantly negative estimates in the other labor regressions. These results weakly suggest that cost reimbursement may result in substitution in the direction of more expensive labor inputs; yet, because this finding is not reflected in the TSCS labor cost regressions of chapter 7, we do not feel it is worth much attention.

Regulatory Effects on Particular Types of Hospitals

In chapter 5 we identified a reservation advanced by some critics of hospital regulation that regulatory programs might not be implemented neutrally.[13]

That is, by virtue of their status in their communities, some hospitals may fare better than others in their dealings with the regulatory agencies, independent of their adherence to formal regulatory criteria and guidelines. As a preliminary investigation of this issue, we have selected certificate of need and prospective reimbursement for further analysis. Specifically, do for-profit hospitals receive more than their fair share of tough treatment by regulatory authorities? Do hospitals with medical school affiliations receive favorable treatment? Although other forces affecting the neutrality of regulation are surely at work, our evaluation provides some tentative evidence.

Both CON and PR require the formation of judgments on the part of regulatory agency personnel. Certificate of need involves determinations of whether hospital capital expansion plans are consistent with community needs, which is *never* a totally unambiguous concept; PR generally involves determinations of the reasonableness of projected hospital expenditures, in addition to evaluating appeals for reimbursement of unexpected expenditure increases not allowed for prospectively. One might argue that this type of decision making should be much less likely under a formula than a budget PR system. However, formula systems require that hospitals be grouped and reimbursement rates be determined according to hospital performance relative to group norms, and hospitals must still contend with appeals processes. Thus, there is some room for nonneutrality of implementation even with formula PR.

Table 8–6 presents parameter estimates pertaining to interaction variables in TSCS input regressions. The interaction variables are computed as the products of regulation variables and binary hospital characteristics variables. To reduce the number of coefficients, we have combined new and mature CON programs. Thus, for example, NCON12 · PROP is the sum of NCON1 and NCON2 multiplied by PROP.[14] Because the variables from which these products are computed have been entered separately, the interaction coefficients measure the *additional* interaction effects between regulatory programs and hospital characteristics. If regulation is "unfair" in the ways just discussed, proprietary hospital regulation coefficients should be negative and their medical school affiliation counterparts positive.[15]

Even after some regulation variables are combined, the parameter estimates in table 8–6 are, in general, very difficult to interpret. On the whole, however, we find no support for the notion that regulatory bodies discriminate against proprietary hospitals or favor those with medical school affiliations. In fact, with regard to CON impact on bed expansion, we find a slight tendency in the opposite direction: all proprietary hospital coefficients are positive and teaching hospital coefficients negative. A plausible, but admittedly *ex post*, explanation of this finding is that because proprietaries are relatively fast responders to changing market circumstances, and teaching hospitals relatively slow, the coefficients reflect varying capabilities for anticipating implementation of CON.[16] However, we would not wish to push this interpretation too far. On the whole, there is very little consistency in the

Table 8-6
Time-Series Cross-Sectional Regression Coefficients—Interactions between Regulation and Hospital Characteristics

Variable	RNs per Bed	LPNs per Bed	Other Employees per Bed	Assets per Bed	Current Nonlabor Expenses per Bed	Beds
PRECON·PROP	-0.108*	-0.041	-0.037	0.384*	-0.082***	0.0088
	(0.038)[a]	(0.074)	(0.030)	(0.070)	(0.042)	(0.020)
PRECON·MEDSCH	0.036	0.055	0.016	0.017	0.0059	-0.013
	(0.022)	(0.043)	(0.017)	(0.041)	(0.025)	(0.012)
NCON12·PROP	-0.135**	0.086	-0.094**	-0.116	-0.148**	0.075**
	(0.055)	(0.102)	(0.042)	(0.111)	(0.059)	(0.035)
NCON12·MEDSCH	0.065*	0.084**	-0.0065	0.010	0.0070	-0.017
	(0.021)	(0.041)	(0.017)	(0.040)	(0.024)	(0.012)
CCON12·PROP	-0.130	-0.214	0.126	0.281	-0.0081	0.106***
	(0.116)	(0.221)	(0.090)	(0.215)	(0.127)	(0.060)
CCON12·MEDSCH	0.107*	0.069	0.014	0.063	0.036	-0.043**
	(0.034)	(0.065)	(0.027)	(0.063)	(0.038)	(0.019)
FPR·PROP	0.028	-0.071	-0.185	1.374*	0.167	-0.019
	(0.156)	(0.270)	(0.115)	(0.424)	(0.159)	(0.192)
FPR·MEDSCH	0.0055	-0.193	-0.033	-0.088	0.097	-0.024
	(0.090)	(0.160)	(0.068)	(0.216)	(0.094)	(0.077)
BPR·PROP	-0.063	0.479	-0.174	-0.224	-0.045	-0.093
	(0.220)	(0.412)	(0.169)	(0.429)	(0.238)	(0.132)
BPR·MEDSCH	-0.058	-0.097	-0.0050	-0.046	-0.067	-0.031
	(0.045)	(0.086)	(0.035)	(0.083)	(0.050)	(0.024)

*Significant at the 1% level (two-tailed test).
**Significant at the 5% level (two-tailed test).
***Significant at the 10% level (two-tailed test).
[a]Figures in parentheses are standard errors.

CON interaction results. We find both positive and negative coefficients scattered throughout, a distinct minority of which are statistically significant.

Our results with PR interactions support the same conclusion. Most of the coefficients for both proprietary and teaching hospitals are negative; however, all but one do not reach conventional levels of statistical significance. Moreover, the single significant parameter estimate, the FPR · PROP coefficient in the assets per bed regression, is unexpectedly positive and implausibly large. We are unable to explain this result, but nevertheless feel, on balance, that the general finding of no consistent relationship is warranted.

Dynamic Properties of the Model

Short-Run Responses

As specified, our input model allows the adjustment of one input in response to an exogenous change to affect the use of other inputs. Table 8–7 presents

Table 8–7
Direction Effect of Adjustment Coefficients

	Dependent Variables					
Lagged Variable	RNs per Bed	LPNs per Bed	Other Employees per Bed	Current Nonlabor Expenses per Bed	Assets per Bed	Beds[a]
RNs per bed (LAGRN)	0.72*	+*	−*	−*	−	0, −*
LPNs per bed (LAGLPN)	+*	0.70*	+	−*	+	0, −*
Other employees per bed (LAGOTH)	−*	−*	0.78*	−*	−	0, +*
Current nonlabor expense per bed (LAGEXP)	+**	+*	−	0.83*	−	0, +*
Assets per bed (LAGASS)	+	+	+	−*	0.60*	0, −
Beds (LAGBED)	−*	+	−*	−	−	0.46, 0.43*

*Significant at the 1% level (two-tailed test).

**Significant at the 5% level (two-tailed test).

***Significant at the 10% level (two-tailed test).

[a]The first and second columns of adjustment coefficients for beds pertain to the first and second TSCS regressions for beds, respectively, in table 8–2. See the text.

own–adjustment coefficients along the diagonal. The two coefficients for beds are taken from the two TSCS beds regressions in table 8–2. The own–adjustment coefficients have the same meaning that they would if each factor adjusted independently (as in the standard Koyck lag formulation). Each of these coefficients represents the proportion of dependent variable response to exogenous changes occurring in the first year. All own–adjustment coefficients are statistically significant, and the pattern of the coefficients is logical. Beds has the slowest speed of adjustment, followed by assets, labor inputs, and current nonlabor expenses.

To simplify table 8–7, only the signs of the cross–adjustment terms are shown. A plus sign indicates that excess demand for the input under the heading "Lagged Variable" increases the short-run demand for the input under the heading "Dependent Variable." Conversely, a minus sign indicates that a surfeit of the lagged variable input would lead to decreased demand for the dependent variable input in the short-run. By using the Nadiri and Rosen (1973) terminology, the inputs are "dynamic substitutes" in the short run if the sign is positive and "dynamic complements" if the sign is negative. Thirteen out of twenty cross-adjustment coefficients in the first four columns are statistically significant. The two sets of adjustment coefficients for beds in table 8–7 correspond to the two TSCS beds regressions in table 8–2, but cross-adjustment terms appear in only the second regression for beds. Four out of five of the adjustment coefficients in the beds column of table 8–7 are significant.

It is worth emphasizing that two inputs may be dynamic substitutes when the hospital is in a disequilibrium state, but complements in equilibrium. Whether inputs are substitutes or complements in the latter sense depends on the signs of coefficients on the cross-price (as opposed to the cross-adjustment) terms.

Our specification provides a technical foundation for questions often posed about markets for the health workforce. For example, there has been considerable policy discussion about a potential RN shortage and its consequences for employment of other hospital inputs and for delivery of health services generally.[17] According to table 8–7, additional LPNs would be hired in the short run in response to excess demand (a shortage) for RNs. The number of other (non-LPN) employees and beds (setup and staffed) would be reduced under such circumstances.

Almost as often as not, the cross–adjustment coefficients are asymmetric in terms of direction of effect. For example, excess demand for RNs leads to a temporary reduction in employment of current nonlabor inputs; by contrast, under conditions of excess demand for current nonlabor inputs (an unlikely situation), additional RNs would be demanded in the short run. Asymmetries of this sort may seem unlikely, but they cannot be ruled out a priori and may, in fact, be quite plausible in many cases.

Long-Run Responses

The dynamic model estimated is of the general form

$$Y_{it} = \beta A X_{it} + (I - \beta) Y_{it-1} \qquad (8.1)$$

By recursion, equation 8.1 becomes

$$Y_{it} = \beta A X_{it} + (I - \beta)\beta A X_{it-1} + (I - \beta)^2 \beta A X_{it-2} +$$
$$(I - \beta)^3 \beta A X_{it-3} + \cdots \qquad (8.2)$$

With four products on the right side, one obtains the response to an exogenous stimulus after four periods, with five products, five periods, and so on. Equilibrium responses are calculated from $[\,I - (\,I - \beta\,)\,]^{-1}\beta A$. The requisite information on βA and $I - \beta$ is supplied by tables 8–1 and 8–2.

With a single-equation Koyck lag structure, such as the one specified for our cost analysis, equilibrium responses are always greater than the initial (first-period) response. With the interdependent lag structure specified for our input analysis, responses need not increase monotonically from the initial reaction to equilibrium. Short-run excess demand for a factor which is not readily varied may, for example, lead to greater use of another factor than in equilibrium. Furthermore, sign reversals are possible—a positive impact multiplier does not necessarily imply positive longer-term and equilibrium responses.

With a data base spanning a period of six years, there is legitimate reason for concern that emphasis on equilibrium responses may be pushing our data too far. Hence, there is merit in examining responses for a shorter period. Furthermore, the political life of most policymakers may fall somewhat short of the time required for equilibrium to be reestablished. We have calculated responses after three years, after five years, and in equilibrium. The latter two sets of results are presented in tables 8–8 through 8–11. Three-year responses, not shown, in general fall somewhere between the one- and five-year responses. The odd-numbered tables, entitled "Simple Lag Structure," use parameter estimates from the first beds regression in table 8–2 and those from the TSCS regressions on other inputs in tables 8–1 and 8–2. The even-numbered tables, entitled "Complex Lag Structure," are based on the second beds regression in table 8–2 and the TSCS structural estimates for the other inputs. The latter specification is both more complex and more general.

Although we do not discuss individual parameters (except for examples), several general features of tables 8–8 through 8–11 are noteworthy. First, as anticipated, the response after a few years is generally much larger (in

Table 8–8
Response after Five Years—Simple Beds Lag Structure

Explanatory Variables	RNs per Bed	LPNs per Bed	Other Employees per Bed	Assets per Bed	Current Nonlabor Expenses per Bed	Beds
PERCAP	0.139	0.235	−0.013	1.333	−0.130	0.054
DENS	−0.012	−0.118	0.039	−0.044	0.039	0.025
POPMD	−0.026	0.024	0.020	0.104	−0.118	−0.022
GPPROP	−0.141	−0.257	−0.069	0.151	−0.143	−0.024
POPBD	−0.003	−0.011	0.017	−0.102	0.012	0.012
MCARE	−0.502	−0.038	0.116	−0.263	−0.189	0.154
MCAID	0.091	−0.098	0.020	0.091	−0.020	0.006
INS	−0.496	0.287	0.241	0.196	−0.087	0.151
RNWG	−1.197	−0.259	0.260	0.020	−0.020	0.000
LPNWG	−0.120	−2.007	−0.001	−0.039	0.101	0.000
OTHWG	−0.270	−0.337	1.035	−0.021	−0.689	0.000
CAP	0.023	0.025	0.020	1.033	−0.045	−0.138
CPI	0.036	0.040	−0.008	−0.008	0.714	0.000
RELRN	−0.096	0.782	0.796	0.863	−0.245	−0.254
RELLPN	0.251	0.076	−0.150	−0.534	0.097	0.181
RELOTH	0.190	−0.010	−0.018	0.743	1.044	−0.167
RELCAP	−0.593	−1.514	0.341	−0.024	−0.102	0.000
ASSETB	0.063	0.001	0.071	−0.003	−0.020	0.000
GOVT	−0.189	−0.016	0.156	−0.216	−0.087	−0.094
PROP	−0.614	−0.229	−0.195	−2.725	0.757	−0.580
MEDSCH	0.033	0.123	0.295	0.125	0.268	0.635
NURSCH	−0.068	−0.329	−0.069	−0.018	0.005	0.363
PRECON	−0.029	−0.029	−0.009	−0.033	−0.032	0.025
NCON1	0.006	0.020	0.068	−0.055	−0.002	−0.0001
NCON2	0.016	0.020	0.069	−0.078	−0.018	0.0007
CCON1	0.003	0.102	−0.055	−0.045	−0.048	0.042
CCON2	0.023	0.240	−0.040	−0.052	−0.066	0.022
S1122	0.228	0.467	0.107	−0.064	−0.123	−0.073
BCPAA	0.037	−0.075	0.114	0.185	−0.124	−0.036
FPR	−0.125	0.521	−0.047	0.112	−0.113	0.076
BPR	0.073	0.061	0.044	0.050	−0.135	0.010
UR	−0.209	0.193	−0.160	−0.226	−0.160	−0.085
COSTB	0.349	−0.321	−0.256	−0.197	0.181	−0.002
ESP	−0.023	−0.098	−0.078	−0.160	−0.036	0.015
TIME	0.084	0.078	−0.028	−0.060	0.211	0.000
CONST	1.518	1.807	−2.038	−0.164	0.108	1.279

absolute terms) than the initial response. For example, the PERCAP elasticity in the RNs per bed regression in table 8–1 is 0.039; in tables 8–8 and 8–9, which give five-year coefficients, the PERCAP elasticities are 0.139 and 0.140, respectively. Second, the five-year coefficients very often are larger than their equilibrium counterparts. Following the PERCAP example for RNs per bed, the equilibrium elasticity is close to the initial (one-year) response, but only about one-third the magnitude of the five-year elasticity.[18] Third, the largest differences between the odd- and even-

Table 8–9
Response after Five Years—Complex Beds Lag Structure

Explanatory Variables	RNs per Bed	LPNs per Bed	Other Employees per Bed	Assets per Bed	Current Nonlabor Expenses per Bed	Beds
PERCAP	0.140	0.233	−0.0098	1.336	−0.130	0.024
DENS	−0.012	−0.117	0.038	−0.044	0.039	0.031
POPMD	−0.026	0.024	0.019	0.103	−0.118	−0.008
GPPROP	−0.142	−0.255	−0.072	0.147	−0.142	0.004
POPBD	−0.003	−0.011	0.017	−0.101	0.012	0.011
MCARE	−0.505	−0.034	0.111	−0.270	−0.188	0.234
MCAID	0.091	−0.098	0.020	0.092	−0.020	0.005
INS	−0.496	0.286	0.243	0.197	−0.088	0.174
RNWG	−1.200	−0.256	0.256	0.014	−0.021	0.092
LPNWG	−0.121	−2.005	−0.003	−0.042	0.101	0.030
OTHWG	−0.281	−0.323	1.016	−0.046	−0.690	0.343
CAP	0.043	−0.008	0.064	1.083	−0.054	−0.510
CPI	0.038	0.037	−0.004	−0.002	0.714	−0.079
RELRN	−0.096	0.778	0.800	0.866	−0.249	−0.175
RELLPN	0.253	0.074	−0.147	−0.530	0.097	0.125
RELOTH	0.196	−0.017	−0.007	0.756	1.043	−0.315
RELCAP	−0.597	−1.509	0.333	−0.033	−0.103	0.135
ASSETB	0.062	0.002	0.070	−0.005	−0.020	0.019
GOVT	−0.195	−0.007	0.143	−0.232	−0.085	0.046
PROP	−0.614	−0.227	−0.197	−2.727	0.758	−0.597
MEDSCH	0.029	0.130	0.287	0.116	0.269	0.718
NURSCH	−0.073	−0.321	−0.080	−0.029	0.008	0.439
PRECON	−0.028	−0.030	−0.008	−0.031	−0.032	0.017
NCON1	0.006	0.021	0.068	−0.055	−0.002	0.012
NCON2	0.015	0.021	0.068	−0.079	−0.018	0.016
CCON1	0.004	0.101	−0.054	−0.044	−0.049	0.023
CCON2	0.023	0.239	−0.038	−0.051	−0.067	0.007
S1122	0.228	0.466	0.109	−0.063	−0.123	−0.073
BCPAA	−0.038	−0.072	0.111	0.181	−0.124	0.014
FPR	−0.125	0.522	−0.048	0.111	−0.113	0.083
BPR	0.072	0.061	0.043	0.048	−0.135	0.030
UR	−0.215	0.204	−0.175	−0.243	−0.157	0.033
COSTB	0.350	−0.322	−0.254	−0.194	0.182	−0.066
ESP	−0.022	−0.101	−0.075	−0.156	−0.036	−0.018
TIME	0.084	0.077	−0.027	−0.059	0.212	−0.021
CONST	1.575	1.735	−1.935	−0.033	0.108	−0.476

numbered tables 8–8 through 8–11 are in the beds column. Otherwise, the longer-run coefficients are quite stable between the two sets of tables. Fourth, there are some sign reversals as one extends the analysis beyond the immediate response. Since there are no standard errors around the estimates in tables 8–8 through 8–11, it is probably advisable to place greater reliance on the structural estimates in tables 8–1 and 8–2.

This last comment notwithstanding, there is some use in looking for sign reversals on the regulation variables, given both their policy relevance and

Table 8–10
Equilibrium Response—Simple Beds Lag Structure

Explanatory Variables	RNs per Bed	LPNs per Bed	Other Employees per Bed	Assets per Bed	Current Nonlabor Expenses per Bed	Beds
PERCAP	0.046	0.052	0.012	0.975	0.007	0.065
DENS	0.009	−0.054	0.020	−0.021	0.028	0.030
POPMD	−0.012	0.021	0.00039	0.068	−0.034	−0.026
GPPROP	−0.071	−0.128	−0.053	0.100	−0.100	−0.028
POPBD	0.004	0.00034	0.009	0.070	0.010	0.015
MCARE	−0.214	0.068	−0.007	−0.170	−0.067	0.185
MCAID	0.056	−0.062	0.025	0.074	0.014	0.007
INS	−0.221	0.240	0.038	0.159	0.036	0.180
RNWG	−0.571	0.065	−0.081	−0.017	−0.053	0.000
LPNWG	0.049	−1.032	0.012	0.022	−0.019	0.000
OTHWG	0.063	0.077	0.407	0.013	0.171	0.000
CAP	−0.018	−0.012	−0.015	0.714	0.004	−0.165
CPI	−0.009	−0.009	−0.00017	0.003	0.240	0.000
RELRN	−0.005	0.566	0.271	0.564	0.251	−0.304
RELLPN	0.130	−0.019	0.005	−0.338	0.010	0.217
RELOTH	0.031	−0.081	−0.008	0.517	0.364	−0.200
RELCAP	−0.167	−0.646	0.073	0.011	0.008	0.000
ASSETB	0.045	0.007	0.041	0.002	0.032	0.000
GOVT	−0.078	0.064	0.024	−0.182	−0.002	−0.113
PROP	−0.386	0.049	−0.246	−2.130	−0.034	−0.696
MEDSCH	0.119	0.047	0.219	0.259	0.294	0.761
NURSCH	0.014	−0.206	0.017	0.080	−0.004	0.435
PRECON	−0.010	−0.013	−0.004	−0.018	−0.017	0.030
NCON1	0.014	0.025	0.030	−0.037	0.028	−0.00017
NCON2	0.020	0.025	0.032	−0.054	0.024	0.00080
CCON1	−0.006	0.042	−0.018	−0.028	−0.034	0.050
CCON2	−0.002	0.117	−0.013	−0.040	−0.031	0.026
S1122	0.106	0.247	0.066	−0.065	−0.033	−0.087
BCPAA	−0.00017	−0.013	0.038	0.128	0.001	−0.043
FPR	−0.092	0.272	−0.038	0.078	−0.054	0.091
BPR	0.046	0.032	0.031	0.039	−0.014	0.012
UR	−0.146	0.118	−0.116	−0.206	−0.159	0.102
COSTB	0.158	−0.258	−0.047	−0.128	−0.014	−0.002
ESP	−0.013	−0.057	−0.032	−0.114	−0.052	−0.017
TIME	0.029	0.020	0.00045	−0.040	0.070	0.000
CONST	0.159	−0.099	−0.496	0.271	3.120	1.533

our statements about their effects earlier in this chapter. However, we find few worth mentioning. Two such reversals involve changes in sign of S1122 and BCPAA from negative in table 8–2 to positive in table 8–11, but the coefficients on these variables had very high standard errors in the first place. As a general statement, we believe we are justified in concluding that tables 8–8 through 8–11 strengthen our earlier statements on the effects of

Table 8–11
Equilibrium Response—Complex Beds Lag Structure

Explanatory Variables	RNs per Bed	LPNs per Bed	Other Employees per Bed	Assets per Bed	Current Nonlabor Expenses per Bed	Beds
PERCAP	0.045	0.053	0.011	0.973	0.0067	0.054
DENS	0.009	−0.054	0.020	−0.022	0.028	0.024
POPMD	−0.013	0.022	−0.00050	0.066	−0.034	−0.038
GPPROP	−0.069	−0.129	−0.051	0.103	−0.098	−0.00034
POPBD	0.004	0.00073	0.0086	−0.071	−0.0093	0.0056
MCARE	−0.213	0.067	−0.0057	−0.166	−0.066	0.210
MCAID	0.055	−0.061	0.024	0.072	0.013	−0.0099
INS	−0.224	0.243	0.034	0.152	0.033	0.123
RNWG	−0.571	0.065	−0.081	−0.018	−0.053	−0.0022
LPNWG	0.046	−1.031	0.0093	0.017	−0.021	−0.037
OTHWG	0.055	0.083	0.395	−0.0056	0.163	0.156
CAP	−0.046	0.010	−0.052	0.653	−0.021	−0.671
CPI	−0.0061	−0.011	0.0031	0.009	0.243	0.045
RELRN	−0.020	0.578	0.252	0.533	0.238	−0.565
RELLPN	0.131	−0.020	0.0066	−0.336	0.011	0.234
RELOTH	0.032	−0.082	−0.0066	0.520	0.365	−0.176
RELCAP	−0.170	−0.643	0.069	0.0037	0.0046	−0.062
ASSETB	0.044	0.0074	0.040	0.0011	0.031	−0.011
GOVT	−0.073	0.060	0.031	−0.172	0.0026	−0.025
PROP	−0.381	0.045	−0.240	−2.120	−0.030	−0.610
MEDSCH	0.124	0.043	0.227	0.272	0.299	0.866
NURSCH	0.023	−0.213	0.028	0.098	0.0041	0.588
PRECON	−0.011	−0.013	−0.0052	−0.020	−0.017	0.017
NCON1	0.013	0.025	0.029	−0.039	0.028	−0.014
NCON2	0.019	0.026	0.031	−0.056	0.024	−0.014
CCON1	−0.0057	0.042	−0.019	−0.028	−0.034	0.047
CCON2	−0.0025	0.117	−0.014	−0.041	−0.031	0.023
S1122	0.103	0.250	0.062	−0.072	0.030	−0.147
BCPAA	−0.00077	−0.012	0.037	0.127	0.00072	−0.054
FPR	−0.089	0.270	−0.035	0.083	−0.052	0.134
BPR	0.046	0.033	0.030	0.037	−0.015	−0.003
UR	−0.135	0.109	−0.102	−0.183	−0.150	0.093
COSTB	0.160	−0.259	−0.044	−0.123	−0.012	0.040
ESP	−0.015	−0.056	−0.034	−0.117	−0.053	−0.0068
TIME	0.031	0.019	0.0025	−0.0037	0.071	0.029
CONST	0.213	−0.141	−0.427	0.387	3.168	2.498

regulation since the coefficients are substantially larger. For example, the substitution of LPNs for RNs attributable to formula PR is much larger in tables 8–8 through 8–11 than in table 8–1.

Finally, we have ascertained whether the dynamic system, once displaced by an exogenous force, would, in fact, converge to a new set of equilibrium values. One way of examining this behavior is to compute the characteristic roots of $I - \beta$. We have calculated the characteristic roots corresponding to the above dynamic systems. All roots are below 1 in absolute value, a sufficient condition for dynamic stability.

Summary

In this chapter we present empirical results on determinants of variation in hospital employment of six inputs: RNs, LPNs, other employees, assets, current nonlabor purchases, and beds. Our findings are contained in eleven tables. Tables 8–1 and 8–2 present structural parameter estimates where the dependent variables (except for beds) are expressed in per-bed form. Tables 8–3, 8–4, and 8–5 give short-run impact multipliers, showing the total effects of the exogenous variables on per-hospital impact levels. Table 8–6 presents structural estimates of interactions between hospital characteristics and regulation variables to test for nonneutralities in regulatory program implementation. Dynamic relationships, indicating the effects of shortages or surpluses of one input on employment of the other inputs, are given in table 8–7. Finally, five–year and equilibrium effects of the explanatory variables on input employment are presented in tables 8–8 through 8–11.

As in chapter 7, the independent variables fall into four categories: product demand, factor price, hospital characteristics, and regulation and reimbursement variables. On the whole, our findings on inputs are consistent with the cost regressions in chapter 7 in most important respects. However, the input analyses provide some insights into hospital behavior not available from cost analysis alone.

Among the product demand variables, those pertaining to health insurance merit the most attention. Our private health insurance measure had a positive effect on all inputs except RNs (an anomalous result). The majority of short-run elasticities relating private health insurance to input use are in the 0.1 to 0.2 range, and some equilibrium elasticities are larger than this. Most of the Medicare and Medicaid variable coefficients are positive in the input regressions. But because there are several negative coefficients as well, the Medicare and Medicaid effects on hospital costs are clearer than those on inputs. Our insurance results are broadly consistent with the view that health insurance expansion increases input intensity in hospitals, but our estimates of specific effects on inputs are imprecise.

Personal per capita income generally has a positive impact on input employment, especially on some nonlabor inputs, but several insignificant coefficients were obtained. As with costs, the evidence does not suggest that variations in real per capita income were an important determinant of variations in input employment during the first half of the 1970s. Similarly, our findings do not indicate important effects of physician availability on input employment, but input intensity does tend to be lower in areas with high proportions of general practitioners.

Factor price effects on input employment in hospitals are consistent with the comparative statics predictions of chapter 2. Our factor price variables are necessarily crude, given the absence of ideal data, but the vast majority of own-price elasticities are negative.

Input use follows expected patterns with regard to hospital ownership and teaching status. Except for current nonlabor purchases, proprietary hospitals tend to use fewer inputs, with other factors held constant, and medical school–affiliated hospitals tend to use more inputs. Our analysis of inter-actions among the hospital characteristic variables and certificate-of-need and PR measures did not reveal the hypothesized negative proprietary hospital and positive medical school affiliation interactions. In fact, pro-prietary hospitals located in certificate-of-need states seem more likely to expand inputs than other hospitals.

In general, results on the influence of regulatory programs on input employment reinforce the findings in chapter 7 on costs. The regressions provide very little support for the view that these programs, as a group, have restrained input growth during the first half of the 1970s, and several perverse results were obtained.

Our analysis has considered three hospital investment control programs: state certificate-of-need laws, section 1122 of P.L. 92–603, and planning agency approval requirements instituted by some Blue Cross plans. The rationale for this form of regulation begins with the notion that certain areas are overbedded. We find no evidence that certificate of need has curtailed bed growth, and comprehensive programs (as defined in chapter 5) appear to have stimulated investment in hospital beds in some areas. The regressions indicate negative effects of the section 1122 and Blue Cross programs on bed expansion, but these are largely offset by positive effects on other inputs.

Results on our certificate-of-need variables indicate both anticipatory and compensatory hospital responses. With other factors held constant, bed growth is increased by 1.4 percent by anticipation of certificate of need in the year prior to implementation. The labor input regressions indicate that certificate of need tends to increase labor employment, an unintended compensatory effect of this type of regulation.

With the exception of RNs, the input regressions give no indication that formula PR has reduced hospital employment of inputs. This result is almost certainly influenced by the fact that the vast majority of our observations on formula PR pertain to hospitals in New York State only. Budget-based PR is far more common. In contrast to the cost regressions in chapter 7, the input regressions showed no constraining influence of this form of PR either. The Economic Stabilization Program had a slight negative effect on inputs. Although no impact on beds was obtained, which is not surprising given

ESP's rather short duration, we did find statistically significant negative effects on assets and current nonlabor purchases. Also ESP coefficients are negative in the labor input regressions, but statistically insignificant in two out of three cases.

In contrast to the simple Koyck lag structure specified for the cost analysis, the input model has a complex (but more flexible) lag structure in which excess demand for one input may lead to short-run substitutions of other inputs. This approach gives a technical meaning to *shortage* and *surplus*, terms that are used rather loosely in many health workforce discussions. Our empirical results on this topic, summarized in table 8–7, point to specific substitutions that hospitals tend to make when confronted with shortages of particular inputs.

Although much of our analysis has concentrated on short-run (one-year) effects of the explanatory variables on inputs, we have also calculated three-year, five-year, and equilibrium responses. In many instances the longer-run effects are larger (in absolute value) than the short-run effects, but this is not always so. Despite the flexibility of the input lag structure, there is only so much that can be gleaned from a time series of cross sections spanning six years. For this reason, estimates of the time shape of input responses should be interpreted cautiously. In any event, the length of the run in response times is not very important to policy implications—normally the direction of effect is far more important.

Notes

1. Substantial intraclass correlations (ρ) have been obtained in all input regressions, an indication that it is indeed important to use a procedure that removes time-invariant hospital or state effects. Estimated values of ρ are as follows: RNs per bed, 0.82; LPNs per bed, 0.78; other employees per bed, 0.80; net plant assets per bed, 0.93; current nonlabor expenses per bed, 0.79; and beds, 0.97. It is quite reasonable that estimated values of ρ for the fixed-capital equations (assets and beds) are relatively high because opportunities to vary capital are very limited in the short run.

2. See, for example, Sloan and Elnicki (1978).

3. For a recent review of these studies, see Hamermesh (1976).

4. For more discussion of this point, see Ehrenberg (1974).

5. See, for example, Davidson (1978).

6. Consider the position of hospital medical staff members who are frustrated by the hospital's inability, because of the presence of CON, to expand beds or to purchase complementary (to their practices) equipment. When queried, physicians often place good nursing service at the top of a list of items of great importance to them. To take nursing as an example, failure

to expand capital because of regulation can be compensated to some extent by improved nursing staffing. A cross-sectional study, based on 1973 data, found that certificate of need had a positive impact on hospital demand for nurses (Sloan and Elnicki 1978). The certificate-of-need coefficient was larger than its standard error, although it was insignificant at conventional levels.

7. For a policy discussion of the excess hospital capacity issue, see McClure (1976).

8. For summaries of evidence pertaining to prospective reimbursement, see Gaus and Hellinger (1976), Hellinger (1976b), and chapter 5 (of this book).

9. Because our data on formula PR pertain predominantly to New York State, past analysis of the New York system can be compared to our FPR results.

10. Abt Associates, Inc., and Policy Analysis, Inc. (1976) found evidence of a shift from RN to non-RN personnel in New York hospitals, although the shift was not pronounced.

11. Because the measure of assets per bed is generated from instruments pertaining primarily to the hospital's facilities-services mix (see Appendix C), it is possible that our result on assets per bed reflects our method of variable creation. These results conflict with those of Berry (1976), but there is reason to question Berry's use of Ohio hospitals as a control group. Moreover, the *ceteris paribus* assumption is difficult to make in one-way tabular analysis.

12. Ginsburg (1978) concluded that ESP reduced wages but not hospital costs. We believe, as noted in chapter 7, that the difference between our two studies lies in the fact that Ginsburg's analysis is in money and ours in real terms.

13. See, for example, May (1967) and Harmon (1977).

14. Recall that NCON1 and NCON2 represent mutually exclusive programs: Therefore NCON12 measures all noncomprehensive certificate-of-need programs. Because PROP and MEDSCH are unchanging over the six-year period, all variations in the interaction variables over time are due to initiation or expansion of regulatory programs.

15. Parameter estimates shown in table 8–6 are taken from regressions with all variables from table 8–1 and 8–2 included. However, tables 8–1 and 8–2, as presented, were estimated without the interaction variables.

16. For further discussion of proprietary hospital responsiveness to changing market conditions, see Steinwald and Neuhauser (1970) and Kushman and Nuckton (1977).

17. Sloan (1975) provides considerable information and analysis of alleged RN shortages based on a survey of hospital directors of nursing conducted at the University of Florida in 1973. The survey included

questions about employment of other hospital inputs in response to perceived RN shortages.

18. We do not wish to imply that year-by-year differences in the elasticity estimates are enormously significant in a policy framework. In the case of the effect of PERCAP on RNs per bed (and in other cases as well), one's advice to a policymaker is not very different if the estimated elasticity is 0.14 or 0.04. Irrespective of the table used, the results imply that per capita income makes some difference in hospital employment of RNs, but not a great deal of difference.

9 Summary, Conclusions, and Implications: Conceptual and Institutional Considerations

In chapters 1 and 6 we presented descriptive evidence on hospital costs, outputs, and input use over the 1970–1975 period. This period was characterized as one of moderate increases in hospital outputs (in terms of patients treated and days of care), substantial increases in gross labor and nonlabor inputs, and alarming increases in costs. Because it inspires policy interest, hospital cost inflation is a motivating force behind this book. One can learn most about this complex inflationary process by identifying its important elements and discovering how they are jointly determined to arrive at the bottom line of increases in hospital costs per admission and per adjusted patient-day. This is why we have devoted considerable attention to hospital input choices in addition to costs.

The 1970–1975 period is well suited for this type of research. Unlike the late 1960s, this period was not dominated by a single event, that is, implementation of the Medicare and Medicaid programs. Yet, 1970 to 1975 was an active period in terms of external forces affecting hospitals, especially the formation and implementation of regulatory programs at the state level. Most of our exogenous explanatory variables exhibit considerable cross-sectional and intertemporal variation. The trends and events occurring during the period and captured, at least in part, by our empirical analysis are ones that are likely to continue or to be replicated in one form or another in the future. For this reason, our findings are relevant to current policy deliberations about the hospital industry.

By and large, this book is empirical rather than theoretical. However, during initial phases of our research, we devoted considerable attention to models of hospital behavior with the hope that this work would improve our empirical specification as well as our interpretation of findings. Conceptual research on hospitals has a long history, and there are several alternative frameworks from which to choose. One important conceptual issue is whether it makes sense to postulate a single decisionmaker for the hospital. Compared to most alternatives, single-decisionmaker models, preferred by the vast majority of economists, are much more easily formalized (cast in mathematical terms). However, as chapter 2 emphasized, there are numerous offsetting effects, even in static models of hospital behavior. When one considers dynamics, as one must for a complete understanding of hospital responses to regulation and other exogenous forces, matters become even more complex.

As seen in the summary tables of chapter 2, only a few unambiguous predictions can be derived from economic theorizing on hospitals; and, to adequately understand hospital behavior, one must leave the chalkboard behind and engage in comprehensive empirical research. Yet, it is useful to know what *cannot* be predicted. Further, to readers who view formal modeling as a strictly academic exercise, we emphasize that formalization is a means of making underlying assumptions and implicit deductive processes explicit. Even though one can easily generate predictions from feelings or commonsense reasoning, ambiguities in the theory should serve as a warning that the hospital decision-making process is too complex to expect such predictions to be reliable.

In some cases it is not necessary to rely on theory to generate hypotheses. For example, from the standpoint of public policy, various regulatory programs are intended to constrain the growth in hospital costs. The null hypothesis that specific regulatory programs have no effect is tested against the alternative outcomes of the (desired) negative effects on costs or perverse positive effects. Theory may be helpful, but it is not essential to formulating these empirical questions. Results of past studies, anecdotal evidence, and conventional wisdom also provide foundations for constructing hypotheses regarding effects of external factors on hospital behavior.

Our institutional descriptions have emphasized third-party reimbursement (chapter 4) and regulation (chapter 5) because a thorough background in these two areas is essential to a full understanding of current issues relating to hospital decision-making as well as outcomes in this sector. We suspect that most serious observers of hospitals would concur with this view; yet, for reasons discussed throughout this book, relatively little concrete evidence exists on the systematic effects of these forces on hospital behavior.

The thrust of chapter 4 was toward developing a private health insurance depth-of-coverage variable for our empirical analysis, and institutional descriptions and findings were largely by-products. Our investigation of health insurance premiums revealed that generosity of hospital inpatient benefits was a major determinant of premium levels, but we were unable to detect systematic influences of factors related to premium loading. In general, despite some thought-provoking and sometimes controversial past empirical research on this topic, health insurance plan administration and insurer-hospital interactions remain very much a "black box" in research on hospital behavior. Our empirical work on health insurance demand identified several characteristics of household heads and geographic areas that influence the likelihood of having private coverage and the amount of insurance once coverage is obtained. Because these results are not central to our primary analyses and were summarized at the end of chapter 4, we do not review them further.

Chapter 5 contained detailed discussions of institutions and findings from studies on the effects of hospital regulation. We identified regulatory programs as falling into three broad categories: investment controls, reimbursement controls, and utilization-quality controls. Despite the fact that the third category has the longest and most diverse history of the three types, attention was focused on the first two categories, which have experienced the greater amount of measurable activity in recent years. Our discussion of regulatory programs was oriented toward the development of variables for empirical testing of hypotheses in chapters 7 and 8.

Background discussions indicated that the development of hospital investment controls is very much tied to the health planning movement in the United States. Such controls, including certificate-of-need and P.L. 92–603, section 1122, programs, represent major attempts to implement "planning with teeth." Proponents of this form of regulation regard it as a most effective cost containment device; unneeded investments are simply disallowed, or their associated current expenses are not compensated under major third-party reimbursement programs. The literature abounds with both enthusiastic endorsement and profound skepticism regarding the ability of planning agencies to implement investment controls fairly and effectively.

Several new regulatory programs use hospital reimbursement as a regulatory tool to control hospital rates, revenues, and both capital and current expenditures. The ultimate in this form of regulation is direct rate setting by an independent authority, a concept which has some support; but by far the most popular program is PR. Prospective reimbursement has graduated from the experimental to the mandatory stage in a growing number of states. There are far more budget-based systems than formula-based ones, largely, it appears, because hospitals, when given a choice, tend to prefer the former version of PR. Prospective reimbursement has been "sold," in part, on the grounds of cost-reducing incentives, but such incentives generally cannot be demonstrated theoretically and are not apparent intuitively when the effects of present costs on future prospective rates are considered. Furthermore, empirical studies of PR before ours revealed mixed outcomes at best. Nevertheless, PR, like certificate of need, represents an attempt to "do something positive" to combat hospital cost inflation and has many enthusiastic supporters, particularly in government.

The major current effort at utilization-quality control is the PSRO program, which we unfortunately were unable to incorporate into our empirical analyses. Utilization review, a concept that has existed in the hospital sector for several decades and which has many variants, is a key component of the PSRO program. The very limited inferences that we can draw about PSRO from our empirical analysis are based on meager data pertaining to UR programs operated by Medicaid and Blue Cross. In terms of cost containment, the literature is generally even less optimistic regarding the impact of PSRO than other major current efforts, such as certificate of need and prospective reimbursement. Yet, in contrast to these programs, PSRO is involved more intimately with the resource allocation decisions of physicians in hospitals. Many experts feel that the ability to intervene in or otherwise influence such decisions is a *sine qua non* for effective hospital cost containment. We have more to say about the hospital-physician nexus below.

In looking at hospital regulation as a whole, it is clear that most current programs have their modern origins in the rather turbulent period immediately following implementation of Medicare and Medicaid. All such programs have hospital cost inflation as a chief motivating influence, even though this problem is attacked from several different directions. Existing evidence, often fragmentary, gives little reason to regard any particular form of regulation, or regulation per se, as "the answer" to hospital cost inflation. The next section includes a review of the contribution of this book to this evidence, which tends to support this overall conclusion.

Empirical Findings

To a considerable extent, rapidly rising hospital costs during the 1970s reflect input price inflation, especially in nonlabor inputs. As stated in earlier chapters and documented more completely in Sloan and Steinwald (1980), real wages of hospital employees rose modestly during the 1970s, and one can find periods in recent years during which real wages have actually declined. From the standpoint of the hospital industry, cost increases attributable to input prices are far more defensible politically than those due to expanded input employment. In this regard, the 1970s can hardly be called a period of retrenchment for the hospital industry as a whole. In our cohort of 1,228 hospitals, beds increased an average of 7 percent over 1970 to 1975, and measurable nonbed inputs, including employees per bed, all displayed increases; RNs, a relatively expensive labor input, increased, on average, 26 percent per hospital.

The growth in current nonlabor inputs over 1970–1975 was even more dramatic. Measured in real (consumer price index) dollar terms, this class of inputs increased an average of 42 percent per bed in our sample hospitals. It may be legitimately argued (see chapter 1) that our price deflator results in an overstatement of growth in real nonlabor inputs over our study period. But, if any reasonable price deflator is used, this growth was substantial.

In recent years, economists have often attributed increases in hospital costs in general and input use in particular to developments on the demand side for the hospital's product (for example, Feldstein 1971b). Underlying the notion that demand factors are responsible is the idea that invention and innovation, especially the latter, do not occur at random, but are somehow responsive to the patient's ability to pay. Associated with innovation are vast expenditures on both capital and workforce. The fact that improved financing mechanisms, including Medicare and Medicaid, have led to better patient access to hospital care is generally regarded as socially desirable. Yet, given the open-ended nature of public financing, such programs have also contributed greatly to inflation in hospital expenditures.

Debates about the relative importance of "demand-pull" versus "cost-push" hospital cost inflation[1] are pertinent to public policy. The relative weight one places on each side of the argument has a definite bearing on the attractiveness of alternative public policies to contain hospital costs. Yet it is essential to remember that times change. For example, the fact that demand-pull inflation characterized the 1960s does not necessarily make it true, at least to the same degree, in the 1970s. The first half of the 1970s saw a relatively low growth in real personal per capita income, and no new public health insurance programs were introduced. However, during the 1970s, private health insurance coverage grew at a steady pace, especially for physicians' and other nonhospital services. The 1970s also saw a substantial growth in the physician-population ratio, a continued decline in the proportion of general practitioners, a rather dramatic growth in hospital regulation, and an increase in unionization, which, as documented in Sloan and Steinwald (1980), had a positive impact on hospital wages.

Despite the differences between the 1960s and the 1970s, we do find that selected demand factors influenced hospital costs and input choices in the 1970s. In our analyses, real per capita income shows an important positive effect on assets per bed and, to a much lesser extent, on hospital demand for labor. Bed expansion is less responsive to changes in income than either assets per bed or labor. We are unable to say much about the impact of income on hospital costs because of collinearity between per capita income and the hospital wage variable in our hospital cost regressions.

We have devoted extensive effort to developing a private health insurance coverage variable because even quasi-adequate measures for small geographic areas are unavailable from other sources. Clearly, given the policy importance of health insurance, the absence of accurate data for research and/or policy purposes is regrettable. Because construction of this variable involved a somewhat complex and indirect estimation method, conclusions regarding the effects of private insurance should be considered tentative. But our caution is more with regard to precise magnitudes of effect than with our general finding that insurance coverage is an important determinant of variations in hospital costs and input employment. Further, the insurance premium regressions in chapter 4 are sufficiently plausible to merit confidence that the variable does indeed measure small-area variations in coverage.

With one exception, our private health insurance variable demonstrated a positive impact on our hospital cost measures with implied short-run and long-run elasticities as high as 0.2 and 0.3, respectively. Effects on hospital input employment were also shown to be positive, with the exception of professional nurses. We are not able to explain the anomaly in the RN equation. With regard to inputs, the largest impact by far was on assets, where the short-run elasticity was 0.17 (table 8-3). Elasticities for other inputs, which with the exception of RNs are in the 0.1 range, are by no means trivial. We conclude from this evidence that private health insurance coverage has stimulated hospital costs in general and input use in particular, and the implied elasticities are sufficiently large for policymakers to take note.

We have also assessed the effects of public insurance, both Medicare and Medicaid, on the dependent variables. In this case, variable construction has been much more straightforward, but, given available data, it is impossible to separate demographic from reimbursement influences. After all, Medicare eligibles are also elderly, and Medicaid recipients are also poor. In both cases, we know that age and income-wealth status affect hospital utilization patterns independent of any effects reimbursement might have. As reported in chapter 7, both public insurance variable coefficients are positive in our cost regressions and generally statistically significant at the 1 percent level.

Parameter estimates on our Medicare and Medicaid variables in the input regressions in chapter 8 are unstable. We detected a positive impact of Medicare on beds and a negative impact on RNs per bed, as well as a positive impact of Medicaid on RNs and assets per bed and a negative impact on LPNs per bed. One can easily devise a plausible *ex post* explanation of this pattern, incorporating both reimbursement and demographic effects. But to truly understand the impact of Medicare and Medicaid on hospital input decisions, it is necessary to develop more fine-tuned measures that allow one to separate reimbursement from demographic influences.

As a result of rapid expansion in government support of medical education and the influx of foreign medical school graduates in recent years, the physician-population ratio has increased dramatically. At the same time, the proportion of general practitioners (GPs) to all physicians has fallen. Since physicians are the gatekeepers in the sense that they admit patients to hospitals and have important roles in hospital decision making, it is reasonable to hypothesize a link between physician availability and various indicators of hospital performance. Our regressions have included measures of physician availability and the proportion GPs in the hospital's county. Of the two variables, the GP proportion is much more important. Not surprisingly, where GPs are relatively numerous, hospital costs per unit of output are lower, as is usually the case with input employment. To the extent that programs aimed at increasing the proportion of physicians engaged in primary care succeed, this may be one of the more positive developments in terms of hospital cost containment. Of course, if the case for primary-care doctors is used as a justification for expanding medical school enrollments, some of the hospital cost savings may be lost.

Considerable attention has been devoted in this book to the measurement of input prices. Unfortunately, given data constraints, our input price variables are necessarily crude. Nevertheless, the fact that virtually all own-input price effects are negative is certainly consistent with the view that hospitals tend to take input prices into account when deciding how much of a specific input to purchase. The magnitudes of own-price effects may be important in other contexts, such as in evaluating the employment effects of a government wage subsidy to firms for hiring the long-term unemployed; however, no such policies are likely to be considered for hospitals in the foreseeable future.

We deemphasized the estimated cross-price effects on input employment in chapter 8; instead, we preferred to concentrate on interrelationships among the inputs in a dynamic sense. Our specification permits a technical interpretation of some statements often made in the health field about the effects of input shortages on the utilization of other hospital inputs. Since the accompanying table (table 8–7) is needed to adequately review these findings, we refer the interested reader to chapter 8. This aspect of our research should be of particular interest to policymakers with responsibilities for health workforce planning.

Our empirical findings pertaining to hospital unionization are confined to the cost analysis presented in chapter 7. As of 1976, 23 percent of all U.S. hospitals had a least one union contract (Frenzen 1978). Given the 1974 amendments to the National Labor Relations Act extending coverage to nonprofit hospitals, this proportion may well rise much further. As stated earlier, a common argument in favor of unions is that their natural tendency to increase wages is offset by productivity improvements and reductions in labor-management costs. If this is true, however, our cost regressions certainly do now show it. The union coefficients are positive and statistically significant without exception. Short-run labor cost responses to acquiring an active union (one willing to engage in strikes or other job actions) are in the 12 to 15 percent range. Equilibrium cost responses are higher than this. The recent amendments may have had political benefits at the time they were passed, but their implications for hospital cost inflation, based on our results, are not encouraging.

Our evidence suggests that, as a group, regulatory programs did not do much to contain hospital costs during the first half of the 1970s. Results on the regulation variables are too numerous to repeat in full; we prefer that readers consult chapters 7 and 8 for particulars. Here we limit the discussion to major findings.

A major effort has been devoted in this book to assessing the effects of certificate-of-need laws on hospital costs and input employment. According to the program's intent, CON should have a negative impact on hospital costs; but on conceptual grounds and from past research, there is good reason to doubt this. We find that, if anything, CON has raised costs per admission and per patient-day, especially the noncomprehensive programs, as we have defined them.

On inputs, we find both an anticipatory effect on bed growth and a compensatory response on labor employment. Hospitals seem to recognize when CON is coming and initiate bed construction earlier than they would have in the absence of this form of regulation. Even if CON is eventually successful in impeding bed growth, it should take some time to offset this anticipatory effect in terms of the number of new beds constructed. We have virtually no information on the long-run "threat effects" of regulation of this sort, but major capital expansion programs clearly span several years from inception to completion. Therefore, some additions to hospital beds, generated by the prospect of future regulation, may not be manifested until long after implementation of a CON program. The solution to this problem is unclear; it is unlikely that "surprise" regulation is a politically viable concept, and in any case, development of CON programs in states which currently do not have them should not surprise anyone, especially since P.L. 93-641 requires states to do so.

The compensatory response on hospital demand for labor, in addition to the anticipatory effect on beds noted above, casts considerable doubt on the usefulness of calculations of CON's effectiveness based on the dollar value of applications disapproved by CON agencies, an approach used by the Health Resources Administration. This method results in an *underestimate* of CON effectiveness in the sense that certain capital projects may be canceled before the hospital even applies. However, anticipatory effects on bed growth, "grandfathering," and compensatory effects on hospital demand for labor mean that such measures *overstate* CON's cost-reducing impact. Our parameter estimates suggest that the discouragement phenomenon is not very important, but the other effects are clearly present.

Other forms of capital-facilities regulation are the section 1122 and Blue Cross planning agency approval programs. Overall, we found that section 1122 has no impact on costs, while the Blue Cross program has small negative effects. In terms of effects on inputs, the section 1122 and Blue Cross programs do not show some of the undesirable features implied by CON's parameter estimates. In both cases, we found negative effects on bed expansion. Section 1122, when implemented by the states, appears to reduce plant asset growth; however, the Blue Cross program has a positive impact on assets. Section 1122 controls show a positive effect on hospital labor, while the Blue Cross program's effects on labor is either negative or nil. In sum, although there are some encouraging signs in the results on these two types of capital-facilities regulation, the overall conclusion must be that no sizable cost reductions are attributable to these programs either.

The descriptive evidence and parameter estimates on ESP, the most comprehensive of the regulatory programs studied, do indicate a slowdown in total cost increases and input employment expansion during the ESP period. This type of global approach to hospital cost containment may not represent an effective long-term solution to inflation in this sector, but it is worth emphasizing that this is one of the few programs implemented to date which clearly has reduced hospital costs and the use of some inputs. The descriptive evidence shows ESP in a more favorable light than does the multivariate evidence. In general, we prefer to rely on the latter type of analysis because it provides a means for holding other variables constant. But certainly the tabulations are impressive and should not be rejected out of hand.

Past research, on the whole, has failed to show that prospective reimbursement contains hospital costs. Our findings also suggest that PR has, at best, a very small negative effect on costs and input use. All we can say is that PR, as currently constituted, has not proved itself to be an effective inflation strategy, and current reliance on PR to hinder future hospital cost increases may be unjustified. Formula PR seems promising, at least on paper, but based on our empirical results, it does not appear to be superior to budget-review PR. Isolated results, such as the substitution of LPNs for RNs attributable to formula PR, are encouraging, but too many coefficients suggest that PR has no impact or even stimulates costs and input employment for us to interpret the weight of the evidence any other way. Still more stringent forms of prospective reimbursement may be effective, but we can only assess empirically what can be observed. As more states adopt PR, more conclusive evaluations of this form of regulation will be possible. Furthermore, some programs may improve with age because PR regulators learn by doing. Preliminary evidence, based on state-level data, presented in a recent report by the Congressional Budget Office (1979), suggest this may be so, but further research is clearly needed.

Given the period covered by our empirical analysis, it has not been possible to assess effects on hospitals of the PSRO program. Analysis of Medicaid and Blue Cross utilization review programs has been undertaken here. We found that these programs have no impact on total expense per adjusted patient-day, but the UR variable had a negative impact on total expense per admission with an associated t value greater than 1. On inputs, all UR impact multipliers, with one exception, were negative. These results suggest that UR may have some cost-reducing influence; however, in view of some of the perverse incentives that utilization reviewers face (Havighurst and Blumstein 1975), we would want to see more evidence before strongly advocating these programs.

As in previous studies, we have evaluated potential inflationary effects of the cost-based reimbursement method. Our evidence is in agreement with past findings that the cost- versus charge-based reimbursement distinction is not important to understand why hospital costs vary. We feel it is time to put this issue to rest; other issues related to third-party reimbursement are far more important.

Dynamic versions of both cost and input equations have been estimated. Parameter estimates on the lagged dependent variables in the cost regressions imply that the effects of changes in the exogenous variables are realized reasonably quickly (over 60 percent in the first year). Because of the estimation technique used in this book, we place more confidence in our estimates of speed of the cost response than in similar estimates reported in past studies. Because the lag structure in our input analysis is far more complex, few, if any, summary statements on input response lags are possible. It is worth emphasizing, however, that the effects of exogenous variables may rise over time and then fall because of a tendency to use inputs in the short run that are readily adjusted.

Early economic studies of hospital costs assessed the existence of economies of scale. After it became evident that parameter estimates alone do not take one very far toward understanding what the optimal size of a hospital truly is, researchers changed their emphasis. Yet this book would not be complete without some reference to scale economies. In our work, estimates of scale economies depend on whether adjusted patient-days or admissions are used as the hospital's output measure. Regressions with adjusted patient-days as the cost deflator imply scale economies, while the reverse is true for regressions based on costs per admission. It would appear that this issue may never be settled, and fortunately it is not a very important one.

Implications

A major policy issue is whether cost increases in hospitals are predominantly due to external forces or to lack of internal cost-consciousness. The evidence supports both points of view to some extent. Certainly, hospital cost inflation is largely a by-product of the general state of the economy during the 1970s. Despite the fact that hospital price increases have been consistently above similar increases in the CPI, inflation in the hospital sector would probably not appear so alarming if the 1970s had not been an inflationary period generally. Moreover, we do observe that hospitals tend to reduce use of an input as its price rises relative to other input prices. Yet, at the same time, hospitals expanded inputs per unit of output during the 1970s. Despite the inflationary times, the trend toward constant upgrading appears to have continued unabated. In addition, although we have not presented much anecdotal evidence on hospital inefficiency, such evidence exists and commands considerable policy interest.[2]

Throughout this book we have referred to inputs per unit of output, measured in terms of cases treated or adjusted patient-days, as service intensity. Some readers may have noticed that this bypasses a very difficult but important issue, that of explicitly defining hospital output and quality. Clearly, a hospital admission or adjusted patient-day is not a constant entity over time, and oft-cited inflation rates fail to adequately account for changes in the nature of the hospital product. Underlying much of the concern over inflation is a tacit consensus that improvements in the hospital product are not worth the price. After all, if greater service intensity in hospitals meant substantially increased cure rates or enhancement of other benefits of medical care, increases in real hospital expenditures might be seen as cause for celebration that more resources were being channeled into an especially productive industry. But this is not a widely held view; in fact, several experts (for example, Carlson 1975; Illich 1976) have quite forcefully expressed the opinion that medical advances at present do very little to improve the health status of the populace.

The other side of this issue is that service intensity often is equated with quality of hospital care. Because quality is difficult to explicitly define and measure, service intensity is often used as a proxy. Moreover, it is widely felt that hospitals devoting relatively large numbers of resources to the production of cases treated or adjusted patient-days tend to be the highest quality hospitals. Very few critics of hospital cost inflation are willing to cite quality as a target for cost-reducing initiatives. Proponents of regulation are far more comfortable with the view that waste and inefficiency alone are the sources of cost problems. This view is somewhat naïve, because it is seldom possible to determine where quality enhancement ends and waste begins and because it sidesteps the very real policy issue of quality-cost tradeoffs.[3] The problem of controlling hospital costs would be illuminated considerably if it were universally recognized that any effective cost-reducing course of action is likely to have some depressing effects on service intensity or quality, and, further, quality reduction is an entirely appropriate strategy *if* we have reached the point where the marginal social costs of increasing hospital quality exceed the associated marginal social benefits.

Historically, planning and regulation have been allies rather than adversaries to quality in health, as in other industries. As stated in chapter 5, many studies of regulated industries have concluded that quality tends to be too high, gauged in terms of social costs versus benefits. The current conventional wisdom about the PSRO program—that it was begun as a cost control initiative but has evolved into a quality enhancement program—is somewhat foreboding. And we cannot help being swayed by the substantial evidence that regulatory agencies are subject to "capture" by regulated industries. At present, there is sufficient ostensible conflict between regulatory agencies and hospitals to doubt that capture has systematically taken place, and our limited analysis of interactions between hospital characteristics and controls revealed no conclusive evidence of favoritism in application of regulatory programs. Yet this phenomenon bears watching in future evaluations.

Our lack of evidence of desirable regulatory effects is disturbing given the magnitude of the regulatory movement during the 1970s. One has only to look at our appendix tables on regulatory program growth to see how rapidly the states adopted controls on hospital behavior during this period. Not shown in the tables are the creation and growth of agencies responsible for implementing the PSRO program and the network of health systems agencies created under P.L. 93-641. To some, this movement is cause for enthusiasm that significant measures are being taken to control hospital costs. To us, the creation of a vast and expensive bureaucracy, without strong theoretical or empirical reasons to believe that these programs will be able to fulfill their missions, is somewhat ominous. We hope that state and federal policymakers will be cautious and attentive to evidence when considering continuance, implementation, and expansion of hospital controls in the future.

As stated earlier, our analysis focuses on responses of individual hospitals rather than hospital service markets. A full analysis of regulatory impact requires measurement of exit, entry, merger activity, and distribution of hospital resources within communities. This is particularly important in the case of hospital investment controls. Do such regulations cause inefficient hospitals to seek mergers or exit from the market? How do they affect entry and propensity toward development of shared services and similar arrangements? Research of this type may have a greater payoff than further microeconomic analysis of regulatory effects on individual hospitals.

A direction toward cost containment that has not been given much active attention involves influencing the physician decision-making process in hospitals. "Every industry has its problems, but nobody else has doctors" is a sentiment that has been stated many times in many different ways.[4] Physicians make many of the resource allocation decisions in hospitals, but seldom do they, or their patients, directly bear many of the financial consequences of these decisions. It is part of the conventional wisdom that much of inflation in hospital expenditures can be traced to this simple fact.[5] Yet, for the purpose of cost control, regulators have not had much success in confronting this decision-making process directly. One of the oft-cited advantages of such programs as CON and PR is that they give cost-conscious hospital administrators leverage in their dealings with medical staff members (see, for example, Altman and Weiner 1978). While this may be true, empirical evidence is currently lacking.

These points do not readily lead to suggestions for new regulatory interventions, particularly in an area where a great deal of resistance can be expected. It may be that if HMOs are ever able to gain a substantial market share of hospital services, some of the inflationary pressure attributable to physician control of hospital resources may be lessened. Also, the PSRO program, once fully implemented, may be able to interject more cost controls than presently exist. But the fact is that we do not know very much about the determinants of physician effects on hospital costs. Very little rigorous theoretical or empirical research has been done on this subject,[6] but it represents one of the potentially most fertile areas in health services research.[7] If systematic associations between medical staff characteristics and hospital performance can be discovered, new policy approaches toward cost containment may emerge. This is not to minimize the political difficulties of implementing public programs that may threaten physicians' incomes and/or power base in the health care industry.

Our prognosis for hospital cost inflation is mixed. We have noted that inflation in this sector is tied in part to the general state of the economy. If federal efforts to control inflation are successful (or if inflation abates on its own), we may expect some fortuitous consequences for the hospital industry. Moreover, as some of the rough edges are worn off relatively new hospital cost control programs, perhaps some evidence of desirable effects will materialize. On the negative side, we do not see much in the way of trends in important explanatory variables to suggest a reduction in inflation. Our evidence of the effects of unions on hospital costs is foreboding, as is the decline of the general practitioner. We can expect additional inflationary pressures on hospitals from these sources in the future.

Notes

1. See Davis (1973) for a summary of these arguments.

2. Anecdotal evidence probably attracts more attention than is warranted. One really cannot tell much about systematic influences on hospital costs and the need for regulation based on isolated instances of waste. For this reason, such evidence has been deemphasized in this book.

3. For a detailed discussion of the quality-cost trade-off, see Havighurst and Blumstein (1975).

4. Quoted without source in Cunningham (1976, p. 61).

5. The extensive literature on prepaid group practice and HMOs, for example, contains detailed discussions and empirical evidence on this issue. A seminal article is by Monsma (1970), and there are many others. This is one of the few areas in health services research where theory and empirical evidence are strongly consistent. And such evidence undoubtedly underlies the opinion of some experts (for example, Havighurst 1973b; Enthoven 1978a, 1978b) that expansion of HMOs is a desirable market-oriented method of combating hospital cost inflation.

6. Exceptions are Pauly and Redisch (1973) and Pauly (1978).

7. In keeping with this view, the authors are currently engaged in research to determine the effects of physician market and medical staff characteristics on hospital costs under Grant No. 18-P-97090/4 from the Health Care Financing Administration to Vanderbilt University. The need for research in this area has been recently emphasized by Fuchs and Newhouse (1978).

Appendix A:
Variable Definitions and
Data Sources

Table A–1

Variable Name[a]	Definition	Source
	Dependent Variables—Inputs	
RNBED	FTE[b] RNs per hospital bed	AHA annual surveys
LPNBED	FTE LPNs per hospital bed	AHA annual surveys
OTHBED	FTE other employees per hospital bed (excludes RNs, LPNs, trainees, and employed MDs)	AHA annual surveys
ASSETB	Net plant assets per bed index, deflated (see Appendix C)	AHA annual surveys
NLEXP	Other nonpayroll expenses per bed, deflated (excludes fringe benefits, interest expense, and depreciation expense)	AHA annual surveys
BDTOT	Total hospital beds (includes long-term-care beds, excludes bassinets)	AHA annual surveys
	Dependent Variables—Costs	
EXPAPD	Total expense per adjusted patient-day, deflated	AHA annual surveys
EXPADM	Total expense per admission, deflated	AHA annual surveys
LABAPD	Labor expense per adjusted patient-day, deflated	AHA annual surveys
LABADM	Labor expense per admission, deflated	AHA annual surveys
	Own Price Variables	
RNWG	Estimated area hourly wage for RNs, deflated (see Appendix D)	U.S. Bureau of the Census (1970); U.S.
LPNWG	Estimated area hourly wage for LPNs, deflated (see Appendix D)	Bureau of Labor Statistics (1971, 1974, 1975, 1976); U.S. Bureau of Health Resources Development (1974)
OTHWG	Estimated area hourly wage for other employees, deflated (see Appendix E)	AHA annual surveys
CAP	National estimate of price of capital, deflated (see Appendix G)	U.S. Bureau of the Census (1976)
COL72	Area cost-of-living index for an intermediate-budget family of four, expressed in 1972 dollars (see Appendix B)	U.S. Department of Labor (1974, 1975)
	Relative Input Price Variables[c]	
RELRN	= RNWG/X; X = LPNWG, OTHWG, CAP, or COL72	See above
RELLPN	= LPNWG/X; X = RNWG, OTHWG, CAP, or COL72	See above

Table A–1 *(continued)*

Variable Name[a]	Definition	Source
RELOTH	= OTHWG/X; X = RNWG, LPNWG, CAP, or COL 72	See above
RELCAP	= CAP/X; X = RNWG, LPNWG, or OTHWG	See above

Demand Variables

PERCAP	Per capita income, by county, deflated	U.S. Bureau of Health Manpower (1976); Sales Management, Inc. (1975, 1976)
DENS	Population per square mile, by county	American Medical Association (1971–1976)
POPMD	Population per office-based, patient-care MD, by county	American Medical Association (1971–1976)
GPPROP	Proportion of patient-care MDs in general practice, by county	American Medical Association (1971–1976)
POPBD	Population per other hospital bed (total county beds minus BDTOT), by county	American Medical Association (1971–1976)
MCARE	Proportion of population age 65 or over, by county	U.S. Bureau of Health Manpower (1976); Sales Management, Inc. (1975, 1976)
MCAID	Proportion of population that is under 65 and eligible for Medicaid, by state	National Center for Social Statistics (1970–1975)
INS	Predicted total insurance coverage index, deflated, based on 1970 estimates of insurance premium determinants (see Appendix H)	CHAS-NORC household survey (1971); various sources for demographic data, 1970–1975

Hospital-Characteristics Variables

GOVT	$= \begin{matrix} 1 \\ 0 \end{matrix}$	for nonfederal, government hospitals otherwise	AHA annual surveys
PROP	$= \begin{matrix} 1 \\ 0 \end{matrix}$	for proprietary hospitals otherwise	AHA annual surveys
MEDSCH	$= \begin{matrix} 1 \\ 0 \end{matrix}$	for hospitals with medical school affiliation otherwise	AHA annual surveys
NURSCH	$= \begin{matrix} 1 \\ 0 \end{matrix}$	for hospitals with professional nursing school otherwise	AHA annual surveys
SIZE1	$= \begin{matrix} 1 \\ 0 \end{matrix}$	if BDTOT < 100 otherwise	AHA annual surveys
SIZE2	$= \begin{matrix} 1 \\ 0 \end{matrix}$	if $100 \leq$ BDTOT < 250 otherwise	AHA annual surveys
SIZE3	$= \begin{matrix} 1 \\ 0 \end{matrix}$	if $250 \leq$ BDTOT < 400 otherwise	AHA annual surveys

Table A–1 *(continued)*

Variable Name[a]		Definition	Source
		Unionization Variables (See Appendix K)	
COLREQ =	1	if hospital has received request for recognition as collective-bargaining agent in current or any preceding year	AHA annual survey (1970); special topics surveys
	0	otherwise	(1973 and 1975)
UNION =	1	if hospital has at least one signed collective-bargaining agreement in current or any preceding year	AHA annual survey (1970); special topics surveys
	0	otherwise	(1973 and 1975)
STRIKE =	1	if hospital has had strike or other work stoppage in current or any preceding year	AHA annual survey (1970); special topics survey (1973)
	0	otherwise	
		Reimbursement and Regulation Variables (See Appendix I)	
NCON1 =	1	for noncomprehensive CON program in effect for 2 years or less, by state	Lewin and Associates (1975a); Erman (1976); Curran (1974)
	0	otherwise	
NCON2 =	1	for noncomprehensive CON program in effect for more than 2 years, by state	Lewin and Associates (1975a); Erman (1976); Curran (1974)
	0	otherwise	
CCON1 =	1	for comprehensive CON program in effect for 2 years or less, by state	Lewin and Associates (1975a); Erman (1976); Curran (1974)
	0	otherwise	
CCON2 =	1	for comprehensive CON program in effect for more than 2 years, by state	Lewin and Associates (1975a); Erman (1976); Curran (1974)
	0	otherwise	
PRECON =	1	for year prior to CON program taking effect, by state	Lewin and Associates (1975a); (1976); Curran (1974)
	0	otherwise	
S1122		Proportion of population served by hospitals subject to P.L. 92-603, section 1122, review of capital expansion, by county	Erman (1976)[d]
BCPAA		Proportion of population served by hospitals subject to a Blue Cross requirement of local planning agency approval for reimbursement of expenses related to capital expansion, by Blue Cross plan area	American Hospital Association (1972, 1976)[d]
COSTB		Proportion of population covered by cost-based hospital reimbursement programs under Blue Cross, Medicare, and Medicaid, by insurer catchment area	American Hospital Association (1972, 1976)[d]
FPR		Proportion of population covered by formula-based hospital programs, by insurer catchment area	Lewin and Associates (1975a); Laudicina (1976)[d]
BPR		Proportion of population covered by budget-based hospital PR programs, by insurer catchment area	Lewin and Associates (1975a); Laudicina (1976)[d]

Table A-1 *(continued)*

Variable Name[a]	Definition	Source
UR	Proportion of population covered by Blue Cross and Medicaid programs requiring utilization review, by state, 1974	Lewin and Associates (1975a)[d]
ESP	Proportion of months in a year that ESP was in effect	

Variables Used to Estimate ASSETB and OTHWG[e]

ICARD	Cardiac intensive care unit (0,1)	AHA annual surveys
ICU	Mixed intensive care unit (0,1)	AHA annual surveys
OPENHRT	Open-heart surgical facilities (0,1)	AHA annual surveys
FARMFT	Pharmacy, with full-time registered pharmacist (0,1)	AHA annual surveys
XRAYT	X-ray therapy program (0,1)	AHA annual surveys
COBLT	Cobalt therapy programs (0,1)	AHA annual surveys
RADISO	Radio-isotope facility (0,1)	AHA annual surveys
HISTO	Histopathology laboratory (0,1)	AHA annual surveys
ORGNBK	Organ bank (0,1)	AHA annual surveys
BLODBK	Blood bank (0,1)	AHA annual surveys
EEG	Electroencephalography (0,1)	AHA annual surveys
INHAL	Inhalation (respiratory) therapy department (0,1)	AHA annual surveys
PRENUR	Premature nursery (0,1)	AHA annual surveys
SLFCR	Self-care unit (0,1)	AHA annual surveys
PT	Physical therapy department (0,1)	AHA annual surveys
OT	Occupational therapy department (0,1)	AHA annual surveys
OPD	Outpatient department (0,1)	AHA annual surveys
EMD	Emergency department (0,1)	AHA annual surveys
SOCWK	Social work department (0,1)	AHA annual surveys
FAMPLN	Family planning service (0,1)	AHA annual surveys
HOMCR	Home-care department (0,1)	AHA annual surveys
AUXIL	Hospital auxiliary (0,1)	AHA annual surveys
CANCER	Cancer program approval (0,1)	AHA annual surveys
PROLTB	Proportion of hospital beds for long-term-care patients	AHA annual surveys
BIRBD	Births per hospital bed	AHA annual surveys
SRGBD	Surgical operations per hospital bed	AHA annual surveys
BDTOT2	Bed size squared	AHA annual surveys
FTERNC	FTERN/(FTERN + FTELPN + FTEOTH)	AHA annual surveys
FTELPNC	FTELPN/(FTERN + FTELPN + FTEOTH)	AHA annual surveys
CD1	Location in New England census division (0,1)	AHA annual surveys
CD2	Location in mid-Atlantic census division (0,1)	AHA annual surveys
CD3	Location in South Atlantic census division (0,1)	AHA annual surveys
CD4	Location East North Central census division (0,1)	AHA annual surveys
CD5	Location in East South Central census division (0,1)	AHA annual surveys
CD6	Location in West North Central census division (0,1)	AHA annual surveys
CD7	Location in West South Central census division (0,1)	AHA annual surveys
CD8	Location in Mountain census division (0,1)	AHA annual surveys
CD9	Location in Pacific census division (0,1)	AHA annual surveys
SMSA1	Location in non-SMSAs and SMSAs under 250,000 popultion (0,1)	AHA annual surveys
SMSA3	Location in SMSAs of 250,000–500,000 population (0,1)	AHA annual surveys
SMSA4	Location in SMSAs of 500,000–1,000,000 population (0,1)	AHA annual surveys

Table A–1 *(continued)*

Variable Name[a]	Definition	Source
SMSA5	Location in SMSAs of 1,000,000–2,500,000 population (0,1)	AHA annual surveys
SMSA6	Location in SMSAs of over 2,500,000 population (0,1)	AHA annual surveys

[a]All monetary variables were divided by COL72 (see Appendix B) and are therefore measured in 1972 dollars, adjusting for interarea price-level differences. This is indicated by the word *deflated*.

[b]FTE = full-time equivalent. Part-time employees are computed as half of a full-time employee.

[c]Denominators of the relative input price variables depend on the dependent variable in the equation estimated. For example, in the LPNBED regression, the denominator of RNWG/X, OTHWG/X, and CAP/X is LPNWG (LPNWG/X is not included in this regression). Because all regressions were estimated in logarithmic form, price ratios Y/X were computed as $\ln Y - \ln X$. See chapters 7 and 8.

[d]Additional data sources are required to estimate population proportions covered by each reimbursement program. See Appendix J.

[e]Variable definitions followed by (0,1) signify binary variables which take the value 1 if the hospital has the indicated program or attribute and the value 0 otherwise.

Appendix B:
Variable COL72

Variable Name: COL72.

Description: Cost-of-living index (1972 metropolitan areas $= 1.00$) for an intermediate-budget family of four.

Methodology

Step 1: Record cost-of-living (COL) index data for available metropolitan areas corresponding to primary sampling units (PSUs) for 1972, using BLS data for each PSU.[1]

Step 2: For PSUs without corresponding BLS metropolitan-area COL data, the following assignment procedure was used (see table B–1): For metropolitan PSUs, data pertaining to nearby metropolitan areas of similar size, for which BLS COL data were available, were assigned; for nonmetropolitan PSUs, BLS data pertaining to nonmetropolitan areas by census region (Northeast, South, Midwest, West) were assigned.

Table B–1
Cost-of-Living Data Assignments for Nonmetropolitan Areas and for Metropolitan Areas without Bureau of Labor Statistics Data Available, by State

State	Nonmetropolitan[a]	Metropolitan[b]
Alabama	South	Atlanta, Ga.
Alaska	Anchorage[c]	Anchorage, Alas.
Arizona	West	Bakersfield, Calif.
Arkansas	South	Baton Rouge, La.
California	West	Bakersfield, Calif.
Colorado	West	Denver, Colo.
Connecticut	Northeast	Hartford, Conn.
Delaware	South	Philadelphia, Pa.
District of Columbia	[d]	District of Columbia
Florida	South	Orlando, Fla.
Georgia	South	Atlanta, Ga.
Hawaii	Honolulu[e]	Honolulu, Haw.
Idaho	West	Denver, Colo.
Illinois	Midwest	Champaign-Urbana, Ill.
Indiana	Midwest	Indianapolis, Ind.
Iowa	Midwest	Cedar Rapids, Iowa
Kansas	Midwest	Wichita, Kans.
Kentucky	South	Nashville, Tenn.
Louisiana	South	Baton Rouge, La.

Table B–1 continued

State	Nonmetropolitan[a]	Metropolitan[b]
Maine	Northeast	Portland, Me.
Maryland	South	Baltimore, Md.
Massachusetts	Northeast	Boston, Mass.
Michigan	Midwest	Detroit, Mich.
Minnesota	Midwest	Minneapolis-St. Paul, Minn.
Mississippi	South	Baton Rouge, La.
Missouri	South	Kansas City, Mo.
Montana	West	Seattle-Everett, Wash.
Nebraska	Midwest	Cedar Rapids, Iowa
Nevada	West	Bakersfield, Calif.
New Hampshire	Northeast	Portland, Me.
New Jersey	Northeast	Philadelphia, Pa.
New Mexico	West	Denver, Colo.
New York	Northeast	Buffalo, N.Y.
North Carolina	South	Durham, N.C.
North Dakota	Midwest	Minneapolis-St. Paul, Minn.
Ohio	Midwest	Dayton, Ohio
Oklahoma	South	Dallas, Tex.
Oregon	West	Seattle-Everett, Wash.
Pennsylvania	Northeast	Lancaster, Pa.
Rhode Island	Northeast	Boston, Mass.
South Carolina	South	Atlanta, Ga.
South Dakota	Midwest	Minneapolis-St. Paul, Minn.
Tennessee	South	Nashville, Tenn.
Texas	South	Austin, Tex.
Utah	West	Denver, Colo.
Vermont	Northeast	Portland, Me.
Virginia	South	Durham, N.C.
Washington	West	Seattle-Everett, Wash.
West Virginia	South	Durham, N.C.
Wisconsin	Midwest	Green Bay, Wisc.
Wyoming	West	Bakersfield, Calif.

[a]Nonmetropolitan cost-of-living index values were assigned by census region (Northeast, South, Midwest, or West).

[b]Metropolitan cost-of-living index values assigned as shown for all metropolitan areas in the state for which BLS data were unavailable.

[c]Anchorage SMSA data assigned to all Alaska.

[d]The District of Columbia is entirely metropolitan.

[e]Honolulu SMSA data assigned to all Hawaii.

Step 3: Cost-of-living index values for years other than 1972 were adjusted according to changes in SMSA-specific consumer price index values. Years prior to 1972 were adjusted downward, and years after 1972 were adjusted upward. The result is an index for use in converting variables measured in nominal dollars to real terms, correcting for interarea variations in price levels. National means of the price index series used to adjust COL72 are as follows: 1969, 0.876; 1970, 0.928; 1971, 0.968; 1972, 1.000; 1973, 1.062; 1974, 1.179; and 1975, 1.287.

Note

1. Direct data are available for the following SMSAs: Boston, Mass.; Buffalo, N.Y.; Hartford, Conn.; Lancaster, Pa.; New York–Northeastern New Jersey; Philadelphia, Pa.–New Jersey; Pittsburgh, Pa.; Portland, Me.; Cedar Rapids, Iowa; Champaign–Urbana, Ill.; Chicago, Ill.–Northwestern Indiana; Cincinnati, Ohio–Kentucky–Indiana; Cleveland, Ohio; Dayton, Ohio; Detroit, Mich.; Green Bay, Wisc.; Indianapolis, Ind.; Kansas City, Mo.–Kansas; Milwaukee, Wisc.; Minneapolis–St. Paul, Minn; St. Louis, Mo.–Illinois; Wichita, Kans.; Atlanta, Ga.; Austin, Tex.; Baltimore, Md.; Baton Rouge, La.; Dallas, Tex.; Durham, N.C.; Houston, Tex.; Nashville, Tenn.; Orlando, Fla.; Washington, D.C.–Maryland–Virginia; Bakersfield, Calif; Denver, Colo.; Los Angeles–Long Beach, Calif.; San Diego, Calif.; San Francisco–Oakland, Calif; Seattle–Everett, Wash.; Honolulu, Haw.; and Achorage, Alaska. See Appendix F for PSU definition and list.

Appendix C:
Variable ASSETB

Variable Name: ASSETB.

Description: Index of hospital plant assets per bed, net of accumulated depreciation, in 1972 dollars.

Methodology

Because the measured dollar value of hospital plant assets is sensitive to asset vintage and depreciation methods, use of a direct asset measure would impart serious errors-in-variables bias to most analyses. Variable ASSETB was created to circumvent this problem. The following procedure was employed:

Step 1: Develop a "standard" vector of variables (that is, available to all sample years) that describe hospital characteristics, including facility and services mix.

Step 2: Using 1975 AHA data, regress net plant assets on the vector of hospital characteristics variables. Parameter estimates are shown in table C–1.

Step 3: Apply the parameter estimates from step 2 to each year separately to compute ASSETB. This effectively makes variations in assets per bed a function of variations in hospital service-mix characteristics over time. The index is not influenced by variations in asset vintage, except insofar as vintage variations influence the single cross-sectional estimates of step 2. However, because the variable is constrained to be a function of service-mix characteristics for which data were available for 1969 to 1975 inclusive, the index does not reflect additions of facilities and services for which data were not available in all years. Thus, overall growth in the index from 1969 to 1975 is likely to be understated. This error was deemed to be less in magnitude than the error involved in using measured asset values. The method used also has the advantage of reducing the frequency of missing values in the asset variable.

Mean values of ASSETB for each year in real (deflated) terms are as follows: 1970, 31,159; 1971, 31,946; 1972, 31,804; 1973, 32,366; 1974, 32, 848; and 1975, 32, 851.

Table C–1
Parameter Estimates of Regression for Net Plant Assets per Bed, 1975

ICARD	3,641	PRENUR	−3,966	GOVT	−2,246
	(1,504)[a]		(1,628)		(1,882)
ICU	4,502	SLFCR	−4,053	PROP	−10,555
	(2,592)		(2,715)		(2,406)
OPENHRT	8,659	PT	3,802	MEDSCH	4,534
	(2,123)		(2,555)		(2,033)
FARMFT	2,942	OT	−1,241	NURSCH	488
	(2,649)		(1,522)		(1,823)
XRAYT	756	OPD	−2,592	CANCER	6,602
	(1,562)		(1,671)		(1,733)
COBLT	5,040	EMD	2,369	PROLTB	102
	(8,858)		(2,706)		(89)
RADISO	2,560	SOCWK	1,318	BIRBD	525
	(2,046)		(1,740)		(290)
HISTO	1,766	FAMPLN	−3,315	SRGBD	257
	(1,846)		(2,050)		(98)
ORGNBK	3,060	HOMCR	4,613	Constant	4,131
	(3,011)		(1,980)		
BLODBK	1,623	AUXIL	3,665		$R^2 = 0.225$
	(1,617)		(1,851)		
EEG	2,111	BDTOT	−26.3	$F(32, 1,050) = 9.6$	
	(1,821)		(12.8)		
INHAL	2,859	BDTOT2	0.013		
	(2,821)		(0.010)		

[a]Standard errors are reported in parentheses below the parameter estimates.

Appendix D:
Variables RNWG
and LPNWG

Variable Names: RNWG and LPNWG.

Description: Estimated area [primary sampling unit (PSU)] RN and LPN hourly wages, in 1972 dollars.

Methodology

Step 1: Construct RN and LPN wage series, 1969–1975, for twenty-two SMSAs using BLS data. Data are available for 1969, 1972, and 1975. Data for missing years are filled in by linear interpolation. Compute percentage increases (base year = 1969) for each SMSA and year.

Step 2: Record data on payroll, hours worked, and number of employees for all PSUs using 1969 census data pertaining to RNs and LPN-aides (combined). Compute mean hours per RN and mean hours per LPN-aide per year.

Step 3: Estimate the LPN wage using census combined LPN-aide payroll data according to the following formulas:

$$\alpha_1 \text{ aide wage} + \alpha_2 \text{ LPN wage} = \text{aide-LPN wage}$$

$$\text{Aide wage/LPN wage} = \alpha_3$$

where $\alpha_1 + \alpha_2 = 1.00$. Also α_1 and α_2 are estimated by using state data on nonfederal LPNs and aides from Bureau of Health Resources Development (1974); α_3 is estimated from BLS data on LPN and aide wages in twenty-two SMSAs. We solve for the LPN wage using the following computational formula:

$$\text{LPN wage} = \text{aide-LPN wage}/(\alpha_1 \alpha_3 + \alpha_2)$$

Step 4: Specify and estimate RN and LPN wages, generating equations using 1969 data corresponding to the twenty-two BLS SMSAs. The Bureau of Labor Statistics RN and LPN wages are the dependent variables, and census wage and hours data are included in the independent variable set. The

213

following specification was estimated:

$$\text{Wage}_{\text{BLS}} = b_0 + b_1 \text{wage}_{\text{census}} + b_2 \text{hours/year}_{\text{census}} + b_3 \text{index}$$

The wage-generating equations yielded the following estimates:

	b_0	b_1	b_2	b_3	
RNs	−1.62	0.325	0.00098	0.0225	$R^2(3, 18) = 0.812$
Standard error		(0.076)	(0.00023)	(0.0062)	
LPNs	0.18	0.563	0	0.0096	$R^2(3, 18) = 0.768$
Standard error		(0.126)	—	(0.0063)	

Step 5: By using the above parameter estimates, estimated RN and LPN wages are calculated for all AHA PSU areas in 1969. Wage estimates for successive years are computed according to the following formula:

$$\text{Wage}_j = \text{wage}_{69}(1 + \text{PCT}_j)$$

where $j = j$th year and $\text{PCT}_j =$ the proportional increase in the wage from 1969 to the jth year. Wage estimates were calculated for all PSUs and years except for PSUs for which actual BLS data were available, in which case the latter were used.

Step 6: The wage estimates were merged to the AHA pooled file for 1970–1975 and divided by COL72 (expressed in 1972 dollars).

Appendix E:
Variable OTHWG

Variable Name: OTHWG.

Description: Estimated hourly wage for other hospital employees (excludes RNs, LPNs, interns and residents, and employed MDs).

Methodology

Because no independent data source exists for area wages paid to hospital employees classified as "other," a wage variable was estimated from AHA data pertaining to the 1,228 sample hospitals. This task encountered the following problems. First, while data are available from the AHA surveys to calculate full-time-equivalent (FTE) other employees, payroll data required to estimate the wage for the other employee include salary expenses pertaining to RNs and LPNs. Second, there are considerable missing values in the payroll data series. Third, even if complete data on payroll pertaining to other employees were available, this measure would be very sensitive to the mix of employees categorized as "other" which, in turn, is dependent on variations in the scope and sophistication of the hospital product. Estimated wages based on such data would be subject to considerable errors in variables as a measure of area "other" employee wage structure.

To circumvent these problems, the following estimation procedure was employed:

Step 1: Construct a "standard" set of variables for each year from 1970 to 1975 (using data available for each year), which describes payroll per FTE other employee (including RNs and LPNs) and hospital characteristics of the following types: facility and service mix, location (census division and community population size), and proportions of RNs and LPNs included in the "other" category.

Step 2: Estimate OLS regressions for each year (1970–1975) of the following form:

$$\text{TOTHSAL} = b_0 + b_{1i}\text{CD}_i + b_{2i}\text{SMSA}_i + b_{3k}X_k +$$
$$b_4\text{FTERNC} + b_5\text{FTELPNC}$$

where TOTHSAL = total other employee + RN + LPN payroll divided by
(FTEOTH + FTERN + FTELPN)
CD_i = dummy variable signifying the ith census division
$SMSA_j$ = dummy variable signifying the jth SMSA size class
X_k = kth variable in a vector of variables representing scope
and sophistication of hospital product
FTERNC = FTERN/(FTERN + FTELPN + FTEOTH)
FTELPNC = FTELPN/(FTERN + FTELPN + FTEOTH)

The New England census division (CD1) and smallest SMSA size class (SMSA1) are held constant in the regressions. Parameter estimates are shown in table E–1.

Step 3: Compute an estimated area salary per other hospital employee for each hospital using the following formula:

$$OTHSAL = b_0 + \sum_{k=1}^{n} (b_{3k}\bar{X}_k) + b_{1j}CD_j + b_{2j}SMSA_j$$

where OTHSAL = estimated annual salary for other hospital employees (excluding RNs and LPNs) and $\bar{X}_k$ = sample mean for the kth variable.

Step 4: Convert OTHSAL into an hourly-wage variable, expressed in 1972 dollars, using the following formula:

$$OTHWG = (OTHSAL/2,080)/COL72$$

The number of working hours in a year is 2,080, assuming 40 hours of work per week and 52 (paid) working weeks per year.

Table E–1
Parameter Estimates Pertaining to Variable OTHSAL
Ordinary-Least-Squares Regressions

Variable Name	1970	1971	1972	1973	1974	1975
CD2	−385	−180	−117	−12	−163	−74
	(118)[a]	(185)	(131)	(139)	(158)	(165)
CD3	−587	−520	−611	−501	−518	−541
	(143)	(221)	(159)	(166)	(188)	(198)
CD4	−280	−247	−158	−114	−127	−120
	(124)	(195)	(138)	(148)	(166)	(175)
CD5	−1,004	−1,093	−908	−970	−911	−1,034
	(204)	(323)	(230)	(242)	(280)	(293)
CD6	−506	−409	−279	−165	−438	−541
	(167)	(264)	(188)	(195)	(223)	(239)
CD7	−989	−884	−982	−978	−1,020	−851
	(163)	(262)	(188)	(196)	(224)	(234)
CD8	−671	−554	−295	−485	−484	−390
	(198)	(310)	(219)	(234)	(263)	(275)
CD9	439	650	487	578	700	613
	(133)	(213)	(148)	(153)	(177)	(185)
SMSA3	−64	−218	−31	−7	−231	−100
	(156)	(232)	(166)	(177)	(205)	(216)
SMSA4	−93	0.115	13	35	165	253
	(120)	(196)	(143)	(163)	(184)	(193)
SMSA5	162	−24	180	142	241	204
	(99)	(160)	(118)	(133)	(151)	(160)
SMSA6	673	821	969	996	1,167	1,145
	(101)	(163)	(119)	(133)	(152)	(161)
ICARD	−114	25	73	−38	−40	117
	(70)	(112)	(75)	(77)	(93)	(99)
ICU	27	113	51	209	−48	337
	(90)	(148)	(108)	(121)	(146)	(159)
OPENHRT	187	−150	77	112	−76	−178
	(106)	(172)	(118)	(118)	(135)	(143)
FARMFT	416	200	85	160	−70	257
	(103)	(157)	(121)	(131)	(155)	(163)
XRAYT	−19	−138	34	−136	−90	−135
	(73)	(116)	(83)	(83)	(95)	(102)
COBLT	26	21	−88	−24	−166	79
	(87)	(139)	(99)	(01)	(117)	(123)
RADISO	69	117	−124	−55	128	−129
	(83)	(128)	(97)	(100)	(121)	(131)
HISTO	74	132	108	65	111	218
	(87)	(127)	(94)	(96)	(114)	(118)
ORGNBK	109	879	−180	188	93	−356
	(146)	(240)	(164)	(161)	(178)	(201)
BLODBK	39	−0.693	31	104	71	21
	(78)	(124)	(91)	(91)	(104)	(107)
EEG	92	158	208	228	128	380
	(75)	(123)	(89)	(95)	(110)	(116)
INHAL	−83	−142	61	83	−114	−637
	(85)	(152)	(125)	(134)	(175)	(177)
PRENUR	−212	114	−84	−44	−253	−169
	(71)	(116)	(86)	(88)	(99)	(107)

Table E-1 continued

Variable Name	1970	1971	1972	1973	1974	1975
SLFCR	−55	−11	−204	−117	−129	−191
	(112)	(188)	(138)	(144)	(170)	(186)
PT	−28	−29	138	−178	−12	−183
	(91)	(153)	(122)	(124)	(149)	(157)
OT	145	−36	−18	116	−80	27
	(83)	(130)	(89)	(90)	(98)	(101)
OPD	116	−30	107	287	270	342
	(72)	(121)	(84)	(88)	(103)	(110)
EMD	−8	−21	−249	−143	175	428
	(129)	(201)	(131)	(136)	(157)	(171)
SOCWK	154	110	273	220	248	256
	(79)	(123)	(87)	(89)	(107)	(114)
FAMPLN	207	220	205	113	275	322
	(101)	(162)	(114)	(114)	(127)	(138)
HOMCR	167	216	319	333	563	340
	(89)	(150)	(108)	(113)	(124)	(136)
AUXIL	54	−4	14	62	−101	−187
	(89)	(132)	(97)	(97)	(113)	(121)
GOVT	1	−62	74	112	40	12
	(88)	(140)	(101)	(102)	(115)	(122)
PROP	116	−96	3	236	−202	−45
	(113)	(188)	(133)	(129)	(155)	(158)
MEDSCH	10	122	241	266	191	177
	(101)	(156)	(112)	(108)	(126)	(136)
NURSCH	−55	51	−56	15	−97	−224
	(83)	(136)	(97)	(101)	(115)	(23)
CANCER	70	39	63	137	112	88
	(82)	(129)	(93)	(95)	(108)	(115)
PROLTB	−14.9	−8.5	−9.7	−16.0	−16.6	−20.7
	(4.6)	(7.2)	(5.3)	(5.2)	(5.3)	(5.5)
BIRBD	3.3	−12.1	−25.4	−30.8	−20.8	−45
	(9.2)	(15.3)	(14.7)	(15.2)	(17.6)	(19)
SRGBD	0.3	4.2	4.2	1.5	6.3	−8.2
	(3.8)	(6.3)	(5.3)	(5.0)	(5.6)	(5.5)
BDTOT	0.27	0.74	0.64	−0.229	1.7	0.992
	(0.64)	(0.85)	(0.71)	(0.711)	(0.807)	(0.885)
BDTOT2	−0.00003	−1.76	0.0003	0.0004	−0.0004	0.00004
	(0.0005)	(5.0082)	(0.0005)	(0.0005)	(0.0006)	(0.0006)
FTERNC	4,121	2,920	3,626	3,265	4,927	5,315
	(457)	(793)	(615)	(657)	(739)	(851)
FTELPNC	2,428	363	923	672	1,406	−462
	(541)	(957)	(663)	(721)	(807)	(839)
Constant	4,374	5,178	5,353	5,705	5,561	6,609

$R^2 = 0.479$ $R^2 = 0.324$ $R^2 = 0.496$ $R^2 = 0.496$ $R^2 = 0.483$ $R^2 = 0.473$

$F(46, 1,034)$ $F(46, 1,000)$ $F(46, 1,026)$ $F(46, 1,040)$ $F(46, 1,010)$ $F(46, 1,030)$
$= 20.7$ $= 10.4$ $= 21.9$ $= 22.3$ $= 20.5$ $= 20.1$

[a]Standard errors are reported below each parameter estimate.

Appendix F:
Variable PSU

Variable Name: PSU.

Description: Primary sampling unit defines geographic areas within which sample hospitals are located.

Methodology: The PSU framework used in this book was developed by the National Opinion Research Center (NORC) and the Center for Health Administration Studies (CHAS) at the University of Chicago for national household surveys. The PSU framework, based on 1970 census data, defines geographic area whose populations are representative of the United States as a whole. Nonfederal, short-term general hospitals which are located in these PSUs and which were recorded by the AHA in all surveys from 1969 to 1975 were selected for analysis. Table F–1 identifies the PSUs, the number of sample hospitals in each PSU, and the number of counties in each PSU.

Table F–1
Nonfederal, Short-Term General Hospital Sample PSU Areas and Number of Sample Hospitals in Each PSU

PSU	Number of Hospitals	Number of Counties
Alabama		
Birmingham SMSA	15	4
Houston Co.	2	1
Washington Co.	1	1
Arkansas		
Little Rock SMSA	5	2
Arizona		
Phoenix SMSA	15	1
California		
Colusa Co.	1	1
Fresno SMSA	9	1
Los Angeles–Long Beach SMSA	114	1
San Bernardino–Riverside–Ontario SMSA	25	2
San Diego SMSA	23	1
San Francisco–Oakland SMSA	43	5
Santa Rosa SMSA	6	1
Yuba Co.	1	1
Colorado		
Denver SMSA	15	7
Mesa Co.	4	1
Connecticut		
Hartford SMSA	5	5
New Britain SMSA	2	1

219

Table F–1 continued

PSU	Number of Hospitals	Number of Counties
District of Columbia		
Washington SMSA	28	7
Florida		
Miami SMSA	16	1
Orlando SMSA	8	3
Pensacola SMSA	4	2
St. Lucie Co.	1	1
Georgia		
Atlanta SMSA	16	15
Illinois		
Chicago SMSA	85	6
Indiana		
Gary–Hammond–East Chicago SMSA	6	2
Indianapolis SMSA	14	8
Iowa		
Des Moines SMSA	5	2
Kansas		
Topeka SMSA	4	3
Louisiana		
New Orleans SMSA	11	4
Maryland		
Baltimore SMSA	22	5
Massachusetts		
Boston SMSA	65	5
Springfield–Chicopee–Holyoke SMSA	32	4
Michigan		
Detroit SMSA	51	6
Flint SMSA	6	2
Gogebic Co.	2	1
Marquette Co.	1	1
Newaygo Co.	2	1
Minnesota		
Minneapolis–St. Paul SMSA	24	10
Rock–Lincoln Cos.	4	2
Missouri		
St. Louis SMSA	34	8
Montana		
Great Falls SMSA	2	1
New Jersey		
Jersey City SMSA	5	1
Long Branch–Asbury Park SMSA	3	1
Newark SMSA	27	4
Sussex Co.	2	1
New York		
Buffalo SMSA	18	2
New York SMSA	102	9
Rochester SMSA	14	5
North Carolina		
Brendell Co.	3	1
Wilkes Co.	1	1
Ohio		
Akron SMSA	5	2
Cleveland SMSA	30	4

Table F–1 continued

PSU	Number of Hospitals	Number of Counties
Columbiana Co.	1	1
Columbus SMSA	11	5
Knox Co.	2	1
Oklahoma		
Oklahoma City SMSA	12	5
Oregon		
Portland SMSA	12	4
Pennsylvania		
Allentown–Bethlehem–Easton SMSA	5	4
Philadelphia SMSA	60	8
Pittsburgh SMSA	31	4
Reading SMSA	3	1
Schuylkill Co.	5	1
South Carolina		
Columbia SMSA	2	2
Florence Co.	3	1
Tennessee		
Knoxville SMSA	6	4
Nashville SMSA	16	8
Texas		
Dallas SMSA	31	11
Houston SMSA	45	6
Victoria Co.	3	1
Wichita Falls SMSA	3	2
Willacy Co.	0	1
Virginia		
Mecklenberg Co.	1	1
Norfolk–Portsmouth–Virginia Beach SMSA	6	1
Smyth Co.	2	1
Washington		
Tacoma SMSA	9	1
West Virginia		
McDowell Co.	2	1
Marion Co.	1	1
Uphur Co.	1	1
Wisconsin		
Appleton–Oshkosh SMSA	9	3
Burnett–Washburn Co.	1	1
Manitowoc Co.	3	1
Racine SMSA	3	1
Total	1,228	250

Appendix G:
Variable CAP

Variable Name: CAP.

Description: National price of capital index ($1972 = 100$).

Methodology: The variable CAP is a composite index based on construction cost and interest rate trends for 1970–1975. The variable was computed as follows:

$$CAP_i = \frac{C_i \cdot I_i}{C_{1972} \cdot I_{1972}}$$

where i represents the ith year, C_i = wholesale construction cost index ($1967 = 100$), and I_i = 20-year bond interest rate. Values of C_i, I_i, and CAP_i are as follows:

	1970	1971	1972	1973	1974	1975
C_i	112.5	119.5	126.6	138.5	160.9	174.0
I_i	7.60	7.12	7.05	7.20	7.80	8.35
CAP_i	95.9	94.9	100.0	111.3	140.6	162.3

Appendix H:
Variable INS

Variable Name: INS.

Description: Predicted expected value, in 1970 dollars, of mean family total health insurance premium, by county.

Methodology

Step 1: Estimate the determinants of health insurance premiums pertaining to family and individual private health insurance policyholders in 1970. Explanatory variables include benefits variables, which jointly describe the services covered, generosity of coverage, and type of insurance programs; loading variables, which describe factors associated with the "price" of insurance (that is, the excess of premium over expectation of dollar benefits paid); regulation variables, which describe state laws and activities governing the sale and administration of health insurance; and other variables which do not fit the first three categories.

Table H–1 presents names and definitions of variables included in the premium-estimating regressions. Variable means and standard deviations, predicted coefficient signs, and parameter estimates and standard errors are presented in table H–2. The estimation process is explained in chapter 4. The Data source is the Center for Health Administration Studies (CHAS)– National Opinion Research Center (NORC) Survey of Households (1971).

Step 2: An estimated insurance premium variable is computed for each sample family by using the parameter estimates from step 1. Compared to actual premiums paid, this procedure "purifies" the premium data of factors influencing the price of insurance without affecting the depth of coverage. Thus, the estimated insurance premium may be viewed as an index of purchasing power of health insurance benefits.

By using household data from the CHAS-NORC survey, regressions are estimated to identify determinants of the probability of having insurance and the expected amount of insurance once insurance is obtained. Explanatory variables are limited to data which are contained on the CHAS-NORC file (for families or family heads) and which are available in analogous form at the county level (in anticipation of step 3). The variables are defined, and the estimation process is explained in chapter 4. Variable means and standard deviations are presented in table 4–3; parameter estimates and standard errors, in table 4–4. Modifications of these regressions were estimated excluding variables pertaining to household heads *without* analogous data

225

Table H–1
Variable Names and Definitions for Health Insurance
Premium Regressions

Variable[a]	Definition
PREMIUM	Total health insurance premium including employer's share, when applicable, deflated by an area cost-of-living index (U.S. 1970 metropolitan average = 1.00)

Benefits Variables[b]

C11B	Inpatient hospital, basic only; intermediate room-and-board benefit[c] (0,1)[d]
C11C	Inpatient hospital, basic only; generous room-and-board benefit[c] (0,1)
C11E	Inpatient hospital, basic only; intermediate days of care covered[e] (0,1)
C11F	Inpatient hospital, basic only; generous days of care covered[e] (0,1)
C12	Inpatient hospital, major medical only (0,1)
C13B	Inpatient hospital, combined; intermediate room-and-board benefit (0,1)
C13C	Inpatient hospital, combined; generous room-and-board benefit (0,1)
C13E	Inpatient hospital, combined; intermediate days of care covered (0,1)
C13F	Inpatient hospital, combined; generous days of care covered (0,1)
C61	MD home and office visits, basic only (0,1)
C62	MD home and office visits, major medical only (0,1)
C63	MD home and office visits, combined (0,1)
C71	X-ray and laboratory tests, basic only (0,1)
C81	Nursing home care, basic only (0,1)
C83	Nursing home care, combined (0,1)
C93	Out-of-hospital prescribed drugs, basic only *or* combined (0,1)
CX2	Out-of-hospital dental care, major medical only (0,1)
CX3	Out-of-hospital dental care, basic only *or* combined (0,1)
CY1	Flat daily payment for hospitalization (0,1)
CY3	Coverage for optical care and/or rare or dread diseases (0,1)
C2X	*No* coverage for hospital outpatient or emergency services (0,1)
C3X	*No* coverage for in-hopital surgery (0,1)
C4X	*No* coverage for surgery in a doctor's office (0,1)
C5X	*No* coverage for in-hospital doctor visits (0,1)

Insurer/ Insurance Variables[f]

CIR	Commercial individual premium, regulated (0,1)
CGN	Commercial group premium, not regulated (0,1)
CGR	Commercial group premium, regulated (0,1)
BIN	Blue Cross individual premium, not regulated (0,1)
BIR	Blue Cross individual premium, regulated (0,1)
BGN	Blue Cross premium, not regulated (0,1)
BGR	Blue Cross group premium, regulated (0,1)

State Regulation Variables

CAP	Commercial insurer capitalization and reserve requirements exceed $1 million (0,1)
HRATE	Regulatory agency has authority to monitor and approve hospital reimbursement rates (0,1)

Table H–1 continued

Variable[a]	Definition
UR	Mandated hospital utilization review program is in effect in state (0,1)
PREX	Regulations limit ability of insurer to exclude preexisting conditions from coverage (0,1)
EDUCP	Regulatory agency sponsors health insurance consumer education program (0,1)
EFPOP	Full-time-equivalent regulatory staff per 1 million insured state population (specific to Blue Cross or commercially insured populations)
TAX	Health insurance premium tax rate (specific to Blue Cross or commercial insurer)

Remaining Variables

EXPAPD	Hospital average daily inpatient expense adjusted for average expense per outpatient visit, by SMSA or by county for nonmetropolitan areas; deflated by an area cost-of-living index (U.S. 1970 metropolitan average = 1.00)[f]
GSIZE	Size of insured group for group policies (individual policies = 0)
MEDSUP	Medicare supplement policy (0,1)
NONYR	Policy provides less than a full year's coverage (0,1)

[a]Data pertain to a sample of household heads with Blue Cross and commercial health insurance covering hospitalization and other benefits in 1970. The CHAS-NORC Survey (1971) is the primary data source, with the following supplements: CIR, CGN, CGR, BIN, BIR, BGN, and BGR identify whether the policy is Blue Cross or commercial and group or individual; identification of whether there is state authority to regulate premiums comes from Lewin and Associates (1975a) (data from the latter source are for 1974); CAP, HRATE, UR, PREX, EDUCP, EFPOP, and TAX are from Lewin and Associates (1975a); EXPAPD is from the American Hospital Association (1971), Table 3, pp. 468–479, and Table 8, pp. 491–492.

[b]Variables indicating covered benefits were given names in the form *Cnpq*. Here *n* signifies which benefit is covered (1 = inpatient hospital care, 2 = hospital outpatient or emergency-room care, 3 = in-hospital surgery, 4 = surgery in a doctor's office, 5 = doctor visits in a hospital, 6 = other doctor visits, 7 = X-ray and laboratory tests, 8 = nursing home care, 9 = out-of-hospital prescribed drugs, X = out-of-hospital dental care, Y = optical and/or rare or dread disease coverage); *p* indicates types of coverage (1 = basic only, 2 = major medical only, 3 = combined basic and major medical); *q*, which pertains to basic and combined coverage for inpatient hospital care, indicates generosity level of benefits. Because of collinearity, many coverage variables were omitted (the omitted variables can be inferred from names of variables included).

[c]Intermediate room-and-board benefits correspond to plans that pay over $25 but less than $55 per day hospitalized *or* pay a fraction (less than 100 percent) of the most common semiprivate room rate. Generous room-and-board benefits correspond to plans that pay over $55 per day *or* pay service benefits equal to or more than the most common semiprivate rate. Low-option daily room-and-board benefits, paying $25 per day or less, were held constant in (omitted from) the regressions.

[d]Variables with definitions followed by (0,1) are dummy variables which take the value 1 if the indicated attribute is present and the value 0 otherwise.

[e]Intermediate days-of-care benefits correspond to plans that cover more than 70 but less than 300 days hospitalized per year. Generous days-of-care benefits correspond to plans that cover 300 days or more. Low-option benefits, covering 70 days or less, were held constant in (omitted from) the regressions.

[f]Our source provided average hospital expense per adjusted patient-day only for states. To obtain estimates of data for SMSAs and counties, we used more thorough 1971 AHA data to perform the necessary adjustments to the 1970 data.

Table H-2
Premium Regression Results: Sample of Insured Household Heads, 1970

Variable	Mean (Standard Deviation)		Predicted Signs	Coefficient (Standard Error)	
	Family Coverage	Individual Coverage		Family Coverage	Individual Coverage
PREMIUM	344.6 (146.5)	116.1 (72.6)		—	—
C11B	0.05 (—)	0.04 ( )	+	*89.9 (21.4)	*58.4 (14.7)
C11C	0.24 (—)	0.12 ( )	+	*145.4 (19.2)	*68.9 (12.8)
C11E	0.17 ( )	0.17 ( )	+	43.3 (15.6)	*40.7 (9.7)
C11F	0.12 ( )	0.07 ( )	+	*109.3 (17.8)	*44.7 (12.7)
C12	0.08 ( )	0.04 ( )	+	17.2 (20.5)	−6.1 (21.9)
C13B	0.14 ( )	0.06 ( )	+	*53.1 (16.9)	18.2 (17.5)
C13C	0.27 ( )	0.08 ( )	+	*81.8 (17.6)	14.4 (16.7)
C13E	0.12 ( )	0.05 ( )	+	42.3 (15.1)	21.6 (15.8)
C13F	0.16 ( )	0.05 ( )	+	*53.9 (14.8)	15.0 (15.7)
C61	0.08 ( )	0.04 ( )	+	*−65.2 (16.2)	**27.8 (13.8)
C62	0.42 ( )	0.16 ( )	+	*70.0 (21.0)	*54.1 (18.8)
C63	0.14 ( )	0.05 ( )	+	*65.5 (23.5)	42.5 (24.0)
C71	0.37 ( )	0.23 ( )	+	3.0 (11.8)	**17.4 (8.1)
C81	0.06 ( )	0.03 ( )	+	*53.0 (16.9)	32.4 (16.7)
C83	0.05 ( )	0.21 ( )	+	*42.4 (19.9)	10.5 (8.0)
C93	0.06 ( )	0.10 ( )	+	0.3 (18.3)	2.1 (9.3)
CX2	0.05 ( )	0.01 ( )	+	*43.3 (19.2)	46.6 (25.4)
CX3	0.05 ( )	0.03 ( )	+	*62.8 (19.4)	16.7 (14.7)
CY1	0.02 ( )	0.11 ( )	?	32.9 (27.4)	**31.8 (11.6)
CY3	0.03 ( )	0.01 ( )	−	26.8 (24.5)	−15.9 (22.5)
C2X	0.03 ( )	0.13 ( )	−	34.0 (26.3)	10.4 (10.1)
C3X	0.04 ( )	0.11 ( )	−	−45.8 (48.9)	26.7 (24.2)
C4X	0.05 ( )	0.12 ( )	−	−81.9 (49.0)	**−50.2 (23.3)
C5X	0.10 ( )	0.21 ( )	−	−34.3 (19.6)	−2.2 (10.7)
CIR	0.07 ( )	0.20 ( )	−	−13.8 (24.6)	−3.5 (10.6)
CGN	0.24 (—)	0.10 ( )	−	**48.1 (24.3)	22.6 (14.1)
CGR	0.14 (—)	0.04 ( )	−	26.6 (26.3)	−16.6 (17.4)

Variable					
BIN	0.01 (—)	0.05 (—)	—	−27.9 (57.9)	9.1 (15.9)
BIR	0.06 (—)	0.24 (—)	—	*113.9 (27.8)	6.5 (12.2)
BGN	0.11 (—)	0.04 (—)	—	14.9 (27.1)	4.4 (17.1)
BGR	0.33 (—)	0.21 (—)	—	31.4 (25.4)	−4.1 (13.7)
CAP	0.36 (—)	0.34 (—)	+	1.74 (10.3)	5.0 (7.5)
HRATE	0.12 (—)	0.15 (—)	—	**−50.5 (18.3)	−13.8 (12.0)
UR	0.45 (—)	0.44 (—)	—	**27.0 (10.5)	*25.4 (7.1)
PREX	0.81 (—)	0.82 (—)	+	15.7 (16.9)	−1.4 (12.7)
EDUCP	0.46 (—)	0.49 (—)	—	−10.3 (10.1)	*−20.3 (7.0)
EFPOP	24.5 (65.5)	38.6 (121.1)	—	−0.07 (21.4)	0.001 (0.02)
TAX	1.34 (0.94)	1.23 (0.99)	+	*−21.9 (6.9)	**−8.9 (4.1)
EXPAPD	70.6 (13.0)	71.7 (13.8)	+	0.46 (0.38)	−0.43 (0.26)
MEDSUP	0.01 (—)	0.36 (—)	?	−51.7 (45.6)	19.7 (11.4)
GSIZE	713.9 (667.8)	331.3 (566.4)	—	−0.13 (0.07)	0.006 (0.07)
NONYR	0.05 (—)	0.05 (—)	—	*−162.4 (17.4)	*−32.7 (12.1)
Constant	—	—		175.4	108.3
				$R^2 = 0.431$	$R^2 = 0.334$
				$F_{(44, 844)} = 14.6^*$	$F_{(44, 582)} = 6.6^*$

*Significant at the 1% level.

**Significant at the 5% level.

All significance tests are two-tailed, even though a few of the parameter estimates are implausible (for example, negative signs of the coefficients of TAX).

available at the county level. The excluded variables are AGE2, FEMALE, EDUC, and FARM. These exclusions reduced the adjusted R^2 from 0.173 to 0.151 in the insured/uninsured regression and from 0.476 to 0.443 in the predicted total premium regression.

Step 3: Parameter estimates from the regressions in step 2 are applied to county data merged to the AHA files for 1970–1975, yielding estimates of the proportion of population with private insurance and expected average amount of insurance, once insured. These two values are multiplied to arrive at an estimated depth-of-coverage variable for each county.

Step 4: The variable computed in step 3 provides substantial intercounty variation in depth of coverage (comparable direct data are not available on a county level), but values for 1970 through 1975 do not accurately reflect secular trends in the growth of health insurance. Therefore, the depth-of-coverage variable for each year was multiplied by an adjustment factor which is computed as follows:

$$A_i = \frac{PR_i/PR_{1970}}{(X_i/X_{1970})(P_i/P_{1970})}$$

where A_i = adjustment factor for ith year

$\quad PR_i$ = total private health insurance premiums paid in ith year, all United States

$\quad X_i$ = medical care component of the consumer price index in ith year (1970 = 1.00)

$\quad P_i$ = U.S. population in ith year

Appendix I:
Variables
NCON1, NCON2,
CCON1, CCON2,
PRECON, S1122,
BCPAA, COSTB, FPR,
BPR, UR, and ESP

Variable Name: All are regulation variables.

Description: Definitions are provided in Appendix A.

Methodology: Tables I–1, I–2, and I–3 provide raw data from which regulation variables were constructed. The following procedures were employed:

Certificate-of-Need Variables (NCON1, NCON2, CCON1, CCON2, PRECON)

1. For states not having a CON program during 1970–1976, all variables take the value 0 for all years.
2. The variable PRECON takes the value 1 for hospitals located in an area where CON is instituted for the year *prior* to the year when CON becomes effective.[1] Thus PRECON can equal 1 for at most one of the six years.
3. An operating CON program is defined as either comprehensive or noncomprehensive. Comprehensive CON programs are those which include service expansion review *and* which have a threshold less than $100,000 for equipment purchase review; CON programs are further distinguished as being either new (first or second year of operation) or mature (greater than two years of operation).
4. Hospitals located in areas where CON programs were established in 1975 or before are assigned CON dummy variables for each year. Although fragmentary evidence exists suggesting that there have been changes in characteristics of CON programs over time, our data treat each program as fixed in terms of comprehensiveness; thus, no states change from noncomprehensive to comprehensive or vice versa. Hospitals in states instituting CON between 1969 and 1973 change from new to mature, however. Table I–4 illustrates how CON variables were coded for example cases.

Reimbursement Variables (S1122, BCPAA, COSTB, FPR, BPR, UR, ESP)

$$S1122 = DS1122_i(MCARE_i + MCAID_i)$$

where $DS1122_i$ is a dummy variable which equals 1 if P.L. 92-603 is in effect in the state in the ith year and which equals $= 0$ otherwise; $MCARE_i =$ proportion of county population age sixty-five or over (Medicare eligibles) in the ith year; and $MCAID_i =$ proportion of state population who are under age sixty-five and eligible for Medicaid benefits in the ith year.

$$BCPAA_i = (DBCPAA_1 \cdot YR_1 + DBCPAA_2 \cdot YR_2)BCP_i$$

where $DBCPAA_1$ equals 1 if Blue Cross plan requires local planning agency approval for capital expansion in hospital contracts in 1971 and equals 0 otherwise; YR_1 equals 1 if year is 1970, 1971, or 1972 and equals 0 otherwise; $DBCPPA_2$ equals 1 if Blue Cross plan requires local planning agency approval for capital expansion in hospital contracts in 1974 and equals 0 otherwise; YR_2 equals 1 if year is 1973, 1974, or 1975 and equals 0 otherwise; and $BCP_i =$ proportion of population in the Blue Cross plan catchment area covered by Blue Cross hospital insurance in the ith year.

$$COSTB_i = BCOST \cdot BCP_i + MCARE_i + MCAID_i$$

where BCOST equals 1 if Blue Cross uses cost-based hospital reimbursement and equals 0 otherwise, by Blue Cross plan area; $BCP_i =$ proportion of Blue Cross plan area population with Blue Cross hospital insurance coverage in the ith year; $MCARE_i =$ proportion of county population age sixty-five or over (Medicare eligibles) in the $i$the year; and $MCAID =$ proportion of state population under age sixty-five and eligible for Medicaid benefits in the ith year.

$$FPR_i = DFPR_i\{BCPR \cdot BCP_i + MCDPR \cdot MCDP_i + COMPR \cdot COMP_i$$
$$+ MCRPR[MCARE_i - (MCDP_i - MCAID_i)]\}$$

where $DFPR_i$ equals 1 if a formula PR program exists in a state in the ith year and equals 0 otherwise; BCPR equals 1 if the PR program governs Blue Cross hospital reimbursement and equals 0 otherwise; BCP_i is defined as above; MCDPR equals 1 if the PR program governs Medicaid reimbursement and equals 0 otherwise; $MDCP_i$ is the proportion of state population eligible for Medicaid benefits in the ith year; COMPR equals 1 if the PR program governs commerical insurer hospital reimbursement and equals 0 otherwise; $COMP_i$ is an estimate of the proportion of county

Table I-1
Hospital Investment Control Programs by State, 1976

	Certificate of Need				1122 Section Agreement		Blue Cross Planning Agency Approval	
	Program Exists	Year Effective[a]	Equipment Threshold[b]	Service Regulated[c]	Program Exists	Year Agreement Signed	Required in 1971	Required in 1976
Alabama	none	–	–	–	yes	1973	no	no
Alaska	none	–	–	–	yes	1974	yes	no
Arizona	yes	1972	15k	yes	none	–	yes	yes
Arkansas	yes	1976	n.d.	n.d.	yes	1973	no[d]	no
California	yes	1970	n.s.	no	none	–	no	no
Colorado	yes	1974	10k	yes	yes	1974	yes	no
Connecticut	yes	1970	25k[e]	yes	none	–	yes	no
Delaware	none	–	–	–	yes	1973	yes	yes
District of Columbia	yes	1971	100k	yes	none	–	no	yes
Florida	yes	1973	100k	no	yes	1973	no	no[f]
Georgia	no	–	–	–	yes	1974	no	n.d.
Hawaii	yes	1975	100k	yes	yes	1973	n.d.	no
Idaho	none	–	–	–	yes	1974	no	no
Illinois	yes	1975	100k	no	none	–	no	no
Indiana	none	–	–	–	yes	1973	yes	yes[g]
Iowa	none	–	350k[h]	–	yes	1973	yes	yes
Kansas	yes	1973	100k	no	none	–	yes	yes
Kentucky	yes	1973	100k	yes	yes	1974	yes	yes
Louisiana	none	–	–	–	yes	1973	no	no
Maine	none	–	–	–	yes	1973	no	yes
Maryland	yes	1971	100k[i]	yes	yes	1974	yes	no
Massachusetts	yes	1972	100k	yes	none	–	no	yes
Michigan	yes	1973	1k × bed size	no	yes	1973	yes	no
Minnesota	yes	1972	50k	yes	yes	1974	no	yes
Mississippi	none	–	–	–	yes	1973	no	no

Table I-1 continued

	Certificate of Need				1122 Section Agreement		Blue Cross Planning Agency Approval	
	Program Exists	Year Effective[a]	Equipment Threshold[b]	Service Regulated[c]	Program Exists	Year Agreement Signed	Required in 1971	Required in 1976
Missouri	none	—	—	—	yes	1973	[j]	yes
Montana	yes	1974	n.d.	n.d.	yes	1974	no	n.d.
Nebraska	none	—	—	—	yes	1973	no	n.d.
Nevada	yes	1973	n.s.	no[k]	yes	1974	no	no
New Hampshire	none	—	—	—	yes	1973	no	yes
New Jersey	yes	1972	40k	yes	yes	1974	no	no
New Mexico	none	—	—	—	yes	1973	no	no
New York	yes	1965	100k	yes	yes	1974	yes	yes
North Carolina	none[l]	—	—	—	yes	1973	yes	yes
North Dakota	yes	1972	50k	yes[m]	yes	1974	no	n.d.
Ohio	none	—	—	—	yes	1974	no	[n]
Oklahoma	none[o]	—	—	—	yes	1974	no	n.d.
Oregon	yes	1972	200k[p]	yes	yes	1974	[q]	n.d.
Pennsylvania	none	—	—	—	yes	1973	yes	yes
Rhode Island	yes	1968	50k[r]	yes	none	—	yes	yes
South Carolina	yes	1971	n.s.	yes	yes	1974	no	no
South Dakota	yes	1973	50k	yes	none	—	yes	no
Tennessee	yes	1973	100k	yes	none	—	no	no
Texas	yes	1976	100k	100k	none	—	no	no
Utah	none	—	—	—	yes	1974	no	n.d.
Vermont	none	—	—	—	yes	1975	no	yes
Virginia	yes	1973	100k	yes	yes	1973	no[s]	no
Washington	yes	1971	100k	no	yes	1974	yes	no[t]
West Virginia	none	—	—	—	none	—	no	—
Wisconsin	none	—	—	—	yes	1973	no	yes
Wyoming	none	—	—	—	yes	1974	no	no

Source: Lewin and Associates, Inc. (1975a); Curran (1974); American Hospital Association (1972, 1977); Erman (1976); unpublished data from David Salkever.

n.s. = not specified; n.d. = no data.

[a]The CON program is regarded as *effective* if it was in effect six months or more in the year shown.

[b]*Equipment threshold* is the dollar amount below which CON review is not required ($k = \$1,000$).

[c]*Service regulated* indicates CON programs that explicitly include change in hospital services as a criterion for CON review.

[d]Los Angeles plan: no; Oakland plan: yes.

[e]Review optional at 25 to 100k; review mandatory for 100k or more.

[f]Atlanta plan: yes; Columbus plan: no.

[g]Des Moines plan: yes; Sioux City plan: no.

[h]350k or 55% of operating expenses in last fiscal year.

[i]100k or 2% of last annual operating expenses, whichever is less.

[j]Kansas City plan: no; St. Louis plan: yes.

[k]Service reviewed if it results in a change in license classification for the facility.

[l]North Carolina had a CON plan that was effective in 1971 and 1972 and repealed afterward.

[m]No certificate required for provision of new medical service involving expenditure for personnel salaries only.

[n]Cincinnati and Cleveland plans: yes; all other plans: no data.

[o]Oklahoma's CON plan covers nursing homes only.

[p]200k or 2% of average annual operating revenue, whichever is less.

[q]Wilkes-Barre plan: yes; all other plans: no.

[r]50k or 3% of institution's asset value, whichever is less.

[s]Richmond plan: yes; Roanoke plan: no.

[t]Bluefield plan: yes; all other plans: no.

Table I-2
Hospital Rate Regulation and Reimbursement Programs by State, 1975

State	State Authority to Regulate Hospital Rates		Blue Cross Reimbursement Basis	Large-Scale Prospective Reimbursement Programs		
	Year Instituted	Population Covered[a]		Year Instituted	Population Covered[a]	Method
Alabama	none	—	cost	none	—	—
Alaska	none	—	cost	none	—	—
Arizona	1972	ALL	charge	1972	BC, COM	budget
Arkansas	none	—	charge[b]	none	—	—
California	1975	ALL		none	—	—
Colorado	none	—	cost	1974	MCD	formula
Connecticut	1974	ALL	cost	1973	BC, COM	budget
Delaware	none	—	charge	none	—	—
District of Columbia	none	—	cost	none	—	—
Florida	none	—	charge	none	—	—
Georgia	none	—	charge	none	—	—
Hawaii	none	—	n.d.	none	—	—
Idaho	none	—	charge[c]	none	—	—
Illinois	none	—		none	—	—
Indiana	none	—	charge	1970	BC	budget
Iowa	none	—	cost	none	—	—
Kansas	none	—	cost	none	—	—
Kentucky	none	—	charge	1970	BC	budget
Louisiana	none	—	charge	none	—	—
Maine	none	—	cost	none	—	—
Maryland	1974	ALL	charge	1974	ALL	budget
Massachusetts	1968	MCD	cost	1975	MCD	formula
Michigan	none	—	cost	none	—	—
Minnesota	none	—	cost	none	—	—
Mississippi	none	—	cost[d]	none	—	—
Missouri	none	—		none	—	—
Montana	none	—	charge	none	—	—
Nebraska	none	—	charge	none	—	—
Nevada	none	—	n.d.	none	—	—

State		Basis	Year		Method
New Hampshire	none	cost	none	—	—
New Jersey	BC, MCD	cost	1970	BC, MCD	budget
New Mexico	none	charge	none	—	—
New York	BC, MCD	cost	1970	BC, MCD	formula
North Carolina	none	charge	1972	BC	budget
North Dakota	none	charge	none	—	—
Ohio	none	[e]	[f]	[f]	[f]
Oklahoma	none	[g]	[g]	[g]	[g]
Oregon	none	charge	none	—	—
Pennsylvania	BC, MCD, MCR	cost	1971	BC, MCD, MCR	budget
Rhode Island	none	cost	none	—	—
South Carolina	none	charge	none	—	—
South Dakota	none	cost	none	—	—
Tennessee	none	charge	none	—	—
Texas	none	charge	none	—	—
Utah	none	charge	none	—	—
Vermont	none	cost	none	—	—
Virginia	none	cost	none	—	—
Washington	none[h]	charge	none	—	—
West Virginia	none	[i]	1972	BC	budget
Wisconsin	none	charge	none	—	—
Wyoming	none	charge	none	—	—

Source: Lewin and Associates, Inc. (1975a); American Hospital Association (1972, 1977); Laudicina (1976).

[a] BC = Blue Cross; MCD = Medicaid; MCR = Medicare; COM = commercial insurer; ALL = all patients.

[b] Los Angeles plan: cost; Oakland plan: charge.

[c] Chicago plan: cost; Rockford plan: charge.

[d] Kansas City plan: charge; St. Louis plan: cost.

[e] Cincinnati plan: charge; all other plans: cost.

[f] Blue Cross of Southwest Ohio (Cincinnati) operates a budget-based hospital PR program. All other hospital reimbursement programs in the state are retrospective.

[g] Oklahoma Blue Cross offers, as an option to hospitals, a budget-based system. As of 1976, roughly 30 percent of Oklahoma hospitals, mostly nonmetropolitan, participated in this system.

[h] Washington has a state hospital rate commission, established in 1973, but it had not begun to exercise authority over hospital rates by 1975.

[i] Wheeling plan: cost; all other plans: charge.

Table I–3
Large-Scale Hospital Utilization Review Programs Operated by
Medicaid and Blue Cross, by State, 1974

	Medicaid[a]	Blue Cross[a]	External Review[b]
Alabama	no	yes	none
Alaska	yes	no	none
Arizona	no	no	—
Arkansas	yes	no	Medicaid
California	yes	no	none
Colorado	yes	no	Medicaid
Connecticut	yes	yes	none
Delaware	no	no	—
District of Columbia	no	no	—
Florida	no	no	—
Georgia	yes	no	none
Hawaii	yes	yes	none
Idaho	no	no	—
Illinois	yes	yes	Medicaid
Indiana	no	no	—
Iowa	yes	no	none
Kansas	yes	no	—
Kentucky	yes	yes	Medicaid
Louisiana	no	no	—
Maine	yes	no	Medicaid
Maryland	yes	no	Medicaid
Massachusetts	yes	no	Medicaid
Michigan	no	yes	none
Minnesota	yes	yes	Blue Cross
Mississippi	yes	no	none
Missouri	yes	yes	none
Montana	yes	no	Medicaid
Nebraska	yes	yes	none
Nevada	yes	no	Medicaid
New Hampshire	yes	no	none
New Jersey	yes	yes	none
New Mexico	no	yes	none
New York	yes	no	none
North Carolina	yes	no	none
North Dakota	yes	yes	none
Ohio	yes	yes	none
Oklahoma	no	no	—
Oregon	yes	yes	Medicaid
Pennsylvania	yes	yes	none
Rhode Island	yes	yes	none
South Carolina	yes	no	none
South Dakota	no	no	—
Tennessee	yes	yes	none
Texas	no	no	—
Utah	yes	no	Medicaid
Vermont	no	no	—
Virginia	yes	yes	none
Washington	no	no	—
West Virginia	no	yes	none

Table I–3 continued

	Medicaid[a]	*Blue Cross[a]*	*External Review[b]*
Wisconsin	yes	no	none
Wyoming	yes	no	Medicaid

Source: Lewin and Associates, Inc. (1975a).

[a]Includes only statewide Medicaid UR programs and planwide Blue Cross programs. Programs that were specified as having only reviewers internal to the provider were also excluded. The Blue Cross data are not totally consistent with data provided in American Hospital Association (1974). The latter source identifies Blue Cross plans which require UR in their contracts with hospitals. The following plans were specified as requiring UR: Arizona, Arkansas, California (Oakland plan), Connecticut, District of Columbia, Indiana, Massachusetts, Michigan, Missouri, New Hampshire, New Jersey, New York, Ohio (Canton plan), Pennsylvania, Rhode Island, South Carolina, Utah, and Virginia. Information regarding UR requirements was missing for several plans—Colorado, Florida, Georgia, Idaho, Illinois, Louisiana (Baton Rouge), Maine, Minnesota, Mississippi, Nebraska, New Mexico, North Dakota, Oklahoma, Oregon, Tennessee, Texas, West Virginia, and Wyoming. Also, the AHA source does not specify whether reviews are performed by reviewers other than provider staff.

[b]This column indicates UR programs with reviewers external to both provider and reviewing agency.

Table I–4
Examples of Construction of Certificate-of-Need Variables by State

Variable	1970	1971	1972	1973	1974	1975
Example 1 = Comprehensive CON Established in 1972 (Arizona)						
NCON1	0	0	0	0	0	0
NCON2	0	0	0	0	0	0
CCON1	0	0	1	1	0	0
CCON2	0	0	0	0	1	1
PRECON	0	1	0	0	0	0
Example 2 = Noncomprehensive CON Established in 1970 (California)						
NCON1	1	1	0	0	0	0
NCON2	0	0	1	1	1	1
CCON1	0	0	0	0	0	0
CCON2	0	0	0	0	0	0
PRECON	0	0	0	0	0	0
Example 3 = Noncomprehensive CON Established in 1976 (Texas)						
NCON1	0	0	0	0	0	0
NCON2	0	0	0	0	0	0
CCON1	0	0	0	0	0	0
CCON2	0	0	0	0	0	0
PRECON	0	0	0	0	0	1

population with commercial hospital insurance coverage in the ith year:

$$COMP_i = 0.95 - BCP_i - MCARE_i - MCAID_i†$$

MCRPR equals 1 if the PR program governs Medicare reimbursement and equals 0 otherwise;[2] and $MCARE_i$ and $MCAID_i$ are defined as above.

$$BPR = DBPR_i\{BCPR \cdot BCP_i + MCDPR \cdot MCDP_i + COMPR \cdot COMP_i +$$

$$MCRPR[MCARE_i - (MCDP_i - MCAID_i)]\}$$

where $DBPR_i$ equals 1 if a budget-based PR program exists in a state in the ith year and equals 0 otherwise; and all other variables are defined as above.

$$UR_i = BCUR \cdot BCP_i + MCDUR \cdot MCDP_i$$

where UR_i = proportion of population in states having large-scale hospital UR programs operated by Blue Cross and/or Medicaid in the ith year; BCUR equals 1 if Blue Cross UR program existed in 1974; MCDUR equals 1 if Medicaid UR program existed in 1974; BCP_i and $MCDP_i$ are defined as above. The ESP values, by year, are: 1970, 0; 1971, 0.25; 1972, 1.00; 1973, 1.00; 1974, 0.25; and 1975, 0.

Notes

1. The year in which CON becomes effective is uniformly defined as first year when the CON program operates for six months or more. It does not pertain to the year when CON legislation was enacted.
2. In all states where MCRPR = 1, MCDPR also = 1.

----

† This is a very crude estimation formula, but because COMPR = 1 in very few areas, a more precise estimation procedure was not undertaken.

Appendix J:
Variables BCP, MCARE, MCDP, MCAID, COMP

Variable names: BCP, MCARE, MCDP, MCAID, COMP.

Description: These variables, which are defined in Appendix I, are measures of area population proportions pertaining to hospital reimbursement programs. They are used in computation of the reimbursement variables S1122, BCPAA, COSTB, FPR, BPR, and UR.

Methodology: All reimbursement variables, excluding ESP, require estimation of area population proportions covered by the different reimbursement programs. With regard to hospital reimbursement, populations are classified in one or more of the following categories (units of observation of area data are also shown): Blue Cross–enrolled by Blue Cross plan area, Medicare-eligible by county, Medicaid-eligible by state, and commercial insurance–enrolled, estimated from above data.

Blue Cross Association publishes annual figures on proportion of plan-area population enrolled in Blue Cross plans. These data were used to construct the area Blue Cross enrollment proportion variable (BCP). The seventy-one Blue Cross plan areas (the United States and Puerto Rico, as of December 31, 1975) are combinations of contiguous counties. In many cases, one Blue Cross plan serves an entire state. In other cases, two or more plans exist within a state, and in a few cases plan areas cross state lines. The value of BCP for a given hospital and year depends on the hospital's location with regard to Blue Cross plan-area boundaries.

Proportion of county population age sixty-five and over (MCARE) is used as our measure of Medicare eligibility. Although some persons age sixty-five and over are not eligible for Medicare, and some under sixty-five are eligible, these cases are sufficiently small in magnitude to be ignored in the area proportion estimates. The variable MCARE is measured directly for 1975 from data published by Sales Management, Inc., and for 1970 from data obtained from the Area Resource File, compiled and distributed by the Bureau of Health Manpower, HEW. In-between years' proportions were estimated via linear interpolation, a process that is subject to very slight estimation error.

Medicaid eligibility data are available by year, but for states only. Two Medicaid variables have been defined: the proportion of state population eligible for Medicaid (MCDP) and the proportion of state population under sixty-five and eligible for Medicaid (MCAID). The latter variable is employed whenever Medicare proportions are added to Medicaid proportions to

Table J–1
Sample Means of Primary Area Population and Reimbursement Proportion Variables, 1970– 1975

Variable	1970	1971	1972	1973	1974	1975	Grand Mean	Percentage Increase 1970–1975
BCP	0.369	0.373	0.380	0.393	0.402	0.408	0.387	10.6
MCARE	0.097	0.098	0.098	0.101	0.102	0.102	0.100	5.1
MCDP	0.095	0.098	0.102	0.100	0.113	0.117	0.104	23.2
MCAID	0.074	0.077	0.081	0.082	0.092	0.096	0.084	29.7
S1122	0.000	0.000	0.000	0.041	0.102	0.105	0.041	—
BCPAA	0.149	0.149	0.150	0.219	0.224	0.226	0.186	51.7
COST	0.479	0.485	0.489	0.502	0.521	0.529	0.501	10.4
FPR	0.088	0.089	0.090	0.092	0.096	0.109	0.094	23.9
BPR	0.029	0.030	0.048	0.061	0.086	0.087	0.057	200.0
UR	0.351	0.357	0.359	0.364	0.380	0.384	0.366	9.4
ESP	0.000	0.250	1.000	1.000	0.250	0.000	0.417	—

avoid double-counting. Because Medicaid variables are computed with state data, they are subject to some errors in variables. Moreover, when Medicaid proportions are combined with other area proportion data (for example, when MCARE and MCAID are summed to obtain county population proportions subject to section 1122 reimbursement regulation), this implicitly assumes that the Medicaid proportion is constant across counties within the state.

The remaining proportion variable, COMP, which measures the proportion of area population with commerical hospital insurance coverage, is very crudely estimated, but used in very few instances. Commercial reimbursement tends to be subject to regulation far less frequently than the Blue Cross and government reimbursement programs. Moreover, when commercial reimbursement is covered by a particular regulation, it is frequently true that *all* reimbursement within a state is covered, such that the area proportion can safely be estimated to be 1.0. The only cases in which nonstatewide regulation includes commercial reimbursement are PR in Arizona and Connecticut. In these cases, the proportion of population with no insurance or with other insurance (nongovernment, non-Blue Cross, noncommerical) was assumed to equal 0.05. The area proportion with commercial insurance was estimated as follows: COMP = 0.95 − BCP − MCARE − MCAID. Because this formula was used so infrequently, a more precise estimating system was deemed unnecessary.

Table J–1 provides estimates of yearly averages of the primary area proportion variables and the reimbursement variables for 1970–1975. Grand means of these variables and percentage increases from 1970 to 1975 are also shown.

Appendix K:
Variables COLREQ,
UNION, STRIKE

Variable Names: COLREQ, UNION, STRIKE.

Description: These variables indicate hospital-specific union activities affecting some of or all the hospital employees. Data for construction of COLREQ and UNION were available for 1970, 1973, and 1975. Data for construction of STRIKE were available for 1970 and 1973 only. In 1970 and 1973, COLREQ indicated that the hospital had " ... received a request for recognition as a collective bargaining agent..." and in 1975 that " ... unions or other employee organizations had conducted any organizing activities for the purpose of collective bargaining among employees of the hospital...." These two questions were treated as equivalent. In each year UNION indicates the presence of a signed collective-bargaining agreement; STRIKE indicates that a strike or other kind of work stoppage had occurred during the previous twelve months.

Methodology: Variables COLREQ, UNION, and STRIKE were constructed as dummy variables. It was necessary to estimate values for these variables for the years for which no data were available. Three assumptions were made: (1) If the data indicated the absence of a unionization "event" for two years, it was assumed to be absent in all intervening years. (2) Once one

Table K–1
Potential Values of Unionization Variables

Variable[a]	1970	1971	1972	1973	1974	1975
COLREQ	0	0	0	0	0	0
	0	0	0	0	0	1
	0	0	0	1	1	1
	1	1	1	1	1	1
UNION	0	0	0	0	0	0
	0	0	0	0	0.5	1
	0	0.33	0.67	1	1	1
	1	1	1	1	1	1
STRIKE	0	0	0	0	0	0
	0	0	0	1	1	1
	1	1	1	1	1	1

[a]The table shows all possible values of each variable for any given hospital for each of the six years. As defined, for any sample hospital, the value of a unionization variable in a given year must be equal to or greater than the value in the preceding year. Sample means of COLREQ, UNION, and STRIKE across all years are 0.25, 0.24, and 0.05, respectively.

of the unionization events took place, it was assumed that its impact would be realized throughout the remainder of the period of the study. (3) For hospitals indicating that they had a signed collective-bargaining agreement in a given year, it was assumed that it was equally likely that the agreement was signed in any prior year following a year when no such agreement was indicated. Potential values of the three variables and means for the sample are shown in table K–1.

Bibliography

Abt Associates, Inc.; Policy Analysis, Inc.; Arthur D. Little, Inc.; and Arthur Andersen and Co. *Evaluation of Nine Prospective Rate Setting Programs.* Mimeograph, 1978.

Abt Associates, Inc., and Policy Analysis, Inc. "Analysis of Prospective Payment Systems for Upstate New York." Final report under contract no. HEW-OS 74-261 to the Social Security Administration, April 6, 1976.

Allison, R.F. "Administrative Responses to Prospective Reimbursement." *Topics in Health Care Financing* 3, no. 2 (Winter 1976):97–111.

Altman, S.H. "The Structure of Nursing Education and Its Impact on Supply." In *Empirical Studies in Health Economics*, edited by H.E. Klarman, pp. 335–352. Baltimore: Johns Hopkins Press, 1970.

Altman, S.H., and Eichenholz, J. "Inflation in the Health Industry—Causes and Cures." In *Health: A Victim or Cause of Inflation?* edited by W. Zubkoff, pp. 7–30. New York: Prodist, 1976.

Altman, S.H., and Weiner, S.L. "Regulation as Second Best." In *Competition in the Health Care Sector: Past, Present, and Future*, edited by W. Greenberg, pp. 421–447. Germantown, Md.: Aspen Systems, 1978.

American Hospital Association. *Hospitals: Guide Issue*, pt. 2, 88, no. 15 (August 1, 1971).

_____. "Statistical Profile of the Nation's Hospitals." In *Hospital Statistics*. 1976 ed. Chicago: AHA, 1976.

American Hospital Association, Bureau of Fiscal Services. "Survey of Provisions of Hospital-Blue Cross Contracts as of September 30, 1971." Chicago: AHA, January 1972.

American Hospital Association, Division of Financial Management. "Blue Cross Contract Provisions as of June 30, 1976." Chicago: AHA, January 1977.

American Hospital Association, Division of Health Economics. "Survey of Provisions of Hospital-Blue Cross Contracts as of February 28, 1974." Chicago: AHA, July 1974.

American Medical Association, Center for Health Services Research and Development. *Distribution of Physicians in the United States, 1970–1973. Chicago: AMA, 1971–1974.*

_____. *Physician Distribution and Medical Licensure in the United States, 1974, 1975.* Chicago: AMA, 1975, 1976.

Andersen, R.; Kravits, J.; and Andersen, O.W. *Equity in Health Services: Empirical Analyses in Social Policy.* Cambridge, Mass.: Ballinger, 1975.

Andersen, R.; Lion, J.; and Anderson, O.W. *Two Decades of Health Services: Social Survey Trends in Use and Expenditure.* Cambridge, Mass.: Ballinger, 1976.

Anderson, O.W. "A Decade of Good Intentions." In *Proceedings of the Eighteenth Annual Symposium on Hospital Affairs*, pp. 3–9. Chicago: University of Chicago Graduate Program in Hospital Administration, April 1976.

Applied Management Sciences. "Analysis of Prospective Reimbursement Systems: Western Pennsylvania." Final report under contract no. HEW OS-74-226 to the Social Security Administration, August 6, 1975.

Arthur Andersen, Inc. "Study of Reimbursement and Practice Arrangements of Provider-Based Physicians." Final report to the Health Care Financing Administration, December 1977.

Averill, R.F., and McMahon, L.F. "A Cost Benefit Analysis of Continued Stay Certification." *Medical Care* 15, no. 2 (February 1977): 158–173.

Bailey, D.R., and Reidel, D.C. "Recertification and Length of Stay: The Impact of New Jersey's AID Program on Patterns of Hospital Care." *Blue Cross Reports* 6 (July 1968): 1–10.

Baron, D.P. "A Study of Hospital Cost Inflation." *The Journal of Human Resources* 9, no. 1 (Winter 1974): 33–49.

Bates, F.L., and White, R.F. "Differential Perceptions of Authority in Hospitals." *Journal of Health and Human Behavior* 2 (1961): 262–267.

Bays, C.W. "Case-Mix Differences between Nonprofit and For-Profit Hospitals." *Inquiry* 14 (March 1977): 17–21.

Bentkover, J., and Sanders, C.R. "Trends in Facility Use: An Evaluation of the Impact of Adverse Economic Conditions on the Health Status of the Poor." Final report under contract no. HRA 230-75-123, August 1977.

Berki, S.E. *Hospital Economics.* Lexington, Mass.: D.C. Heath, 1972.

Berman, L.T. *Utilization Review in Connecticut Hospitals: Three Years After Medicare.* New Haven, Conn.: Yale University, 1969.

Berry, R. "Product Heterogeneity and Hospital Cost Analysis." *Inquiry* 7, no. 1 (March 1970): 67–75.

―――――. "Prospective Rate Reimbursement and Cost Containment: Formula Reimbursement in New York." *Inquiry* 13, no. 3 (September 1976): 288–301.

―――――. "Returns to Scale in the Production of Hospital Services." *Health Services Research* 2 (Summer 1967): 123–139.

Bicknell, W.J., and Walsh, D.C. "Certification of Need: The Massachusetts Experience." *New England Journal of Medicine* 292 (May 15, 1975): 1054–1061.

Blair, R.D., and Vogel, R.J. *The Cost of Health Insurance Regulation.* Lexington, Mass.: D.C. Heath, 1975.

Blue Cross Association. "Utilization Review and Control Activities in Blue Cross Plans." *Blue Cross Reports* 4 (January–March 1966).

Blue Cross Association, and National Association of Blue Shield Plans. *Fact Book, 1971–1976.* Chicago: BCA and NABSP, 1971–1976.

Blum, J.D.; Gertman, P.M.; and Rabinow, J. *PSROs and the Law.* Germantown, Md.: Aspen Systems, 1977.

Blumstein, J.F. "Inflation and Quality: The Case for PSROs." In *Health: A Victim or Cause of Inflation?* edited by M. Zubkoff, pp. 245–295. New York: Prodist, 1976.

Blumstein, J.F., and Calvani, T. "Antitrust and State Regulation of Medical Care Services: The Doctrine of *Parker v. Brown.*" *Duke Law Journal* 1978, no. 2 (1978): 389–441.

Blumstein, J.F., and Sloan, F.A. "Health Planning and Regulation through Certificate of Need: An Overview." *Utah Law Review,* no. 1 (1978): 3–38.

Brian, E. "Foundation for Medical Care Control of Hospital Utilization: CHAP, PSRO Prototype." *New England Journal of Medicine* 288 (April 26, 1973): 878–882.

———. "Government Control of Hospital Utilization." *New England Journal of Medicine* 286 (June, 22, 1972): 1340–1344.

Carlson, R.J. *The End of Medicine.* New York: Wiley, 1975.

Carroll, M.S. "Private Health Insurance Plans in 1976: An Evaluation." *Social Security Bulletin* 41, no. 9 (September 1978): 3–16.

Carroll, M.S., and Arnett, R.H. "Private Health Insurance Plans in 1977: Coverage, Enrollment, and Financial Experience." *Health Care Financing Review* 1, no. 2 (Fall 1979): 3–22.

Cleverley, W.O. "The Relationship of Hospital Cost Measurement to Hospital Cost Control Programs." In *Hospital Cost Containment,* edited by M. Zubkoff, I. Raskin, and R.S. Hanft, pp. 489–513. New York: Prodist, 1978.

Congressional Budget Office. *Controlling Rising Hospital Costs.* Washington: Government Printing Office, September 1979.

Cooper, B.S.; Worthington, N.L.; and McGee, M.R. *Compendium of National Health Expenditure Data.* DHEW Publication no. (SSA) 76-11927. Washington: Government Printing Office, January 1976.

Coser, R.L. "Authority and Decision-Making in a Hospital: A Comparative Analysis." *American Sociological Review* 23, no. 1 (February 1958): 56–63.

Cromwell, J.; Ginsburg, P.; and Hamilton, D. "A Study of the Factors Underlying Capital Equipment Decision Making in Hospitals." Under contract to NCHSRD, contract no. HSM 110-73-513. Cambridge, Mass.: Abt Associates, Inc., September, 1975.

Cunningham, R.M. *Governing Hospitals: Trustees and the New Account-*

abilities. Chicago: American Hospital Association, 1976.

Curran, W.J. "A National Survey and Analysis of State Certificate-of-Need Laws for Health Facilities." In *Regulating Health Facilities Construction,* edited by C.C. Havighurst, pp. 85–111. Washington: American Enterprise Institute, 1974.

Davidson, G.B. "Manpower Substitution and Hospital Efficiency." Paper presented at the 1978 Allied Social Science Association Meeting, Chicago. Mimeograph.

Davis, K. "Economic Theories of Behavior in Nonprofit, Private Hospitals." *Economic and Business Bulletin* 24 (Spring 1972): 1–13.

_____. "The Role of Technology, Demand and Labor Markets in the Determination of Hospital Costs." In *The Economics of Health and Medical Care,* edited by M. Perlman, pp. 283–301. London: MacMillan, 1974.

_____. "Theories of Hospital Inflation: Some Empirical Evidence." *Journal of Human Resources* 8, no. 2 (Spring 1973): 181–201.

_____. "A Theory of Economic Behavior in Non-Profit, Private Hospitals." Ph.D. dissertation, Rise University, May 1969.

Davis, K., and Reynolds, R. "The Impact of Medicare and Medicaid on Access to Medical Care." In *The Role of Health Insurance in the Health Services Sector,* edited by R. Rosett, pp. 391–425. New York: National Bureau of Economic Research, 1976.

Davis, K., and Russell, L. "The Substitution of Hospital Outpatient Services for Inpatient Care." *Review of Economics and Statistics* 54, no. 2 (May 1972): 109–120.

Decker, B., and Bonner, P. *PSROs: Organization for Regional Peer Review.* Cambridge, Mass.: Ballinger, 1973.

Domar, E. "The Soviet Collective Farm as a Producer Cooperative." *American Economic Review* 56, no. 4 (September 1966): 734–757.

Donabedian, A. "Evaluating the Quality of Medical Care." *Milbank Memorial Fund Quarterly* 44, no. 3 (July 1966): 166–206.

Dowling, W.L. "Prospective Reimbursement of Hospitals." *Inquiry* 11, no. 3 (September 1974): 163–180.

Dowling, W.L.; House, P.J.; Lehman, J.M.; Meade, G.L.; Teague, N; Trivedi, V.M.; and Watts, C.A. *Prospective Reimbursement in Downstate New York and Its Impact on Hospitals—A Summary.* Discussion Paper no. 3. Center for Health Services Research, Department of Health Services, University of Washington, December 1976.

Drake, D. "The Hospital as a Public Utility." In *Regulating the Hospital, A Report of the 1972 National Forum on Hospital and Health Affairs.* Durham, N.C.: Duke University, Graduate Program in Hospital Administration, 1973.

Dumbaugh, K., and Neuhauser, D. "The Effect of Pre-admission Testing on Length of Stay." In *Organizational Research in Hospitals*, edited by S.M. Shortell and M. Brown, pp. 13–28. Chicago: Blue Cross Association, 1976.

Ehrenberg, R.G. "Organizational Control and the Economic Efficiency of Hospitals: The Production of Nursing Services." *The Journal of Human Resources* 9, no. 1 (Winter 1974): 21–32.

Elnicki, R.A. "Effect of Phase II Price Controls on Hospital Services." *Health Services Research*, Summer 1972, pp. 106–117.

Enthoven, Alain C. "Consumer-Choice Health Plan" (first of two parts). *New England Journal of Medicine* 298, no. 12 (March 23, 1978a): 650–658.

_____. "Consumer-Choice Health Plan" (second of two parts). *New England Journal of Medicine* 298, no. 13 (March 30, 1978b): 709–720.

Erman, D. "Working Paper on Certificate of Need." Mimeograph, 1976.

Evans, R.G. "'Behavioural' Cost Functions for Hospitals." *Canadian Journal of Economics* 4, no. 2 (May 1971): 198–215.

_____. "Efficiency Incentives in Hospital Reimbursement." Ph.D. dissertation, Harvard University, 1970.

Evans, R.G., and Walker, H.D. "Information Theory and the Analysis of Hospital Cost Structure." *Canadian Journal of Economics* 4, no. 3 (August 1972): 398–418.

Feldman, R.D., and Scheffler, R.M. "The Effect of Labor Unions on Hospital Employees' Wages." Mimeograph, 1977.

Feldstein, M.S. "An Econometric Model of the Medicare System." *The Quarterly Journal of Economics* 85, no. 1 (February 1971a): 1–20.

_____. "Econometric Studies of Health Economics." In *Frontiers of Quantitative Studies, II,* edited by M.D. Intriligator and D.A. Kendrick, pp. 377–433. Amsterdam: North-Holland Publishing Company, 1974.

_____. *Economic Analysis for Health Service Efficiency*. Amsterdam: North-Holland Publishing Company, 1967.

_____. "Hospital Cost Inflation: A Study of Nonprofit Price Dynamics." *American Economic Review* 61, no. 5 (December 1971b): 853–872.

_____. "Quality Change and the Demand for Hospital Care." *Econometrica* 45, no. 7 (October 1977): 1681–1702.

_____. "The Welfare Loss from Excess Health Insurance." *Journal of Political Economy* 81, no. 1 (March/April 1973): 251–280.

Feldstein, M.S., and Taylor, Amy K. *The Rapid Rise of Hospital Costs*. Discussion Paper no. 531. Harvard Institute of Economic Research, January 1977.

Flashner, B.A.; Reed, S.; Coburn, R.W.; and Fine, P.R. "Professional Standards Review Organizations—Analysis of Their Development and

Implementation Based on a Preliminary Review of the Hospital Admission and Surveillance Program in Illinois." *Journal of the American Medical Association* 223 (March 26, 1973): 1473–1484.

Fottler, M.D. "The Union Impact on Hospital Wages." *Industrial and Labor Relations Review* 30, no. 3 (April 1977): 342–355.

Frech, H.E. III, and Ginsburg, P.B. "Competition among Health Insurers." In *Competition in the Health Care Sector: Past, Present, and Future,* edited by W. Greenberg, pp. 167–187. Germantown, Md.: Aspen Systems, 1978.

_____ and _____. "Imposed Health Insurance in Monopolistic Markets: A Theoretical Analysis." *Economic Inquiry* 13, no. 1 (March 1975): 55–70.

Frenzen, P.D. "Survey Updates Unionization Activities." *Hospital* 52, no. 15 (August 1, 1978): 93–104.

Fuchs, V.R. "The Supply of Surgeons and the Demand for Operations." *The Journal of Human Resources* 13, supplement (1978): 35–56.

_____. *Who Shall Live? Health, Economics, and Social Choice.* New York: Basic Books, 1974.

Fuchs, V.R., and Newhouse, J.P. "The Conference and Unresolved Problems." *Journal of Human Resources* 13, supplement (1978): 5–18.

Furst, R.W., and Dunkelberg, J.S. "Study Shows ESP Reduced Hospitals' Profitability." *Hospital Progress*, August 1978, pp. 59–63.

Gaus, C.R., and Hellinger, F.J. "Results of Prospective Reimbursement." *Topics in Health Care Financing* 3, no. 2 (Winter 1976): 83–96.

Geomet, Inc. "Analysis of the New Jersey Hospital Prospective Reimbursement System: 1968–1973." Final report under contract no. HEW OS-74-268 to the Social Security Administration, February 27, 1976.

Gibson, R.M., and Mueller, M.S. "National Health Expenditures, Fiscal Year 1976." *Social Security Bulletin*, April 1977, pp. 3–22.

Ginsburg, P.B. "Impact of the Economic Stabilization Program on Hospitals: An Analysis with Aggregate Data." In *Hospital Cost Containment,* edited by I. Raskin, and R.S. Hanft, pp. 293–323. New York: Prodist, 1978.

_____. "The Impact of the Economic Stabilization Program on Hospitals and Hospital Care." Final report to DHEW under contract HSM 110-73-467, October 15, 1976.

_____. "Price Controls and Hospital Costs." Prepared for presentation to AEA-HERO session of Allied Social Science Association meetings, San Francisco, December 29, 1974.

Goldberg, G.A., and Holloway, D.C. "Emphasizing 'Level of Care' over 'Length of Stay' in Hospital Utilization Review." *Medical Care* 13, no. 6 (June 1975): 474–485.

Goss, M.E.W. "Influence and Authority among Physicians in an Outpatient Clinic." *American Sociological Review* 26, no. 1 (February 1961): 39–50.

Gottlieb, S.R. "A Brief History of Health Planning in the United States." In *Regulating Health Facilities Construction*, edited by C.C. Havighurst, pp. 7–26. Washington: American Enterprise Institute, 1974.

Greenfield, H.I. *Hospital Efficiency and Public Policy.* New York: Praeger, 1973.

Grimes, T.F. *The Effectiveness of Utilization Review since the Advent of Medicare.* Washington: George Washington University, 1970.

Grossman, M. *The Demand for Health: A Theoretical and Empirical Investigation.* New York: National Bureau of Economic Research, 1972.

Guest, R.H. "The Role of the Doctor in Institutional Management." In *Organization Research on Health Institutions*, edited by B.S. Georgopoulos, pp. 283–300. Ann Arbor: University of Michigan Press, 1972.

Hadar, J. *Mathematical Theory of Economic Behavior.* Reading, Mass.: Addison-Wesley, 1971.

Hamermesh, D.S. "Econometric Studies of Labor Demand and Their Application to Policy Analysis." *The Journal of Human Resources* 11, no. 4 (Fall 1976): 507–525.

Harmon, C. "The Efficiency and Effectiveness of Health Care Capital Expenditures and Service Controls: An Interim Assessment." In *Health Regulation: Certificate of Need and 1122*, edited by H.H. Hyman, pp. 27–52. Germantown, Md.: Aspen Systems, 1977.

Harris, J.E. "The Internal Organization of Hospitals: Some Economic Implications." *Bell Journal of Economics* 8, no. 2 (Autumn 1977): 467–482.

Havighurst, C.C. *Public Utility Regulation for Hospitals.* Reprint no. 17. Washington: American Enterprise Institute, 1973a.

———. "Regulation of Health Facilities and Services by 'Certificate of Need.'" *Virginia Law Review* 59, no. 7 (October 1973b):1142–1225.

Havighurst, C.C., and Blumstein, J.F. "Coping with Quality/Cost Trade-offs in Medical Care: The Role of PSROs." *Northwestern University Law Review* 70 (March-April 1975): 6–68.

Hays, R.D. "Regulatory and Administrative Determinants of Health Insurance Premiums." Mimeograph, 1978.

Health Insurance Institute. *Source Book of Health Insurance Data.* New York: HII, various years since 1973.

Hefty, T.R. "Returns to Scale in Hospitals—A Critical Review of Recent Research." *Health Services Research* 4 (Winter 1969): 267–280.

Hellinger, F.J. "The Effect of Certificate-of-Need Legislation on Hospital Investment." *Inquiry* 13, no. 2 (June 1976a): 187–193.

_____. "Prospective Reimbursement through Budget Review: New Jersey, Rhode Island, and Western Pennsylvania." *Inquiry* 13, no. 3 (September 1976b): 309–320.

Illich, I. *Medical Nemesis*. New York: Pantheon Books, 1976.

Ingbar, M.L., and Taylor, L.D. *Hospital Costs in Massachusetts*. Cambridge, Mass.: Harvard University Press, 1968.

Kinzer, D.M. "Straws in a Wind of Change." In *Proceedings of the Eighteenth Annual Symposium on Hospital Affairs*, pp. 10–17. Chicago: University of Chicago, Graduate Program in Hospital Administration, April 1976.

Klarman, H.E. "Comment." In *Empirical Studies in Health Economics*, edited by H.E. Klarman. Baltimore, Md.: Johns Hopkins Press, 1970.

_____. *The Economics of Health*. New York: Columbia University Press, 1965.

Kolb, J., and Sidel, V.W. "Influence of Utilization Review on the Hospital Length of Stay." *Journal of the American Medical Association* 203 (January 8, 1968): 117–119.

Kovner, A.R. "The Hospital Administrator and Organizational Effectiveness." In *Organizational Research on Health Institutions*, edited by B.S. Georgopoulos, pp. 355–376. Ann Arbor: University of Michigan Press, 1972.

Kushman, J.E., and Nuckton, C.F. "Further Evidence on the Relative Performance of Proprietary and Nonprofit Hospitals." *Medical Care* 15, no. 3 (March 1977): 189–204.

Laudicina, S.S. *Prospective Reimbursement for Hospitals: A Guide for Policymakers*. New York: Community Service Society, October 1976.

Lave, J.R., and Lave, L.B. "Hospital Cost Function Analysis: Implications for Cost Controls." In *Hospital Cost Containment*, edited by M. Zubkoff, I. Raskin, and R.S. Hanft, pp. 358–571. New York: Prodist, 1978.

_____. and _____. "Hospital Cost Functions." *American Economic Review* 60, no. 3 (June 1970): 379–395.

Lave, J.R.; Lave, L.B.; and Silverman, L.B. "Hospital Cost Estimation Controlling for Case-Mix." *Applied Economics* 4 (September 1972): 165–180.

_____; _____; and _____. "A Proposal for Incentive Reimbursement for Hospitals." *Medical Care* 11 (March–April 1973): 79–89.

Law, S. *Blue Cross: What Went Wrong?* New Haven, Conn.: Yale University Press, 1974.

Lee, M.L., and Wallace, R.L. "Problems in Estimating Multi-product Cost Functions: An Application to Hospitals." *Western Economic Journal*, September 1973, pp. 350–363.

Leibenstein, H. "Allocative Efficiency vs. X-Efficiency." *American Economic Review* 56, no. 3 (June 1966): 392–415.

_____. *Beyond Economic Man.* Cambridge, Mass.: Harvard University Press, 1976.

Levine, H.D., and Phillip, P.J. *Factors Affecting Staffing Levels and Patterns of Nursing Personnel.* Washington: U.S. Public Health Service, Division of Nursing, 1975.

Lewin and Associates, Inc. "An Analysis of State and Regional Health Regulation." Final report to the Health Resources Administration under contract no. HEW-OS-73-212, February 1975a.

_____. "Evaluation of the Efficiency and Effectiveness of the Section 1122 Review Process." Report to the Health Resources Administration under contract no. HRA-106-74-183, September 1975b.

Lightle, M.A. "'70s See New Approaches to Capital Financing for Hospitals." *Hospitals* 52, no. 12 (June 16, 1978): 135–141.

Link, C.R., and Landon, J.H. "Monopsony and Union Power in the Market for Nurses." *Southern Economic Review* 41, no. 4 (April 1975): 649–659.

Lipscomb, J.; Raskin, J.E.; and Eichenholz, J. "The Use of Marginal Cost Estimates in Hospital Cost-Containment Policy." In *Hospital Cost Containment,* edited by M. Zubkoff, I. Raskin, and R.S. Hanft, pp. 514–537. New York: Prodist, 1978.

Long, M.F. "Efficient Use of Hospitals." In *The Economics of Health and Medical Care,* pp. 211–226. Ann Arbor: University of Michigan Press, 1964.

MACRO Systems, Inc. *The Certificate of Need Experience: An Early Assessment.* Silver Spring, Md., 1974.

Marcom, E. *Medical Staff Utilization Committees: Development and Effectiveness.* Durham, N.C.: The Duke University Press, 1965.

May, J.J. *Health Planning: Its Past and Potential.* Chicago: University of Chicago, Center for Health Administration Studies, 1967.

_____. "The Impact of Health Planning on the Hospital Industry." Presented at the American Economic Association annual meeting, December 29, 1974a.

_____. "The Planning and Licensing Agencies." In *Regulating Health Facilities Construction,* edited by C.C. Havighurst, pp. 47–68. Washington: American Enterprise Institute, 1974b.

McClure, W. "Reducing Excess Hospital Capacity." Prepared for the Bureau of Health Planning and Resources Development, DHEW, under contract no. HRA-230-76-0086. Excelsior, Minn.: InterStudy, October 15, 1976.

McMahon, J.A., and Drake, D.F. "The American Hospital Association

Perspective." In *Hospital Cost Containment*, edited by M. Zubkoff, I. Raskin, and R.S. Hanft, pp. 76–102. New York: Prodist, 1978.

Medical Care Review. Report on "PSRO Program Scored for Slow Development." *Washington Developments* 6, no. 4 (April 27, 1977); *Medical Care Review* 34 (May 1977): 504–505.

Michael, R.T. *The Effect of Education on Efficiency in Consumption.* New York: National Bureau of Economic Research, 1972.

Monsma, G.S. "Marginal Revenue and the Demand for Physicians' Services." In *Empirical Studies in Health Economics*, edited by H.E. Klarman, pp. 145–160. Baltimore, Md.: Johns Hopkins Press, 1970.

Mueller, M.S. "Private Health Insurance in 1975: Coverage, Enrollment, and Financial Experience." *Social Security Bulletin*, June 1977, pp. 3–21.

Nadiri, M.I., and Rosen, S. *A Disequilibrium Model of Demand for Factors of Production.* New York: Columbia University Press, 1973.

National Center for Health Statistics. *Utilization of Short-Stay Hospitals: Annual Summary for the United States, 1974.* DHEW publication no. (HRA) 76-1777. Rockville, Md., September 1976.

National Center for Social Statistics, Social and Rehabilitation Service. *Numbers of Recipients and Amounts of Payments under Medicaid.* DHEW, NCSS Report Series B-1, 1970–1976.

Nerlove, M. "Further Evidence on the Estimation of Dynamic Economic Relations from a Time Series of Cross Sections." *Econometrica* 39, no. 2 (March 1971): 359–382.

Newhouse, J.P. "Inflation and Health Insurance." In *Health: A Victim or Cause of Inflation?* edited by M. Zubkoff, pp. 210–224. New York: Prodist, 1976.

————. "Toward a Theory of Nonprofit Institutions." *American Economic Review* 60, no. 1 (March 1970): 64–74.

Newhouse, J.P., and Phelps, C.E. "New Estimates of Price and Income Elasticities of Medical Care Services." In *The Role of Health Insurance in the Health Service Sector*, edited by R. Rosett, pp. 261–312. New York: National Bureau of Economic Research, 1976.

"1975 Survey of Buying Power." *Sales Management* 115 (July 21, 1975): A7–C148.

"1976 Survey of Buying Power." *Sales Management* 117, no. 2 (July 26, 1976): A7–C214.

Noll, R.G. "The Consequences of Public Utility Regulation of Hospitals." *Controls on Health Care*, pp. 25–48. Washington: National Academy of Sciences, 1975.

O'Donoghue, P. *Evidence about the Effects of Health Care Regulation.* Denver, Colo.: Spectrum Research Inc., 1974.

Oi, W., and Clayton, E. "A Peasant's View of a Soviet Collective Farm." *American Economic Review* 58 (March 1968): 37–59.

Palmiere, D. "Health Facility Planning Councils Evaluation Project." Mimeograph. University of Michigan, School of Public Health, 1970.

Pauly, M.V. "Medical Staff Characteristics and Hospital Costs." *Journal of Human Resources* 13, supplement (1978): 77–111.

Pauly, M.V., and Drake, D.F. "Effect of Third-Party Methods of Reimbursement on Hospital Performance." In *Empirical Studies in Health Economics*, edited by H.E. Klarman, pp. 297–314. Baltimore, Md.: Johns Hopkins Press, 1970.

Pauly, M.V., and Redisch, M. "The Not-for-Profit Hospital as a Physician's Cooperative." *American Economic Review* 63, no. 1 (March 1973): 87–100.

Perrow, C. "The Analysis of Goals in Complex Organizations." *American Sociological Review* 26, no. 6 (December 1961): 854–865.

Pfeffer, J. "Size and Composition of Corporate Boards of Directors: The Organization and Its Environment." *Administrative Science Quarterly* 17, no. 2 (June 1972): 218–228.

Phelps, C.E. *Demand for Health Insurance: A Theoretical and Empirical Investigation*. Santa Monica, Calif.: The Rand Corporation, 1973.

Porter, R.D. "On the Use of Survey Sample Weights in the Linear Model." *Annals of Economic and Social Measurement* 2, no. 2 (1973): 141–159.

Posner, R.A. "Certificates of Need for Health Care Facilities: A Dissenting View." In *Regulating Health Facilities Construction*, edited by C.C. Havighurst, pp. 113–121. Washington: American Enterprise Institute, 1974.

Priest, A.J.G. "Possible Adaptation of Public Utility Concepts in the Health Care Field." *Law and Contemporary Problems* 35, no. 839 (Fall 1970): 839–848.

Rafferty, J., and Schweitzer, S.O. "Comparison of For-profit and Nonprofit Hospitals: A Re-evaluation." *Inquiry* 11 (December 1974): 304–309.

Reder, M.W. "Some Problems in the Economics of Hospitals." *American Economic Review* 55 (May 1965): 472–481.

Redisch, M.A. "Physician Involvement in Hospital Decision Making." In *Hospital Cost Containment*, edited by M. Zubkoff, I. Raskin, and R.S. Hanft, pp. 217–243. New York: Prodist, 1978.

Reinhardt, U.E. "Comment on Sloan and Feldman, 'Competition among Physicians.'" In *Competition in the Health Care Sector: Past, Present, and Future*, edited by Warren Greenberg, pp. 121–148. Germantown, Md.: Aspen Systems, 1978.

_____. *Physician Productivity and the Demand for Health Manpower.* Cambridge, Mass.: Ballinger, 1975.

Roemer, M., and Friedman, J. *Doctors in Hospitals: Medical Staff Organization and Hospital Performance.* Baltimore, Md.: Johns Hopkins Press, 1971.

Roos, N.L.P.; Schermerhorn, J.R.; and Roos, Jr., L.L. "Hospital Performance: Analyzing Power and Goals." *Journal of Health and Social Behavior* 15 (June 1974): 78–92.

Rosenthal, G. *The Demand for General Hospital Facilities.* Chicago: American Hospital Association, 1964.

Rothenberg, E. *Regulation and Expansion of Health Facilities: The Certificate of Need Experience in New York State.* New York: Praeger Publishers, 1976.

Salkever, D.S. "Competition among Hospitals." In *Competition in the Health Care Sector: Past, Present, and Future,* edited by W. Greenberg, pp. 149–161. Germantown, Md.: Aspen Systems, 1978a.

_____. "A Microeconomic Study of Hospital Cost Inflation." *Journal of Political Economy* 80, no. 6 (November/December 1972): 1144–1166.

_____. "Will Regulation Control Health-Care Costs?" *Bulletin of the New York Academy of Medicine* 54, (January 1978b): 73–83.

Salkever, D.S., and Bice, T.W. "The Impact of Certificate-of-Need Controls on Hospital Investment." *Milbank Memorial Fund Quarterly* 54 (Spring 1976a): 185–214.

_____ and _____. *Impact of State Certificate-of-Need Laws on Health Care Costs and Utilization.* NCHSR Research Digest Series, DHEW publication no. (HRA) 77–3163, 1976b.

Salkever, D.S., and Seidman, R.L. "A Comparison of OLS and Two-Limit Probit Estimates for Models with Ordered Trichotomous Dependent Variables." Mimeograph. Johns Hopkins University, 1978.

Shortell, S.M., and Brown, M., eds. *Organizational Research in Hospitals.* Chicago: Blue Cross Association, 1976.

Sigmond, R.M. "How Should Blue Cross Reimburse Hospitals? 'Costs!'" *Modern Hospital* 101, no. 1 (July 1963): 91–94.

Sloan, F.A. *The Geographic Distribution of Nurses and Public Policy.* DHEW publication no. (HRA) 75–53. Bethesda, Md., May 1975.

_____. "A Model of State Income Maintenance Decisions." *Public Finance Quarterly* 5, no. 2 (April 1977): 139–173.

Sloan, F.A., and Bentkover, J.D. *Access to Physicians and the U.S. Economy.* Lexington, Mass.: Lexington Books, D.C. Heath, 1979.

Sloan, F.A.; Cromwell, J.; and Mitchell, J. "Physician Participation in State Medicaid Programs." *The Journal of Human Resources* 13 supplement (1978).

Sloan, F.A., and Elnicki, R.A. "Professional Nurse Staffing in Hospitals."

In *Equalizing Access to Nursing Services, The Geographic Dimension*, edited by F.A. Sloan, pp. 27–56. DHEW publication no. HRA 87–51. Washington: Government Printing Office, 1978.

Sloan, F.A., and Feldman, R. "Competition among Physicians." In *Competition in the Health Care Sector: Past, Present, and Future*, edited by W. Greenberg, pp. 45–102. Germantown, Md.: Aspen Systems, 1978.

Sloan, F.A., and Steinwald, B. *Hospital Labor Markets: Analysis of Wages and Work Force Composition*. Lexington, Mass.: Lexington Books, D.C. Heath, 1980.

_____ and _____. "The Role of Health Insurance in the Physicians' Services Market." *Inquiry* 12, no. 4 (December 1975): 275–299.

Somers, A.R. *Hospital Regulation: The Dilemma of Public Policy*. Princeton, N.J.: Princeton University Press, 1969.

Somers, H.M., and Somers, A.R. *Doctors, Patients, and Health Insurance*. Washington: The Brookings Institution, 1961.

State of Michigan, Department of Social Services. *Rising Medical Costs in Michigan: The Scope of the Problem and the Effectiveness of Current Controls*. Lansing, Mich., July 1973.

Steinwald, B., and Neuhauser, D. "The Role of the Proprietary Hospital." *Law and Contemporary Problems* 35 (August 1970): 817–838.

Taylor, A.K. "Government Health Policy and Hospital Labor Costs: A Study of the Determinants of Hospital Wage Rates and Employment." Mimeograph. Harvard University School of Public Health, December 1977.

Tekolste, E. "How Should Blue Cross Reimburse Hospitals? 'Charges!' " *Modern Hospital* 101, no 1 (July 1963): 90, 92–94.

Theil, H. *Principles of Econometrics*. New York: John Wiley & Sons, Inc., 1971.

Thornberry, H., and Zimmerman, H. *An Analysis of the Voluntary Experiment with Prospective Rate Setting in Rhode Island: Phase I, 1971 and 1972*. Providence, R.I.: SEARCH, November 1976.

U.S. Bureau of the Census. Public Use Sample of the U.S. Census. 1970.

_____. *Statistical Abstract of the United States, 1976*. 97th ed. Washington, 1976.

_____. *Statistical Abstract of the United States, 1977*. 98th ed. Washington, 1977.

U.S. Bureau of Health Manpower, Department of Health, Education, and Welfare. *The Area Resource File: A Manpower Planning and Research Tool*. Data from various sources on computer tape. October 1976.

U.S. Bureau of Health Resources Development, Division of Nursing. *Source Book of Nursing Personnel*. DHEW publication no. (HRA) 75–43. Washington: Government Printing Office, December 1974.

U.S. Bureau of Labor Statistics (BLS), U.S. Department of Labor. *Industry Wage Surveys: Hospitals, March 1969*. Bulletin No. 1688 (1971). *Hospitals, August 1972*. Bulletin No. 1829 (1974). Various unnumbered issues by city for 1975 (August 1975–October 1976).

U.S. Council on Wage and Price Stability. *The Rapid Rise of Hospital Costs*. Washington: January 1977.

U.S. Department of Health, Education, and Welfare, Bureau of Health Planning and Resources Development. *Status of Certificate of Need and 1122 Programs in the States*. Washington, 1978.

U.S. Department of Health, Education, and Welfare, Bureau of Health Resources Development. *The Supply of Health Manpower: 1970 Profiles and Projections for 1990*. Washington: Government Printing Office, 1974.

U.S. Department of Labor. *Handbook of Labor Statistics*. Bulletin No. 1825. Washington, 1974.

————. *Handbook of Labor Statistics*. Bulletin No. 1865. Washington, 1975.

Weiner, S.M. "Reasonable Cost Reimbursement for Inpatient Hospital Services under Medicare and Medicaid: The Emergence of Public Control." *American Journal of Law and Medicine* 3 (Spring 1977): 1–47.

Wendorf, C.E. "Survey on the Medicaid Program." Chicago: American Hospital Association, October 1977.

Williamson, O.E. *The Economics of Discretionary Behavior*. Chicago: Markham, 1967.

————. *Markets and Hierarchies: Analysis and Antritrust Implications*. New York: The Free Press, 1975.

Worthington, P.N. "Prospective Reimbursement of Hospitals to Promote Efficiency: New Jersey." *Inquiry* 13, no. 3 (September 1976): 302–308.

Yett, D.E. "Comment on F.A. Sloan and R. Feldman, Competition among Physicians." In *Competition in the Health Care Sector: Past, Present, and Future*, edited by W. Greenberg, pp. 103–120. Germantown, Md.: Aspen Systems, 1978.

————. *An Economic Analysis of the Nurse Shortage*. Washington: Government Printing Office, 1970.

Zimmerman, H.; Buechner, J.; and Thornberry, H. "Prospective Reimbursement in Rhode Island: Additional Perspectives." *Inquiry* 14, no. 1 (March 1977): 3–16.

Zubkoff, W. "Hospital Cost Containment and the Administrator." In *Hospital Cost Containment*, edited by M. Zubkoff, I. Raskin, and R.S. Hanft, pp. 244–262. New York: Prodist, 1978.

Index